Praise for *The Allergy Solution*

'*Leo Galland and Jonathan Galland unite two
how to use science to heal the body of allergies
how to live in true harmony with nature. Reading
personal and environmental transformation.*'

— **Dr Deepak Chopra**, author of 22 *New York Times* bestselling
books, including *Super Brain*

'*The Allergy Solution is a game changer! Finally we have a scientifically
validated approach to our ever-expanding allergy problems that focuses
on actual causes as opposed to relying on potentially dangerous drug
remedies. The Gallands' user-friendly text is a long-awaited answer
for the countless allergy sufferers who can now regain immune balance
and bid their allergy problems good-bye.*'

— **Dr David Perlmutter**, #1 *New York Times* bestselling author
of *Grain Brain* and *Brain Maker*

'*Dr Leo Galland is one of the most important medical thinkers of the 21st
century. He has pioneered a new model of practice that is followed by
thousands of physicians, called Functional Medicine. It is medicine WHY!
And in* The Allergy Solution, *Dr Galland and Jonathan Galland dig deep
into why we are in an epidemic of allergic disorders and provide a clear
road map to recovery for millions of sufferers. If you have allergies, have
any chronic disease, or just feel lousy, this book is your way toward renewed
health. It will be a must-read for doctors and patients for years to come!*'

— **Dr Mark Hyman**, #1 *New York Times* bestselling author
of *The Blood Sugar Solution*

'*Dr Galland takes us on a fantastic voyage to an uncharted understanding of
ourselves and our personal environment that will change many readers' lives.*'

— **Dr Mehmet Oz**, Professor of Surgery, Columbia University; host
of *The Dr. Oz Show*

'*The Allergy Solution is a godsend for the millions of people worldwide
who are increasingly suffering from allergies. The Gallands ask the big,
important question: "Why are you allergic?" Not only "what are you
allergic to?". That's the game changer. And once you know why, they show
you exactly what you need to do to live a life free of the drugs that just
treat symptoms and never get to the real cause. Bravo to the Gallands!*'

— **I**   estselling author
of   *lesses Never Age*

'This is the book I have been waiting for! In a masterful piece of investigative reporting, Dr Leo Galland and Jonathan Galland uncover the shocking truth about what is making us so allergic and sick. They present the science that shows how our environment and our health are threatened by air pollution, chemicals, fast food, and global warming. The Allergy Solution *gives you a detailed map to take control of your health and your life.'*

— **Dr Amy Myers,** New York Times bestselling author of
The Autoimmune Solution

'Dr Leo Galland and Jonathan Galland *have put together a masterful and critically important discussion about allergies. Underappreciated, misunderstood, and misdiagnosed, allergies are common and growing in importance. This book provides astounding wisdom about the world of allergies to the reader searching for health answers. I truly enjoyed reading it and picked up a lot of information I had not heard before. Terrific job!'*

— **Dr William Davis**, #1 New York Times bestselling author
of Wheat Belly

'Dr Leo Galland, *a board-certified internist, was classically trained at one of New York's finest medical schools. In* The Allergy Solution, *he gives readers a clear, comprehensive, and effective approach to remedying the ubiquitous allergies that cause us to wheeze, sneeze, gain weight, feel exhausted, foggy, and depressed, and perturb our lives in too many other ways. Before you pick up your next prescription for allergies, asthma, or a host of other common disorders, see what he has to say!'*

— **Dr Lloyd I. Sederer**, Adjunct Professor, Columbia University
Mailman School of Public Health; Medical Editor for Mental Health,
The Huffington Post

'Leo Galland and Jonathan Galland *reveal the true cause of our worldwide allergy epidemic and provide a desperately needed solution for millions with allergy symptoms. A must-read for anyone with allergies!'*

— **Dr Steven Masley**, bestselling author of
The 30-Day Heart Tune-Up and Smart Fat

'This book is a blessing. The Allergy Solution *is a practical toolkit for patients, as well as a scientific source for clinicians to breathe easier, decrease suffering, and help enliven the long-lost you!'*

— **Dr Patrick Hanaway**, Medical Director, Center for
Functional Medicine at the Cleveland Clinic

'In this highly revealing book, Dr Galland goes beyond conventional Western medicine and offers readers the knowledge they need to reverse their allergies and start to feel vibrantly well. Bringing Dr Galland's clinical experience together with Jonathan Galland's wealth of scientific research on why we have become so allergic, The Allergy Solution attacks this new epidemic at its source and helps us restore our bodies to balance.'

— **Dr Frank Lipman**, *New York Times* bestselling author of *The New Health Rules* and *10 Reasons You Feel Old and Get Fat*

'The research in The Allergy Solution *is a revelation. If you want to uncover what's behind your mystery symptoms, or how to thrive in a toxic world, this book is the answer. Discover how to fix your stomach, heal your headaches, beat stress, improve your mood, and conquer pain. Leo Galland and Jonathan Galland provide the scientific validation of something that traditional healing practices, East and West, have understood for millennia, that living in harmony with nature is essential for healing ourselves and the planet.'

— **Dr Vijay Vad**, Assistant Professor, Weill Cornell Medical College; author of *Stop Pain: Inflammation Relief for an Active Life*

'The Allergy Solution *is a must-read for anyone who has suffered from any type of allergy or hasn't felt quite themselves, either intermittently or on an ongoing basis. As a patient of Dr Galland, and a health and fitness professional who has suffered from seasonal allergies my entire life, I have gotten tremendous relief from following Dr Galland's advice and as a result feel much better year round.'

— **Joe Dowdell**, co-author, *Ultimate You*

'While allergy is common in the modern world, few address the ways in which modern living may be causally implicated. Dr Leo Galland does just that, and changes the conversation entirely by asking why allergy happens rather than just what the allergens are. He blends deep scientific understanding with a holistic perspective to offer a powerful approach, rooted in lifestyle, addressing this modern scourge at its very origins and offering allergy sufferers enlightened help and renewed hope.'

— **Dr David L. Katz**, Director, Yale University Prevention Research Center; Founder, True Health Initiative

'Dr Galland's wisdom has changed my life.'

— **Susan Sarandon**, Academy Award–winning actress

'Another masterpiece by one of the intellectual founders of functional medicine. Dr Galland's encyclopedic understanding of the real causes of allergy and many illustrative case histories make this book a wonderful resource for those suffering this once uncommon illness. Strong recommendation for everyone wanting to stop being allergic.'

— **Joseph Pizzorno ND**, Editor in Chief, *Integrative Medicine: A Clinician's Journal*; co-author of *Encyclopedia of Natural Medicine*

'Allergic diseases are plaguing one-quarter of our planet from the onslaught of our gut flora by over-sanitation and the Westernization of nations. Dr Leo Galland is a pioneer of functional medicine, master clinician, and thought leader whose wisdom and experience make his latest home run—The Allergy Solution—a must-read for everyone afflicted with allergies.'

— **Dr Gerard E. Mullin,** Associate Professor of Medicine, The Johns Hopkins University School of Medicine; author of *The Gut Balance Revolution*

'The Allergy Solution *will be of enormous help to people struggling to understand what triggers their allergies and sensitivities. It offers tools to uncover your specific triggers, as well as practical advice on how to avoid and relieve the problem.'*

— **Dr Lawrence J. Cheskin,** Associate Professor, Johns Hopkins Bloomberg School of Public Health and School of Medicine

'As I was reading this book I kept thinking about "Amazing Grace", where after enlightenment a person was no longer blind. The song speaks of finding the spirit of the Lord. I felt much the same way when reading The Allergy Solution, that I was blind and now I can see. Dr Leo Galland and Jonathan Galland open our eyes to the invisible and offer insight and knowledge with very practical solutions that can change lives.'

— **Dr Lloyd Saberski,** Faculty, Yale University School of Medicine

'I love Dr Galland's work.'

— **JJ Virgin,** *New York Times* bestselling author of *The Virgin Diet*

THE
allergy
solution

ALSO BY DR LEO GALLAND

The Fat Resistance Diet (with Jonathan Galland JD)

Power Healing

Superimmunity for Kids

THE
allergy
solution

Unlock the Surprising, Hidden Truth
about Why You Are Sick and
How to Get Well

Dr Leo Galland,

Jonathan Galland JD

HAY HOUSE

Carlsbad, California • New York City • London • Sydney
Johannesburg • Vancouver • Hong Kong • New Delhi

First published and distributed in the United Kingdom by:
Hay House UK Ltd, Astley House, 33 Notting Hill Gate, London W11 3JQ
Tel: +44 (0)20 3675 2450; Fax: +44 (0)20 3675 2451; www.hayhouse.co.uk

Published and distributed in the United States of America by:
Hay House Inc., PO Box 5100, Carlsbad, CA 92018-5100
Tel: (1) 760 431 7695 or (800) 654 5126
Fax: (1) 760 431 6948 or (800) 650 5115; www.hayhouse.com

Published and distributed in Australia by:
Hay House Australia Ltd, 18/36 Ralph St, Alexandria NSW 2015
Tel: (61) 2 9669 4299; Fax: (61) 2 9669 4144; www.hayhouse.com.au

Published and distributed in the Republic of South Africa by:
Hay House SA (Pty) Ltd, PO Box 990, Witkoppen 2068
info@hayhouse.co.za; www.hayhouse.co.za

Published and distributed in India by:
Hay House Publishers India, Muskaan Complex, Plot No.3, B-2,
Vasant Kunj, New Delhi 110 070
Tel: (91) 11 4176 1620; Fax: (91) 11 4176 1630; www.hayhouse.co.in

Distributed in Canada by:
Raincoast Books, 2440 Viking Way, Richmond, B.C. V6V 1N2
Tel: (1) 604 448 7100; Fax: (1) 604 270 7161; www.raincoast.com

Text © 2016 by Dr Leo Galland and Jonathan Galland JD

Indexer: Jay Kreider • Cover design: Angela Moody
Interior design: Nick C. Welch

The moral rights of the authors have been asserted.

The information given in this book should not be treated as a substitute for
professional medical advice; always consult a medical practitioner. Any use of
information in this book is at the reader's discretion and risk. Neither the authors
nor the publisher can be held responsible for any loss, claim or damage arising
out of the use, or misuse, of the suggestions made, the failure to take medical
advice or for any material on third party websites.

A catalogue record for this book is available from the British Library.

ISBN: 978-1-78180-626-5

Printed and bound by CPI Group (UK) Ltd, Croydon, CR0 4YY

A Note to the Reader

This publication contains the opinions and ideas of its authors. It is intended to provide helpful and informative material on the subjects addressed in the publication. It is sold with the understanding that the authors and publisher are not engaged in rendering medical, health, or any other kind of professional services in this book. The reader should consult his or her medical, health, or other competent professional before adopting any of the suggestions in this book or drawing inferences from it. The authors and publisher specifically disclaim all responsibility for any liability, loss, or risk, personal or otherwise, that is incurred as a consequence, directly or indirectly, of the use or application of any of the contents of this book.

*To Christina Galland, beloved wife and mother,
whose passion for healing and helping
others inspires us every day*

CONTENTS

INTRODUCTION

The New Mystery Disease

The phone rang in the middle of the night. I reached over to the nightstand and fished around for the receiver. "Hello," I said in a low voice.

The connection was eerily quiet; then it crackled with static. It sounded very long-distance. "Dr. Galland? Sorry to bother you at this hour. It's Vivian. We're in Denmark for the Copenhagen International Film Festival." Vivian is an independent filmmaker who has been my patient for several years.

I switched on the light. "Vivian, how are you?"

"Not good. I've been here one day and I'm having a terrible headache, my muscles ache, and my throat itches, making me want to cough. I tried aspirin, but it made my throat worse and didn't do anything for the headache."

Her voice was weak. It was midnight in New York, 6 A.M. in Copenhagen. Her film was due to be shown in 12 hours and she didn't know what to do.

As I talked with Vivian, several aspects of her story jumped out at me. I had treated her successfully for migraines several years earlier. I knew she had pollen allergies, but they had never been severe. Still, her itchy throat without fever suggested allergy rather than a viral infection.

April is birch pollen season in Denmark, as it is in much of northern Europe and America. The active ingredient in aspirin, acetyl salicylate, was originally derived from tree bark, with birch and willow being the main sources. Research has linked birch pollen allergy with sensitivity to salicylates.[1]

I told Vivian to stop taking aspirin and asked her what she'd been eating since her arrival. With her hectic schedule she had been snacking on trail mix and fruit to get through the day. This was the clincher: Many foods are known to aggravate allergic reactions to birch pollen. Apples, peaches, cherries, and most nuts are high on that list.

Strongly suspecting birch pollen as the trigger for Vivian's sudden mystery symptoms, I made two recommendations: First, I told her to avoid fruit and nuts, as well as raw carrots and celery, which are also birch pollen–related foods, and to stay indoors as much as possible. She'd have to leave the sightseeing for another visit. Second, I suggested she remove any traces of pollen on herself by taking a hot shower and shampooing her hair. This was to be followed by a cold shower, as brisk as she could stand it.

This advice was based on my own experience. Years ago, when I first developed hay fever from ragweed pollen, I was camping with my family on the Mohawk Trail in Massachusetts. I was terribly congested. The only relief came when I went swimming in the ice-cold waters of the Deerfield River. My head would clear instantly. One night I woke up so horribly congested that my wife told me to "go jump in the river." I did—and it worked better than any medication I'd taken.

Since then, I've often recommended cold showers as an initial step for people like me who have hay fever. It is a practical and easy solution to gain immediate relief without medications.

It worked for Vivian, too. When she returned to New York after the festival, she called me to say she felt much better after following the steps I had recommended.

The Allergy Epidemic

Your eyes itch and your nose runs. Then it clogs up with congestion. Your skin itches so much from eczema that you want to scratch it hard. You have asthma and keep an inhaler in arm's reach at all times. You have peanut allergy. Or wheat allergy. Or milk allergy.

Skyrocketing asthma, runaway rhinitis, spreading eczema, and spiking food allergies—the epidemic of allergies is bigger than you've ever imagined. Just 50 years ago, one person in thirty had allergies. Today that number is one in three. One billion people worldwide now have asthma, hay fever, eczema, allergic rhinitis, sinusitis, and food allergies.

But that's just the tip of the iceberg. There is another, *hidden* epidemic of allergies that could be making you sick.

Do you have:

- Weight gain?

- Fatigue?

- Depression?

- Anxiety?

- Muscle aches?

- Joint pain?

- Headaches?

- Insomnia?

- Stomachaches?

- Bloating?

- Constipation or diarrhea?

- Brain fog?

Allergy could be the culprit.

Few people realize that allergy can play a critical role in these and many more conditions. So if you have unexplained weight gain, no one suspects allergy. But in my clinical experience, helping thousands of patients overcome unexplained symptoms, I have discovered that allergy is often the cause of these common complaints.

It may be hard to imagine that an obscure food allergy could make weight loss almost impossible, or that mold could cause debilitating fatigue and inability to work. In fact, research shows that allergies are often the cause of seemingly unrelated symptoms. Allergy often contributes to migraine headaches, depression, mood swings, joint and muscle pain, and irritable bowel syndrome. In this book, I will reveal the science that can explain what you may have already sensed: that something in your body chemistry is blocking the path to healing. And I'll show you a natural way to uncover the root cause of your allergies and recover your health.

But first, let's take a look at how we got here.

A Perfect Storm

The origins of the allergy epidemic are environmental and nutritional. There are three levels at which environment impacts allergy: outdoor, indoor, and internal (the world inside your body). Toxicity in each of these areas is a one-two punch. First it damages your body's surfaces—the skin, or the lining of the respiratory tract or the GI tract—and then it promotes an allergic reaction to substances that ordinarily would be tolerated. What you eat and your nutritional status affect your body's response at each of these levels.

Today, going to the supermarket is like navigating a minefield. As you push your cart down the aisle, you rapidly scan the shelves for the words *gluten-free* or *dairy-free*. Your beloved pizza or favorite pasta dish is off the menu if you are allergic to wheat. It seems the basic things that used to sustain us have turned against us, and a new threat lurks around every corner. This is indeed a strange new world, one that would be unrecognizable to earlier generations.

How did it get this way?

In the film *The Perfect Storm*, George Clooney's character is the captain of a fishing boat that sails out from Gloucester, Massachusetts. In search of a great catch of fish, their boat winds up heading straight into a combination of a hurricane and other storm fronts, the proverbial "perfect storm." The violent seas and high waves prove too much for the captain and crew, and the boat is lost at sea.

Like the fishing boat in the movie, we have been hit by the perfect storm of pollution, unhealthy eating habits, stress, lack of exercise, and overuse of antibiotics, all of which are throwing our immune systems way off balance and giving us more allergies than ever before.

If you're among the millions of allergy sufferers, *The Allergy Solution* is a lighthouse that will guide you safely back to shore.

A New Understanding of Allergy

Most people look at allergies as symptoms that get treated with drugs. I'm here to help you think of allergies in a new way, so you overcome them by *understanding their root causes.*

I developed this unique program to empower you to overcome allergies, even the hidden allergies that may be causing your unexplained health problems. Instead of suppressing symptoms with drugs year after year, you can reverse your allergies by getting to the source of the allergic reaction.

I will provide you with the powerful tools you need to support the body's immunity, reverse your allergies, and transform your health. As you follow my plan you will feel healthier, slimmer, more focused, and more energetic.

In the chapters ahead, I will share with you the fascinating science of how allergies happen in your body and walk you through the simple steps you can take to feel better than you have in years.

This book reveals, for the first time, knowledge that has been buried in the medical journals for far too long. In universities and medical centers around the world, amazing scientific research has been done that can transform the way we think about and approach allergy—but like a hidden treasure, it has remained mostly unknown. Until now.

The Origins of the Allergy Solution

Let me share with you my own story. As a child, growing up in a suburb of New York City, I didn't know anyone with allergies.

No one thought twice about bringing peanut butter and jelly to school. You never saw kids with asthma inhalers. If you went into a drugstore, you weren't greeted by an entire aisle devoted to different types of antihistamines and decongestants.

One day when I was ten, our music teacher, Mr. Sorensen, brought his son to school for a concert. The gym floor had just been washed with a strong cleaning solution, and this poor kid began wheezing and coughing and could not catch his breath. His father tried to give him an asthma inhaler, but the boy was so short of breath he could barely breathe in the medication. He looked terrified and started turning blue. I thought he was about to die. I had never been so frightened. The school nurse called an ambulance, they sped off to the hospital, and the boy survived. The next year, Mr. Sorensen moved his family to Arizona, hoping to find a less allergenic environment.

Over the next several decades, so many people moved to the desert hoping to escape from allergies that Phoenix and Las Vegas became the allergy getaway capitals of the United States. But you can't easily escape allergies by moving away. They usually follow you, because the secrets to reversing allergy are on the *inside* of you, not the outside.

I always thought of myself as being energetic and productive. If you asked me for one word that most reflected how I saw myself, that word would have been *stamina*. I was able to study all night through college and medical school. Then one day, during my medical residency, I could barely get out of bed, much less go for my morning run.

I thought the fatigue would go away, but it didn't. After a few weeks I started to get worried. I went to one of my professors, who examined me, ran some blood tests, and shrugged his shoulders.

Then, just as suddenly, one day I woke up feeling fine again. So I forgot about the episode—until it happened again, the same time the following year. And the next year, and the year after . . . this fatigue would hit me like a truck.

When I analyzed the cycle of my illness, I realized that I had hay fever caused by allergy to ragweed pollen and that I could control my symptoms with cold water and exercise. I'd take a vigorous run and then an ice-cold shower. That cleared my allergies much better than antihistamines.

I didn't have pollen allergies as a child. So how did I suddenly develop them as an adult? It started with air pollution. Scientists have studied the effects of urban air pollution on ragweed. They planted ragweed seeds in the inner city of Baltimore and in the countryside. The urban plants grew to be twice as large and produced five times as much pollen as the rural plants.

While science fiction movies often show the future of our planet as a barren wasteland, more likely it will be overgrown with allergenic weeds and vines that thrive on polluted air!

I did my medical residency in the middle of New York City. There was a vacant lot next to the apartment building where I lived, and each summer it would be overgrown with ragweed. Certain kinds of pollen—ragweed included—are actually toxic. They contain an enzyme called NOX, which damages the lining of your nose and lungs. Heavy exposure to toxic pollen was one trigger for my illness.

There was another trigger: the freshly baked baguettes I picked up every day in a French bakery near the hospital, pretending this was Paris. My wife suggested I stop eating them. Eliminating all wheat—bread, pasta, and cookies—added to the benefits of exercise in controlling my hay fever. I stayed away from wheat products beyond the ragweed season, and found that my energy and productivity were greater than they'd ever been.

When I began teaching at a medical school after I finished my training, I realized there were a lot of patients with symptoms like mine: unexplained fatigue, dizziness, lightheadedness. I wondered how many of them had allergies. It took me several years to crack the code that would allow me to recognize that most of them did have allergies—that they were, in fact, unknowing victims of the allergy epidemic.

In my quest to help my patients I developed the innovative new approach to allergies that I present here in *The Allergy Solution*.

A Bold New Approach

Conventional medicine asks, *to what* are you allergic? If you have allergies, you probably know about the standard treatments: avoidance of the allergen and suppression of symptoms with medications. You are also probably familiar with the antihistamines, steroids, bronchodilators, and immune suppressants that are most often used to control allergy symptoms. While they may provide some relief of symptoms, these drugs don't reverse allergy and may have side effects that range from fatigue to impairment of immunity.

I believe in a more natural and yet powerful approach to allergies. From my decades of clinical experience practicing integrated medicine, I understand that we need to ask not just *what* you are allergic to, but *why*.

Solving the problem means looking at all your details, asking what in your life is making you sick or healthy. My mission is to help people recognize the impact of allergy in their own lives and achieve optimal health by reversing the root causes of allergy, not just suppressing symptoms.

This blows the lid off the conventional, limited view of allergy that zooms in on one symptom or area of the body and treats that in isolation. My approach—the Allergy Solution—exposes allergy for what it really is, an imbalance of the immune system that involves the whole body.

As I'll explain, allergic reactions are self-amplifying chain reactions in which your immune system amplifies the effect of something called a trigger. Allergy occurs when the part of your immune system that controls unwanted immune responses fails to function properly. It is actually an immune deficiency state that results in excessive inflammation.

What You'll Get in The Allergy Solution

As you dive into this book, you will meet people and read about their cases. People much like you, who have faced symptoms and problems a lot like your own. Most often, when they came to my office, they had already been to many specialists, but the tests and treatments had not worked. I will explain how the Allergy Solution unlocked these previously impossible-to-crack cases, using remarkably simple methods that you can learn from.

I'll offer plenty of tools and tips that can get you started in not only reversing your allergies, but also restoring your health so you can lose those extra pounds, gain energy, and sleep better.

My collaborator on *The Allergy Solution* is my son Jonathan Galland, J.D., a leader in integrated health education as well as a passionate advocate for the environment. He is the creator of www.pilladvised.com, which is dedicated to transforming health by presenting the wisdom of an integrated approach to medicine.

Combining my knowledge with his expertise, we will trace the origins of the allergy epidemic to the modern Western diet, industrial pollution, the proliferation of toxic chemicals in household, workplace, and personal care products, and the disruption of gut microbial balance by antibiotics and pesticides. And we'll teach you simple, actionable steps for turning back this modern epidemic with nutrition, mind-body practices, and an all-natural way of life that will contribute to your well-being and the health of the planet.

In the pages ahead, you'll learn the Allergy Solution way to address the challenges that allergies pose in our modern world:

Challenge #1

Allergy is directly linked to eating fast foods and nutritionally depleted processed foods.

The Allergy Solution

A nutrient-dense, whole-foods diet, rich in vegetables and fruits, has been shown to prevent or reverse allergy by improving immune function and antioxidant status. *The Allergy Solution* features a whole-foods diet with powerful phytonutrients to improve detoxification and antioxidant status.

At the center of the program is the Three-Day Power Wash, which consists of a delicious smoothie, a satisfying soup, and an aromatic tea. I am excited to share these recipes that I developed and enjoy making every day. The goal is to provide a high level of nutrients that help support detoxification and immune function. The Power Wash is rich in natural substances called flavonoids that inhibit allergic responses, and it's the first step in the unique program that I provide in these pages.

Challenge #2

Depletion of beneficial intestinal microbes, by exposure to antibiotics and pesticides in food and by lack of dietary fiber, is an emerging factor in the rise of allergies.

The Allergy Solution

I will teach you how to support healthy gut flora with prebiotic foods and probiotics. I will reveal the exciting science that shows how fixing the gut can help prevent the development of eczema and reduce symptom severity in people with allergic rhinitis, sinusitis, or asthma.

Challenge #3

Both indoor and outdoor pollution contribute to the rising tide of allergic diseases. Ozone, nitric oxide, and diesel exhaust particles damage the respiratory lining, increase oxidative stress, and act in synergy with allergen exposure to create or aggravate allergic reactions.

The Allergy Solution

First I will explain the role of pollution and chemicals in allergy and provide tips for limiting exposure. Next, I will discuss the research that shows how eating cruciferous vegetables, such as broccoli, and foods high in vitamin C can help protect against allergic reactions, so you can benefit from this knowledge.

I will empower you to overcome these challenges, and many others, by presenting the cutting-edge science that is illuminating the field of allergy. By the time you finish this book, you will have a better understanding of nutritional therapies for a variety of allergic disorders. You'll also understand how to make your homes and workplaces more environmentally friendly and how to heal the immune system by healing the gut.

I strongly recommend that you bring this book with you when you go to see your doctor. Tell her or him about the things you have learned in these pages and about any ideas you may want to try. Working in partnership with your doctor, see how the ideas here may support the treatment plan he or she provides. The professional opinion of your doctor takes precedence over anything you may read in this book.

The Long-Lost You

I am excited to be at the forefront of a powerful movement that is changing how the world looks at allergies and health. And I'm excited to guide you through the program I've developed in my clinical practice for controlling, reversing, and preventing allergies so that you can take a fresh look at your own health.

Read this book and you will rediscover a long-lost friend, the other you. Gone are the dark circles under your eyes. You have new energy. Your nose no longer runs. You breathe easier. Your skin is smooth and comfortable, not red and itchy. Perhaps you have lost those few extra pounds or are sleeping better.

It is the same you that you have always been, of course, only you feel so much better. You are empowered, on the road to robust good health, and ready to take on the world.

Learn more about natural health by joining our community at www.drgalland.com and following us on Facebook (facebook.com/leogallandmd) and Twitter (@leogallandmd).

CHAPTER 1

THE MANY FACES OF ALLERGY

The elevator slid open and I stepped out onto the polished floor of the lobby. I had just finished my interview on the *Today* show and was going to my office. Pushing through the revolving doors, I exited Rockefeller Center Plaza, strode through the crowds, and crossed Fifth Avenue. I walked quickly along 51st Street, past the fashion-filled windows of Saks on my right, while glancing up at the stone spires of St. Patrick's Cathedral on my left. Another day in New York City.

Turning left on Park Avenue, I headed uptown and gained momentum going up the incline past the Armory. At 73rd Street I turned the corner toward my office.

My first patient of the day was sitting in the waiting room.

Julia had consulted 13 specialists in three years. Despite her efforts, she still had received no definite diagnosis. One doctor suspected rheumatoid arthritis, another suggested fibromyalgia. She was told she had irritable bowel syndrome, migraine headaches, Lyme disease, and depression. When she came to my office for her first appointment, she brought a file of medical records two inches thick that was full of normal test results.

When I took her medical history, Julia told me her symptoms: pain in her joints, head, neck, and abdomen, tingling in her arms and legs, fatigue and problems with mental focus—brain fog.

These symptoms had appeared suddenly about three years earlier, when she was 38, and had gotten steadily worse.

When I asked Julia what her health had been like before that, she revealed that she'd never really enjoyed great health. She had experienced asthma in childhood. Then gastrointestinal symptoms started in her teens: abdominal pain and diarrhea with various foods, but following no clear pattern.

Just as troubling, she began gaining weight, about 40 pounds over 20 years, despite numerous attempts at dieting. I saw a pattern emerge that would explain all of her mysterious symptoms.

My clinical experience helped me recognize that Julia's problems were caused by a hidden allergy, almost certainly to something in her diet. Although she was not complaining of asthma, I did a simple breathing test in my office, because I thought that chronic asthma was likely contributing to her fatigue and perhaps other symptoms, like the tingling in her hands and feet. The test indicated that she did indeed have asthma. Then I ordered blood tests to check the level of inflammation in her body.

I also asked her to try a method that I've found very useful for finding hidden allergies to food. I call it the Power Wash, because it not only cleanses your body of allergenic foods, but also enhances your body's ability to eliminate toxins. You will learn more about the Power Wash a little later in the book.

Julia was absolutely determined to get well, so she followed my instructions. For three days she had only the refreshing Smoothie, the delicious Soup, and the mellow Tea that make up the first phase (the elimination phase) of the Power Wash. For the next phase, Re-entry, she started to add back some of her favorite foods.

The results were dramatic. At the end of a week most of her joint pain was gone, her mind felt much clearer, and she'd lost five pounds. Over the next month, she lost another ten, even as she continued expanding her diet to include a wide variety of foods—chicken and fish, oatmeal, potatoes, various fruits and vegetables, eggs, spices, tea, and coffee—so that she didn't feel deprived.

Her headaches disappeared almost completely, her digestion was the best it had been in 20 years, and her energy was great. But she still had occasional attacks of joint pain, headaches, or diarrhea, which could last for a day or two. These occurred only when she ate food she had not prepared herself. One occurred after drinking white wine, another after eating potato salad.

When I reviewed the foods that still made Julia feel unwell, I concluded that her problems were not primarily with foods themselves, but with sulfites, which are common food additives and preservatives known to cause allergic reactions. (You'll find a list of foods that often contain added sulfites at www.drgalland.com.) In addition to being added to food as preservatives, sulfites may occur naturally in foods such as garlic and onions in very small amounts. The typical allergic reaction to sulfites is asthma, but headaches, intestinal symptoms, and joint pain can also result.[1]

There are two nutrients that help your body detoxify sulfites, vitamin B12 and a mineral called molybdenum. Your body makes an enzyme, sulfite oxidase, that breaks down sulfites, and molybdenum is necessary for the enzyme to do its work and lower the level of sulfites in the body.[2] Vitamin B12, in turn, sucks up sulfites so they can be eliminated. In one study, when children with sulfite-sensitive asthma were given vitamin B12 supplements, 80 percent of them experienced an improvement in tolerance for sulfites.[3] So I told Julia to supplement her diet with 1 milligram per day of vitamin B12 and 300 micrograms per day of molybdenum.

Within a month she noticed that when she ate dried fruits or vinegar, both preserved with sulfites, she could tolerate them without having symptoms. And although her initial lab tests had revealed numerous signs of inflammation in her body, when the same tests were repeated three months later, all evidence of inflammation was gone along with her symptoms.

Four Game-Changing Truths about Allergies

I've been treating patients with a wide variety of allergic problems for my entire medical career. People come to see me from around the world with mysterious conditions for which they haven't yet found answers. Frequently the culprit is a hidden allergy.

My clinical experience and my search for answers to common but previously undiagnosed conditions have propelled my quest. I've seen chronic conditions that were previously diagnosed as autoimmune diseases or psychiatric disorders turn out to be allergic in nature, and I've found studies published in research journals that validate my observations. I've reviewed the medical literature, searched the scientific databases, and read the obscure textbooks. Like a detective, I've scrutinized symptoms and clues that have been overlooked, piecing together the evidence. What I have discovered has been fascinating.

Conventional treatment of allergy has two components: 1) try to determine what you're allergic to, so you can avoid it or get desensitized to it with allergy shots, and 2) suppress the symptoms of allergy with drugs. This conventional approach is incomplete because it doesn't ask these questions: Why are you allergic? Why have your allergies gotten worse? What are the underlying imbalances in your body that allow troubling allergic symptoms to occur? These questions unlock the hidden clues that are so critical to solving a case.

Julia's story illustrates four key truths about allergies that are at the core of *The Allergy Solution*. I believe these concepts are so game-changing that they will transform how we approach our health. First, allergies can produce a huge range of common symptoms that trouble millions of Americans but are not ordinarily thought of as allergic. Second, allergies often mimic other diseases. Third, the allergens that trigger your symptoms may not be obvious. Fourth, nutritional therapies can reverse allergies. Let's take a closer look at each of these paradigm-shifting truths.

1. Hidden Allergies Can Lead to Many Common Complaints

As Julia's case makes clear with her pain, fatigue, and brain fog, allergies can cause all sorts of misery—not just the symptoms that we ordinarily think of as allergic, like itchy skin, a runny nose, watery eyes, and wheezing. The symptoms that allergies can produce go well beyond these classic symptoms. Numerous studies have documented the connection between allergies and a profusion of different symptoms.

Scan the list of some common symptoms on the next few pages and see if a hidden allergy could be harming your health.

Feeling Fatigued?

There is a strong link between allergy and fatigue. Though it often goes unrecognized, this is a common problem, called allergic tension-fatigue syndrome.[4] Food allergy, often to wheat, corn, milk, or chocolate, is frequently considered to be the cause. I first read about the research on this when I was teaching medicine at Stony Brook University. The findings explained the vague symptoms of so many patients who are unwell but have no diagnosis.

Packing On the Pounds?

In my clinical experience, allergies have often been the cause of unexplained weight gain. The association between obesity and allergy has been documented in people with asthma.[5] A long-term study found that having asthma increased the propensity to later weight gain among women.[6]

Data from the U.S. National Health and Nutrition Examination Survey found that use of antihistamines is linked to increased body weight.[7] It's possible that antihistamines cause weight gain as a side effect, and people using them are more likely to have allergies than people not using them. I'll discuss this problem in more detail in Chapter 9.

Do Your Muscles Ache?

Many people suffer from mysterious muscle aches and pains. Hidden allergies are very likely contributing to this unexplained pain. The growing evidence on this link between muscle pain and allergy in the journals is confirming what I have seen time and again in my patients.

An association between severe muscle aches and chronic nasal congestion was first described in 1992.[8] Since then researchers have described allergic reactions to foods and to metals (nickel in particular) as a cause of muscle pain.[9] Norwegian scientists found an association between asthma, eczema, and muscle pain and concluded that allergy is a whole-body disorder involving organs that are not typically included in the diagnosis of allergy.[10]

In my own practice, I've observed a high frequency of mold allergy among patients with severe muscle aches. This connection has been documented in people exposed to water-damaged buildings that are contaminated by mold.[11]

Got Joint Pain?

Allergic arthritis was described at least 25 years ago, with specific foods as the major triggers. The allergy-arthritis connection has been confirmed with blinded food challenges.[12] ("Blind" in a scientific experiment means that the subject of the experiment doesn't know what's being done. "Double blind" means that neither the scientists nor the subjects of the experiment know which treatment is being given to which subject.) Cow's milk is the most common trigger food for allergic arthritis. Different allergic mechanisms have been found in different people, even when the allergen is the same.

Suffer from Headaches?

Food allergy as a cause of headache has been known for decades and is well reported in the scientific literature. Allergy can cause both migraine and non-migraine headaches.[13]

Have Stomach Pain and Bloating?

Recurrent abdominal pain may have many causes, allergy among them. Food allergy is linked to inflammation in the stomach or intestines, leading to pain.[14] The allergic response in the gut has been found to be associated with pain and bloating.[15]

Suffer from Heartburn?

Food allergy leads to heartburn by contributing to a condition called eosinophilic esophagitis, which is increasing in prevalence around the world. Eliminating dietary allergens can cure it.[16]

Have Trouble Sleeping?

Various allergies can keep you awake and prevent a good night's sleep. Difficulty falling asleep and maintaining sleep occurs in infants with milk allergy, independent of other symptoms such as colic.[17] In adults with allergy and in older children, poorly controlled or undiagnosed asthma, as well as nasal obstruction or itching from allergic eczema, are important factors that contribute to insomnia.[18]

Feel Depressed or Have a Mood Disorder?

The link between allergies and mental health issues is well established in the medical literature. Adolescents with asthma are three times more likely to develop depression or bipolar disorder later in life than their classmates without asthma.[19] A German study demonstrated an increased incidence of psychiatric disorders of all types among people with physician-diagnosed allergy. This effect was diminished by allergy treatment, so that treated allergy sufferers were 35 percent less likely to experience psychiatric symptoms when compared with those who were not treated.[20]

This leads to two possible conclusions: allergies themselves produce psychiatric symptoms, or psychiatric symptoms lead people with allergies to avoid treatment. In my clinical experience, either conclusion may be right, depending on the person. Another study (double-blind and placebo-controlled) of 30 people suffering from both allergies and psychological symptoms demonstrated that exposure to an allergen but not to a placebo produced significant symptoms of psychological distress, indicating that for some people allergy may be a direct cause of their mood disorders.[21]

Losing Hair?

Alopecia areata is a condition marked by small areas of hair loss on the scalp. Its prevalence is increased among people with allergic disorders. Having a history of allergy increases the risk of relapse after treatment is completed, suggesting that allergy in some way contributes to the condition.[22]

Have Vaginal Itching or Discharge?

I've observed many patients with chronic vaginitis or vulvitis who did not respond to treatment for vaginal infection because their symptoms were actually the result of allergy. Sometimes the proper diagnosis was vulvar eczema or contact dermatitis, an allergic skin reaction like poison ivy. Often women with these types of symptoms have allergic vaginitis, which is provoked by the same variety of triggers as other types of allergic reactions. Gynecologic researchers have confirmed this finding.[23]

Have Painful or Frequent Urination?

Russian scientists have identified allergy as a contributing factor in overactive bladder syndrome.[24] I've made the same observation in many patients with frequent, urgent urination. Treating the allergy often relieves the urinary problem.

Got Brain Fog?

Brain fog can be rapidly caused by exposure to an allergen. Problems with focus, concentration, and memory are very common. They may occur as a late reaction to respiratory allergens in people with allergic rhinitis.[25] I frequently observe them among my patients with allergy to food or mold when allergen exposure occurs.

These unsuspected symptoms of allergy are just as common as the classic allergic symptoms and often coexist with those more familiar symptoms. The more symptoms you have, the more likely that allergy is the cause, especially if the symptoms fluctuate in severity.

The Allergy Solution is here to help you overcome your allergies, whether they are obvious or obscure. I encourage you to bring this book with you when you go to see your doctor, and have an eye-opening discussion about the role allergies can play.

2. Allergies Often Mimic Other Diseases

Allergies are all too easily mistaken for different conditions altogether. That is what we saw in Julia's case, where all her specialists seemed to have their own diagnoses for her problems.

Allergies may mimic inflammatory disorders like arthritis, bronchitis, nephritis (inflammation of the kidneys), or colitis.[26] Allergy can also mimic disorders of unknown cause like migraine headaches, irritable bowel syndrome, fibromyalgia, chronic fatigue syndrome, attention deficit disorder, canker sores, burning mouth syndrome, interstitial cystitis, vulvodynia, anxiety, and depression.[27]

For each of these disorders, only a small percentage of patients diagnosed with it may be sick because of allergy, but if that small percentage happens to include you or someone you love, that's 100 percent. In my medical practice I've treated thousands of patients whose allergies manifest in one of these forms.

3. The Allergens That Trigger Your Symptoms May Not Be Obvious

Here's the third truth about allergies revealed in Julia's story: the triggers may not be obvious. It often takes careful medical detective work to find them. Blood tests and skin tests may not tell the real story. In Julia's case, as in many others, I couldn't rely on laboratory testing, in large part because there are multiple mechanisms of allergy and the available tests measure only one mechanism. A perfect example of this is a story I like to call the Case of the Nightshade Plant Allergy.

Cora was 52 when she first came to my office, a successful attorney with a problem that really hindered her work. At least once a week she would develop mouth sores and painful swelling of the glands in her neck. On a few occasions the symptoms were so bad that she went to a hospital emergency room. Each time she was checked for infection but none was found. Treatment with prednisone, a steroid, had been suggested, but the symptoms usually subsided within two days, and Cora was reluctant to take steroids because of their many side effects.

I met her for the first time a day after one of her worst attacks. My examination revealed that the swollen glands in her neck—right at the angles of her jaw, actually—were not lymph nodes but major salivary glands called parotids, which produce much of the saliva that lubricates your mouth. The name for Cora's symptoms was recurrent parotitis (parotid gland inflammation), a fairly unusual condition.

When we went over Cora's medical and dietary history, she told me that she avoided eating bell peppers and eggplant, because they not only gave her mouth sores but upset her stomach, causing diarrhea. She was also very sensitive to cigarette smoke. Being around a smoker would cause sores in her nose and on her lips. These clues about food and tobacco alerted my Allergy Solution radar that allergies were a likely cause.

Peppers, eggplant, and tobacco all have something in common. They are nightshade plants. Other members of that family include tomatoes and potatoes. Cora often ate foods seasoned with salsa or tomato paste, so I recommended that she totally avoid tomatoes and potatoes. This was a little challenging, because tomato products are so widely used in sauces and potatoes are the most commonly consumed vegetable in the United States. But Cora needed no convincing, because her symptoms had made her so miserable so often. By eliminating nightshades, we healed her mouth sores and she never again suffered an attack of parotitis.

I decided to run some allergy tests, just to see if any of them would identify Cora's sensitivity to any members of the nightshade family. They did not. Tip to take home: a negative allergy test does not rule out an allergy.

4. Nutrition Is a Powerful Tool Against Allergies

For Julia, taking vitamin B12 and molybdenum supplements prevented the sulfite reactions that had made her so sick. Over the years, I've developed many different nutrition treatments that have decreased allergic reactivity in my patients, and you'll read more about them as the book goes on.

I have reviewed a large body of research published in medical journals that shows the important role of nutrition in allergy. Two key areas are 1) the demonstrated link between nutritional deficiency and allergy and 2) the critical role of nutrients in detoxification. These two areas form the foundation of the nutritional therapies in *The Allergy Solution.*

Several nutrients affect immune function. Highly regarded studies have demonstrated how deficiency in these nutrients is directly linked to the development of allergy:

- Vitamin D. Deficiency contributes to the occurrence and severity of asthma and the development of food allergies and eczema, nasal allergies (allergic rhinitis), and allergy in general.[28]

- Zinc. This has been found to be reduced in some people with asthma and eczema.[29]

- Selenium. Levels have been found to be low in some patients with asthma.[30]

- Magnesium. Low consumption is associated with increased risk of asthma and total allergic sensitization.[31]

- Vitamin E. This is reduced in asthmatics, and lower vitamin E intake is associated not only with asthma but with allergic sensitization in general.[32]

- Vitamin C. Higher intake is associated with decreased risk of asthma in children, and reduced intake from food or lower levels in the blood are each associated with asthma in adults.[33]

- Essential fats. Higher omega-3 intake is associated with reduced incidence of asthma in young adults. Increasing a child's intake of omega-3 oils to improve immune function was the theme of my book *Superimmunity for Kids.* Research has confirmed the

importance of adequate omega-3 consumption for
improving immunity and decreasing inflammation
and allergy.[34]

I'll be discussing nutrients and how they may help reverse
your allergic burden in the chapters to come.

The nutritional therapies in *The Allergy Solution* are designed
to help in another important way as well: by enhancing detoxification. This is how vitamin B12 helped Julia's sulfite allergy. Your
body is constantly exposed to toxic substances, either from the
environment or generated from within. You have many mechanisms for eliminating toxins. Most of them are driven by enzymes,
and they work continuously—24/7—to cleanse your body.

Research shows that people with allergy have difficulty detoxifying from heavy metals like lead and mercury as well as environmental pesticides and other pollutants.[35] Your burden of toxicity
depends on your level of exposure to toxins and your ability to
detoxify. The right nutrients can greatly enhance that ability.

Antioxidant Defense Against Allergy

One of your body's most important enzymes for detoxifying
is glutathione-S-transferase, but you can call it GST. It works by
attaching the powerful antioxidant glutathione to a toxin so they
both can be carried out of the body together. That is one way
you detox.

Scientists at UCLA showed that eating broccoli sprouts
increases the levels of GST in people. Broccoli sprouts are rich in
a natural substance called glucoraphanin, which is very stable but
not active in your body. When you crush raw broccoli sprouts, an
enzyme also present in the sprouts converts glucoraphanin to its
active derivative, sulforaphane. Sulforaphane is very active but very
unstable, so it has to be eaten immediately.

The UCLA researchers had healthy volunteers eat ground-
up broccoli sprouts over the course of three days. They found a
significant increase of GST and other detoxifying enzymes in the
subjects' nasal cells. For people exposed to diesel exhaust, broccoli

sprout extract decreased the amount of allergic inflammation found in their nasal secretions.

Broccoli sprouts can enhance GST, and GST can help fight allergy. That's why I've included broccoli sprout powder in the Power Wash program in Chapter 6.

Remember the term *glutathione.* It's so important to your ability to detox. And glutathione depends on GST. Like all enzymes, GST is made in your cells according to a genetic blueprint. There are several different forms of GST, and children with asthma often have a defective gene for one of them. And here's something very significant: children with defective GST develop asthma only if they're also exposed to cigarette smoke or other types of airborne pollution. It's the combination of environmental toxins and impaired ability to detoxify that produces the disease. So take away the tobacco smoke and reduce the pollution from cars, trucks, and other sources, and we can cut the risk of asthma for children. Now that is an idea that could help us all breathe a little easier.

The Mysterious Case of Hives

One bright February morning, Bruce, a professional baseball player, strode into my office like he was rounding second base. He and his wife had flown into town the night before. He was all pent-up energy and looked even more intense in person than on TV or staring out from the magazine covers. But he had a problem. His skin was so itchy it was driving him to distraction, which wasn't helping his game. So he made an appointment to see me.

Bruce's story illustrates the subtleties of allergies and how the Allergy Solution approach goes beyond the limits of conventional medicine to unravel the mysteries of allergies and get to the root causes.

He could barely sit still in his chair across the desk from me in my office. He had greeted me with his trademark smile and a casual "Hi, Doc" and shaken my hand with a viselike grip. Now he got right to the point: "These hives are driving me nuts." Hives are medically known as *urticaria,* and Bruce's case had been going on for two years. That is a long time to be itchy, but it is all too typical for chronic allergic skin conditions. Unless he took two different kinds of antihistamine every day, his body was covered by a carpet of red, itchy lumps that made his life miserable. "It's either the pills, which make me groggy, or the hives, Doc, and I can't take it much longer," he pleaded.

In search of relief, Bruce had seen three dermatologists and two allergists. They agreed that he suffered from hives and that they were the result of an allergic reaction. But pinpointing the underlying allergy that causes hives is often challenging, and nobody was able to identify what the allergens were. The medications Bruce was taking did not fully prevent the hives from appearing, and they made him drowsy, even though they were not supposed to.

On two occasions the hives had broken through the drug therapy so badly that he had been forced to take a short course of prednisone, an immune-suppressing steroid. This is the fate of many patients who suffer from chronic urticaria. Triggers are identified in only 10 to 20 percent of patients, so the mainstay of treatment is suppression of hives with drugs.[36]

When Bruce consulted me, I asked him a question I ask all my patients: *What was happening in your life right before this problem began?* Bruce's answer was immediate, because it was quite a memorable time for him: "After we won the big game, we were celebrating in the locker room, the champagne was flowing, the whole team got a little carried away. All the guys and our wives went downtown for a big dinner, steaks and fine wine." After that, he spent a weekend relaxing postseason, watching TV and drinking beer.

His answer—that he was drinking champagne, wine, and beer—was a red flag for me. This important clue that Bruce provided shows why asking questions, and listening closely to the answers, is at the core of the type of medicine I practice. Like a diligent detective, I want to know all the details of a case so I can deduce the underlying cause. Drinking alcohol increases the permeability of the intestinal lining, creating a condition known as "leaky gut." The leaky gut lets foreign substances penetrate the wall of the intestine, which allows allergic sensitization to food proteins to occur.[37] For example, the major allergens in beer come from barley and yeast.

I've treated a number of patients with chronic hives for whom yeasts were the main trigger. This phenomenon has been described in published studies by European researchers.[38] I told Bruce directly, "If you really want to get rid of these hives, you are going to have to strictly avoid alcohol—no more wine or beer." He looked a little surprised, then played it cool, saying, "Looks like spring training is starting for me today."

In fact, I recommended that Bruce avoid all dietary sources of yeast, like beer, wine, vinegar, bread, dried fruit, and commercial fruit juices. I also suggested he try an herbal extract called berberine, which has been shown to kill intestinal yeasts.[39]

Bruce followed my advice and his hives disappeared within two weeks. He was able to stop antihistamines and has not experienced a recurrence of hives over the past seven years. By carefully examining the circumstances under which Bruce had developed his hives, I was able to go beyond the limits of conventional medicine. By realizing the interplay between nutrition, gut health, allergy, and skin symptoms, I developed a therapy that worked on each of these interconnected areas. These are the principles I am excited to share with you in *The Allergy Solution*. For Bruce it was enough to know that I had relieved his hives and prevented their recurrence.

Allergies on the Brain

There's no topic in the field of allergy as controversial among doctors as the notion that allergic reactions can have a direct impact on your brain. I'm amazed at the controversy, because I've seen the effects of brain allergy in so many of my patients, children and adults alike. The reactions have ranged from spaciness and lack of concentration to depression, anxiety, and mental confusion. Patients of mine with brain allergy have often been previously diagnosed with attention deficit disorder, hyperactivity, autism, and bipolar disorder. For these patients, eliminating the allergic trigger can often help relieve the mental disorder.

Research on Brain Allergy

The earliest published report on brain allergies appeared in the *Southern Medical Journal* in 1943. Dr. Hal Davison, an Atlanta physician, made the following observations:

> For a long time it has been noted that symptoms of bizarre and unusual cerebral disturbances occur in allergic patients. . . . Later it was observed that when the allergic symptoms improved, the cerebral symptoms improved also. . . . Further observations and experiments showed that at times the cerebral symptoms could be produced at will, by feeding patients certain foods. It was also observed in rarer instances, that ingestion of a drug, inhalation of powdered substances or even odors would produce these symptoms.[40]

Davison then described 87 patients seen in his allergy practice over an eight-year period with symptoms that included blackouts, insomnia, confusion, and changes in personality, all clearly provoked by specific foods or inhalants. As is always the case with allergy, different triggers affected different people. One of the patients, a lawyer, had a progression of symptoms that would start with a headache, followed by itching and hives, then blurred vision, drowsiness, and impaired speech, ending with loss of consciousness. The food triggers were eggs, crab, oysters, and strawberries. Avoiding these foods completely resolved his symptoms.

Medical journals today rarely publish the kind of detailed clinical observations made by Dr. Davison, although they are real and reproducible. In 1985 I spent a day with Professor Roy John, founder of New York University's Brain Research Laboratory and a pioneer in the creation of electronic maps of brain activity. He told me that when patients were connected to his brain mapping device and then injected with extracts of foods, molds, or chemicals to which they were allergic, the injections produced dramatic changes in brain electrical activity, accompanied by the symptoms for which the patients had initially sought care.

Later in this book, in the chapter on nasal and sinus allergies, I'll describe experiments done in Europe in which pollen exposure provoked impairment of brain function comparable to the effects of sedative drugs or alcohol.

Allergy and ADHD

Important scientific research on food allergy and the brain comes from England. Dr. Josef Egger, a neurologist, found that food allergy could lead to ADHD.

Dr. Egger and his colleagues identified 40 children with severe ADHD whose behavior improved when they avoided specific foods.[41] Half the children then underwent an allergy desensitization procedure designed by a colleague of mine, Dr. Len McEwen. They received injections of low doses of food allergens mixed with an enzyme that stimulates an immune response. The other half received injections of the carrier solution without the allergens; this was the placebo control.

At the end of six months, 80 percent of the children receiving the allergen injections were no longer reactive to the foods that had caused behavioral changes. Only 20 percent of the children receiving placebo had become nonreactive to the foods they'd been avoiding. This clearly indicates that allergy—a reaction in which your immune system amplifies the response to a trigger—is an important mechanism of food-induced ADHD. Egger's study was published in *The Lancet*, which is the oldest medical journal in the world and the leading medical journal in the United Kingdom.

If you experience neurologic or psychiatric symptoms that you believe may be provoked by a dietary or environmental exposure, know that science is on your side. Find a doctor who respects your observations—and who understands that allergy comes in more guises than ever in our rapidly changing world.

Conclusion

In this chapter, I revealed the many and surprising ways allergy can impact health. Julia's case showed us how a hidden allergy, in her case an allergy to sulfites found in food, can lead to unexplained joint pain, stomach pain, fatigue, and difficulty with mental focus.

For Cora, the attorney, an allergy to nightshade plants (tomatoes, peppers, and potatoes) turned out to be the surprising cause of her mouth sores, which healed when she avoided eating these foods.

A mysterious case of hives was a real curveball for Bruce, the professional baseball player, until we discovered that the yeast in beer and wine was the cause.

These cases illustrate the Four Game-Changing Truths about Allergies that I believe can transform how we approach health. That is why it is so important that you bring this book with you to see your doctor, to share this information with him or her. Ultimately, it is for your doctor to evaluate and decide how the ideas in this book may inform your journey of healing.

CHAPTER 2

HOW DID WE GET SO SICK?

A sunny September afternoon on Long Island, New York.

It's 1956, a simpler time. Neat houses, all identical, are lined up in a row; the recently planted trees are still young. Children play outdoors on green lawns while large American cars glide slowly by. The sun shimmers on the freshly poured concrete driveways. A dog barks in the distance. Nobody is in much of a rush, and this little patch of America is tranquil.

Back in that simpler time, everyone shopped at the grocery store. There were no superstores. No health food stores. No Starbucks, not yet. That would have to wait. If you wanted coffee, you made it yourself or had it in a restaurant, poured into a ceramic cup. To-go cups? Not a chance.

It was a time, too, when allergies were out of the ordinary. Allergies were something you had heard of. Perhaps you knew someone who was allergic to pollen. Perhaps you knew someone who was allergic to cats. Perhaps you didn't know anyone who had allergies at all. Allergies were rare—and this was only 50 or 60 years ago, a very short time from an evolutionary perspective.

Fast-forward to today. There are a growing number of people allergic to an expanding number of things. One billion people worldwide now suffer from allergies, according to the European Academy of Allergy and Clinical Immunology.[1] The rate of allergies is rising in both the developed and developing world, the World Allergy Association has announced.[2]

And the classic allergens such as pollen and dust have been joined by a whole new bunch of allergens. Ordinary, everyday food items that once seemed safe have become a major problem for millions of people. Wheat. Milk. Eggs. Peanuts. And numerous other foods.

Leading medical journals have proclaimed an epidemic of asthma, and rhinitis has been on the rise. Millions suffer from wheezing, coughing, congestion, burning eyes, and itchy skin. Many more have brain fog, fatigue, weight gain, insomnia, and other symptoms linked to the sorts of hidden allergies we discussed in the last chapter. One thing is clear: people are responding in a vigorous allergic way to the changing world in which we live. And this is only the beginning.

Why Are We So Allergic?

So when, you may wonder, did everything become something we had to worry about? When did so many of us become so dangerously allergic to so many things?

Scientists seeking answers to these questions agree that the rise of allergies is not the result of genetic changes. The period of time we're looking at, about half a century, is too brief to allow for changes in our DNA.[3] Instead, they are exploring how the environment we live in and our modern way of life are responsible for the allergy epidemic.

As I said in the Introduction, allergy arises from your nutrition and your environment—and environment impacts allergy on three levels: outdoors, indoors, and inside your body. The food you eat affects your body's response to allergic triggers at each of these levels. Throughout this book I'll note ways in which the modern Western diet promotes inflammation and allergy by undermining the function of T-reg cells, key players in your body's immune response.

Lunch with a Side of Allergy?

The research has been done. The data has been analyzed. Science has once again told us that the food we put in our mouths has a huge impact on our health. And when we frequently eat at fast-food places, we may be getting more than we ordered.

While fast food has long been considered a hallmark of life in America, this form of eating, with its typically high-fat, high-sodium, and high-carbohydrate meals, has spread around the world. Now a major international study by 144 researchers—the International Study of Asthma and Allergies in Childhood (ISAAC)—reveals that rising consumption of fast food could be contributing to the rise of allergies in children and adolescents.

Data was collected from more than 181,000 children from 31 countries and more than 319,000 adolescents from 51 countries to look at the role of eating patterns in asthma, rhinoconjunctivitis, and eczema. The results include both males and females, in countries that are developed and those that are less developed.

The researchers found that for adolescents, eating fast food three times per week or more was associated with:

- Current wheeze and severe asthma
- Current or severe rhinoconjunctivitis
- Current or severe eczema

For children, eating fast food three times per week or more was associated with the same symptoms, with the exception of current eczema, for which no link was identified in the study.

The study went on to explain the nutritional components that make fast food such a problem. The link between fast food and allergic diseases and asthma is probably due to fast food's typically higher levels of:

- Trans fats (which have been linked to asthma in previous research)
- Saturated fats
- Carbohydrates
- Sugars
- Salt
- Preservatives

On the bright side, the study found that eating fruit three or more times per week was associated with a protective effect in asthma and rhinitis for the adolescents and for all three conditions—asthma, rhinitis, and eczema—in the children.[4]

Changes in your body's inner ecology play a part as well. Each of us is naturally colonized even before birth by an army of microbes— bacteria, yeast, viruses—that stay with us throughout life, shaping the function of our immune systems. Each person's characteristic population of microbes is so distinct, in fact, that criminologists are beginning to use this pattern the way they use fingerprints to identify perpetrators. And abnormalities in your resident microbes have been linked to the development of allergy. Swedish researchers followed children from birth to five years of age and found that the absence of certain bacterial species preceded the development of allergic disorders.[5] Research in this area is just getting started. Later in the book I'll discuss studies on the use of beneficial bacteria— probiotics—to improve different allergic conditions, and I'll discuss some cases where probiotics were part of the allergy treatment.

What about the outer environment? We all have to breathe, and every one of us is affected on the most profound biological level by what is in the air. To explain the rise of allergies and asthma, science points toward rising levels of air pollution and exposure to toxic chemicals and pesticides, alongside poor eating habits, smoking, lack of exercise, and increased stress.

Ambient air pollution due to motor vehicle exhaust, cigarette smoke, and manufacturing produces oxidative stress that harms the lining of your respiratory tract and sensitizes you to airborne allergens. People living near heavy-traffic roadways are particularly vulnerable.[6]

Synthetic chemicals found in food and water act on your cells to shift the way in which your immune system responds to stress, so that your immune responses favor allergic reactivity. And there is more. Greenhouse gases such as carbon dioxide, primarily from coal-burning power plants, cars, trucks, and industry have made the earth warmer, producing a greenhouse effect that affects all forms of life—including increasing the growth of allergenic plants and those plants' production of allergenic pollen.

Dr. Maria Neira, director of the Department of Public Health and the Environment at the World Health Organization, urges us to realize the scope of the problem: "Consider air pollution, the single greatest environmental health risk we face. In 2012 alone, exposure to indoor and outdoor pollutants killed more than seven million people—one in eight deaths worldwide." She adds, "Since 2007, I have described climate change as the defining issue for public health in this century."[7]

Mother Nature's Allergic Reaction

Scientists are working hard to understand how global warming is making conditions worse for allergies and asthma. Two examples are through an extended pollen season and through plants that produce more pollen than before.

Perhaps the postwar economic expansion of the 1950s, the time I mentioned at the start of this chapter, held the seeds of the problem. A never-before-seen boom of industrialization and rapidly changing ways of living caused a vast array of dramatic shifts in a very short time.

In the postwar era, we began to see not just a few more cars and trucks, but millions more cars and trucks. In 1960 there were already 74 million vehicles on the road in the United States, and 5 million vehicles in Canada. By 2002 the number of vehicles in the United States had increased to 233 million, and Canada had 18 million.[8] The number of cars on the road around the world in 2010 surpassed one billion.[9]

Thanks to the millions of barrels of oil being pumped out of the ground, gas was cheap, and new products were born from oil, like plastics and chemicals. The chemical industry took off, producing hundreds of thousands of new substances. New houses sprang up like mushrooms in empty fields that had been productive farmland. Supermarkets spread across the country, and we were introduced to mass marketing of thousands of new processed foods. Bread, which had from time immemorial been baked by hand, was now produced in a factory, sliced and wrapped in plastic, and sent out to stores.

An unbelievable assortment of cookies, candies, ice creams, and sodas became available. So we began indulging our collective sweet tooth with not just a little more sugar, but tons more sugar. The use of margarine increased dramatically as it replaced butter for baking pies and spreading on toast, with consumers totally unaware that the artificial trans fats it contained were dangerous to their health.

Pollen Forecast: Double Trouble on the Way

Lush green grass is a big part of the American dream. Cutting the lawn, watering the lawn, is a shared experience. But the tall wild grasses that grow like weeds in any empty space produce a lot of pollen. You may have seen them; they have a big flower head that looks like a dust wand. The pollen from this grass is highly allergenic; it causes allergic reactions in 20 percent of the general population and in 40 percent of people predisposed to grass allergy.

Now scientists from Harvard University and the University of Massachusetts–Amherst have forecast how much more grass pollen we can expect when more carbon dioxide gets pumped into the air in the coming decades. They have concluded that carbon dioxide, which comes from burning fossil fuels, will double by 2100, and that doubling the carbon dioxide will have the effect of a giant greenhouse, doubling the number of pollen-producing grass plants. In addition to more plants, the experiment revealed that the amount of pollen per flower will be boosted by 50 percent.

"The implications of increasing CO_2 for human health are clear," the study authors explain. "Stimulation of grass pollen production by elevated CO_2 will increase airborne concentrations and increase exposure and suffering in grass pollen–allergic individuals."[10]

Our Environmental Crisis Is a Health Crisis

From the places we live and work to the air we breathe to the food we eat, everything has changed. The world we live in, what seems normal to us, is now remarkably artificial. We live in an environment that has been completely transformed by the actions of humankind. Most of us now live in cities and suburbs; you would have to go to a cabin far off in the country to approximate something natural. But even there you would be breathing air that contained pollution blown in from thousands of miles away.

It seems that the earth, having been pushed too far, for too long, by too many people, has finally had enough. With record-setting high temperatures, rising seas, mass extinctions of wildlife, and fertile land turning into desert, Mother Nature is having a vigorous response to the environmental assaults humankind has delivered. You could say, in fact, that Mother Nature is having a vast allergic reaction. It has turned the world into a more chaotic place with direct implications for our health.

Air Pollution Gives Rise to Asthma and Allergies

Our health problems didn't come out of the blue. Instead, they came from the increasingly polluted skies. A review article by Dr. Gennaro D'Amato, professor of respiratory medicine and respiratory allergy at the University of Naples, in Italy, titled "Effects of climatic changes and urban air pollution on the rising trends of respiratory allergy and asthma," lays the scientific groundwork for this critically important area.[11] Based on work done by the European Academy of Allergy and Clinical Immunology, the European Respiratory Society, and the World Allergy Organization, Professor D'Amato's masterful review explains the connections between climate change, air pollution, allergy, and respiratory diseases.

The review tells us that rhinitis and asthma have increased over the past several decades. Studies have sought to understand what is causing the increase, and indoor and outdoor air pollution, as well as climate change, have been blamed. Much attention and research have focused on the negative impacts of air pollution on respiratory health. For those with allergies, air pollution dials up the airway response to allergens. Air pollution also makes asthma worse, causing greater bronchial hyperresponsiveness, greater use of medication, more hospital admissions, and more visits to the emergency room.[12]

A recent review by researchers from the Johns Hopkins University School of Medicine, Imperial College London, and the National Health Research Institutes of Taiwan sought to find out just *how* air pollution is leading to asthma and allergies. The researchers point out that increasing rates of allergic diseases could be directly caused by air pollution that increases inflammation, oxidative stress, and the immune response.[13]

Let's look at some major pollutants that contribute to this problem.

Particulate Matter or Soot

Particulate matter is soot and dirt that is suspended in the air. It is a major component of air pollution. Particulate matter is linked to exacerbation of allergic asthma, chronic bronchitis, respiratory diseases, cardiovascular disease, and hospital admissions. Studies have confirmed that particulate matter enters the lungs and causes inflammation, leading to cardiovascular and respiratory events.

The World Health Organization estimates that inhaling particulate matter is responsible for 500,000 deaths around the world each year.[14]

Diesel Exhaust

Exhaust from diesel engines, mostly from trucks and buses, accounts for up to 90 percent of the particulate matter in many cities. Many diesel vehicles are so dirty that they produce approximately 100 times more black particle soot per mile than gasoline engines do.[15]

Breathing diesel exhaust changes lung function; burns the eyes, nose, and throat; and causes nausea, fatigue, and headache. Long-term exposure is linked to coughing, decreased lung function, and production of sputum.[16]

A study from the University of California–Los Angeles School of Medicine found that diesel exhaust combined with exposure to ragweed pollen produced stronger allergic reactions in lab experiments. The researchers conclude that "this synergy between DEP [diesel exhaust particles] and natural allergen exposure is suggested as a key feature in increasing allergen-induced respiratory allergic disease."[17] Living in New York City, I can tell you that the throat-burning exhaust from diesel buses and trucks is a problem every single day.

Ozone and Smog

Ozone is the main component of smog, the visible haze that sits heavily over many major cities—including, famously, Los Angeles. Ground-level ozone is created by a chemical reaction when radiation from sunlight interacts with hydrocarbons and nitrogen dioxide from cars and other vehicles.[18] A study from Yale University and the Johns Hopkins Bloomberg School of Public Health explains that ozone was first discovered in the smog of Southern California and now is a recognized air pollution problem across the United States and in many other countries.

Writing in the *Journal of the American Medical Association*, the Yale and Hopkins researchers point out the negative impacts of short-term exposure to ozone: increased emergency room visits and hospital admissions, decreased lung function, and exacerbation of asthma and other respiratory conditions. They explain that in the United States, more than 100 locations exceed the government's limit on ozone, and that the high levels of ozone are a result of both the sheer number of cars and other vehicles on the road today and the high number of miles that those vehicles are driven.[19]

Sulphur Dioxide

Sulphur dioxide comes from burning coal and oil that are high in sulfur. Breathing in this chemical causes acute bronchoconstriction in asthmatics. This effect has been observed after periods of exposure as brief as two minutes. Sulphur dioxide has also been found to increase allergic responses to other allergens in lab studies.[20]

A Sizzling Earth Is Making Us Sick

Global warming may seem like a far-off problem, like when rising seas in the future leave the Statue of Liberty in New York Harbor up to her neck in water. But the consequences of rising temperatures for our health are being felt right now.

The majestic glaciers on the Rocky Mountains that provide much-needed water to millions of people in the American West are shrinking. Droughts are drying out the amazingly productive farmland of California. Massive glaciers on the world's tallest mountain range, the Himalayas, are also retreating, putting at risk a key source of fresh water for Asia. Warming oceans, super droughts, melting glaciers, and extreme weather events like hurricanes and heat waves measure the effects of a warming world—and its real impact on our health.

We are not talking about some problem that may happen in the distant future. We have already crossed over into the danger zone, where hotter temperatures are risking our health today. People with asthma are particularly vulnerable to the worsening air quality. Those with hay fever are vulnerable to the longer and more severe pollen seasons that warmer temperatures are bringing. This is happening in North America and around the world, right now.

Climate Change Worsens Respiratory Illnesses

Since the early 1960s scientists have studied the role that global warming plays in the rising asthma rates in adults and children in a wide range of countries. Today, the serious consequences for health from global warming are a major concern of the medical and scientific communities, as the following examples show.

A study from Macquarie University, in Australia, found that a significant portion of the growing prevalence and severity of asthma is the result of man-made climate change. The Australian researchers also note the increasing rates of allergic rhinitis, hives, and atopic eczema throughout the world and reiterate that higher temperatures have been reported to make the pollen season longer.[21]

The European Respiratory Society is a professional organization that seeks to alleviate the suffering of respiratory disease and to promote lung health through research and medical and public education. The American Thoracic Society is a professional organization dedicated to advancing research, clinical care, and public health in respiratory disease. Both of these bodies have published papers voicing their concerns about the impact of global warming on the health of people with respiratory conditions, including asthma.

Higher ozone concentrations from global warming gases lead to more cardiovascular and respiratory events, the European paper explains. Distribution of allergens, molds, infectious diseases, and smoke from forest fires undermines health and worsens respiratory diseases. The paper states: "The key climatic change factors that could potentially influence respiratory disease are extreme temperature events (both hot and cold), changes in air pollution, flooding, damp housing, thunderstorms, changes in allergen disposition and consequent allergies, forest fires, and dust storms, the effects either being short or long term."[22]

The Thoracic Society paper is titled "Global Warming: A Challenge to All American Thoracic Society Members." It notes that billions of tons of carbon dioxide are being pumped into the atmosphere, mostly from the burning of coal to generate electricity and the burning of gasoline and diesel for transportation. It quotes the director-general of the World Health Organization, Dr. Margaret Chan, who has warned that "climate change will ride across this landscape as the fifth horseman. It will increase the power of the four horsemen that rule over war, famine, pestilence, and death."

Building on Dr. Chan's comments, the Thoracic Society paper notes that the fifth horseman of climate change will impact respiratory patients "through the direct effects of heat, extreme weather events, air pollution, allergic diseases, water- and food-borne infections, and vector-borne and zoonotic diseases.[23]

"Health is inextricably linked to climate change," proclaims an article published in the *Journal of the American Medical Association*. The authors, from the Global Health Institute at the University of Wisconsin–Madison, look at the ill health effects of rising temperatures—heat stress, respiratory disorders including asthma, infectious diseases, and mental health issues such as depression and post-traumatic stress disorder—that are linked to natural disasters. They note that "substantial health and economic co-benefits could be associated with reductions in fossil fuel combustion." The article urges health care providers to communicate the health impacts of climate change and the benefits of reducing greenhouse gases, and concludes by saying that reducing greenhouse gases must happen quickly and at a substantial level.[24]

The U.S. Environmental Protection Agency (EPA), in its turn, states that global warming will likely lead to more severe and longer heat waves that occur with greater frequency. The EPA explains that children, older adults, and those with medical conditions are the most vulnerable to heat waves.[25] Heatstroke and dehydration caused by heat waves are dangerous and can be deadly: during the summer of 2003, a severe heat wave in Europe led to 70,000 deaths in 16 countries.[26]

The United States has warmed by more than 2 degrees Fahrenheit over the past 50 years, notes a report by Physicians for Social Responsibility and the National Wildlife Federation titled *More Extreme Heat Waves: Global Warming's Wake Up Call*. The report states that heat waves increase the risk of asthma attacks, heart attacks, and strokes. The Chicago heat wave of 1995, when temperatures peaked at 106 degrees, was made worse by high humidity and air pollution; a total of 739 people died.[27] The report urges comprehensive cuts in greenhouse gases to limit heat waves in the future and encourages a switch from burning fossil fuels to using renewable sources of energy such as solar power.

The European Respiratory Society spells out the connection between climate change and respiratory disease in no uncertain terms. With regard to the impact of climate change, it states: "The main disease areas of concern are asthma, rhinosinusitis, chronic obstructive pulmonary disease (COPD), and respiratory tract infections."[28] Let's take a closer look at how some of these problems arise.

Turning Up the Heat on Asthma

Higher air temperatures combine with air pollution to form ozone, which exacerbates asthma. The EPA states that warming from climate change is expected to raise the number of days with unhealthy levels of ozone at ground level. Ozone inflames and damages the lungs and exacerbates asthma.[29] In the cities, the urban heat island effect, in which hot air sits above highly populated areas night and day, makes conditions for asthma even worse.

A Longer Pollen Season

Ragweed plants like the higher temperatures and higher levels of pollution that go along with global warming. Ragweed plants thrive and produce more pollen, and the pollen is even more potent than before, the EPA points out.[30]

Smoke from Forest Fires

Forests are particularly vulnerable to temperature variation. For example, warmer temperatures are allowing tree-eating insects to thrive at higher elevations and in more locations than ever. These insects have been chewing their way through entire forests in the western United States and Canada. The dead trees they leave behind contain resin that fuels forest fires. These enormous forest fires cause loss of life among residents and firefighters and give off thick black smoke that can travel hundreds or even thousands of miles—smoke that is directly toxic to everyone and exacerbates asthma as well.

The Rising Tide of Mold

Extreme weather events like hurricanes and floods are increasing. Warmer oceans fuel more powerful hurricanes, which not only threaten the coasts but can also leave a path of destruction far inland. Mold thrives as houses and other buildings fall victim to water damage in the wake of the storms and flooding. Damp housing is associated with cough, wheeze, and asthma.[31]

In the original Netflix TV series *Orange Is the New Black,* mold contamination is a continuing theme. In one episode, an activity room could not be used because of mold. A ceiling collapse in another episode released toxic dust and mold in the chapel room. Mold even showed up on a meal tray, growing on the food. As a recurring guest star on TV, mold has definitely entered the popular imagination.

Cutting Greenhouse Gases—What Will It Take?

The American Thoracic Society's call for a reduction in greenhouse gases is framed as a challenge to the society's members, but it reads like a call to action for all of us. The paper states:

Mitigation of the consequences of global warming and climate change will require dedication and prioritization by the public, governments, and professional and scientific societies, such as the American Thoracic Society (ATS). The United States emits 25% of CO_2 and other greenhouse gases and has 4% of the world's population.

The Kyoto Treaty has been ratified by all of the major nations of the world except the United States; it mandated that the United States reduce CO_2 to levels 7% below 1990 levels by the time period 2008–2012. Promotion of environmentally sound policies in the energy, transportation, land development, and agriculture sectors has great potential both to mitigate climate changes and improve public health for all. To avoid the worst impacts of global warming, the United States needs to achieve an 80% reduction of greenhouse gas emissions from 1990 levels by 2050. This requires transforming our economy to one that is efficient and green compared with the present carbon-based economy.

The post-Kyoto era needs vision and political activism across the political spectrum to achieve ambitious goals of reducing CO_2. In addition to advocacy for local, state, and national policies to mitigate CO_2 emissions, we need to reduce our own individual and worksite carbon footprints, and educate our patients and colleagues of the public health and societal threats posed by climate change.[32]

A Tsunami of Toxins

An array of environmental toxins that assault our health has been implicated in the rise of allergies, explains an article in the journal *Allergy, Asthma & Immunology Research*. More than 100,000 new chemicals have been used in consumer products in the past few decades, and they have made their way into the environment. This wave of toxins places a tremendous burden on the environment and has disastrous consequences for our health, in particular for allergies. "Exposure to environmental toxicants," the authors explain, "not only contributes to the increasing prevalence of asthma and allergies, it also affects disease outcomes, many of which are due to an underlying immune and inflammatory dysfunction."[33]

Chemicals That Interfere with Hormones

One key group of environmental toxins that the scientists implicate in allergies and asthma is the category called endocrine disrupting chemicals (EDCs).[34]

EDCs, chemicals found in everyday products, have made their way into the water, food, and soil all around us. In our bodies, these chemicals mimic or interfere with female and male hormones, as well as the thyroid.[35] They trigger inflammation and can be involved in immune and allergic responses.[36] In addition to being a health concern for people, EDCs are a threat to wildlife. As pesticides and other materials containing EDCs have entered the environment, they have harmed fish, birds, and other wildlife.

"There is mounting concern in the scientific, environmental, private, and governmental sectors on a wide range of substances, known as endocrine disruptors, that may interfere with the normal functioning of a living organism's hormone system,"[37] the Environmental Quality website of the U.S. Fish and Wildlife Service states.

So where do all these EDCs come from? The U.S. National Institute of Environmental Health Sciences tells us that EDCs are found in products such as detergents, plastic bottles, metal food can liners, cosmetics, and toys.[38] EDCs are all around us: we consume them in food and water, inhale them in dust and airborne particles, and absorb them through our skin, according to the WHO. EDCs are found in some pesticides as well, and people who are exposed to pesticides in their work commonly experience wheezing, coughing, and inflammation of the airways. The association between working with pesticides and asthma has also been demonstrated.[39]

Phthalates, a type of EDC, have come under particular scrutiny for their adverse health effects. One phthalate, called diethyl hexyl phthalate (DEHP), which gets into the air and hitches a ride on dust, is linked to wheezing in children.[40] DEHP is used to soften plastics and is found in adhesives, coatings, resins, toys, childcare products, and cosmetics, notes the Australian Government Department of Health.[41] DEHP is also found in consumer food packaging.[42]

In a study of more than 10,000 children, exposure to DEHP and butyl benzyl phthalate was associated with asthma, rhinitis, and eczema.[43] Butyl benzyl phthalate is used in plastics, vinyl floor tile, and carpet backing, and people can be exposed when the chemical is released into the air, according to a report from the WHO.[44]

Another type of EDC, called alkylphenols, have been found to be active in the allergic response that could contribute to the development of asthma. Alkylphenols tend to build up in the body, raise inflammation, and contribute to or worsen allergic conditions.[45]

Indoor Air Pollution

It's not only our outdoor air and water that carry harmful toxins. Science has identified a major health problem in air pollution that occurs indoors—at home, at the office, in schools, in stores, and in many other places where we spend our time.

Tobacco smoke, a highly dangerous source of toxic chemicals, is considered the main culprit in indoor air pollution. Tobacco is a public health disaster for asthma. Wheezing and asthma in children are linked to their exposure to tobacco smoke, and 40 million children are exposed to tobacco smoke each year. Passive smoking—secondhand and even thirdhand—raises the risk of wheezing and asthma for children and young people by at least 20 percent. In children admitted to the hospital for these conditions, blood and saliva tests commonly show exposure to tobacco smoke. Researchers emphasize that "stopping parents smoking is crucially important to the prevention of childhood asthma."[46]

Another major source of indoor air pollution is formaldehyde, a very pervasive chemical that has been found to cause and contribute to nasal allergy, dermatitis, and asthma.[47] Formaldehyde is a volatile organic compound (VOC), which means it becomes a gas at room temperature.[48] Products containing VOCs release these compounds in a process called off-gassing, and this is how formaldehyde gets into the air that we breathe.

This chemical is found in a multitude of products that make their way into homes, offices, schools, retail stores—just about any indoor environment. It's commonly used in composite wood products such as plywood and in the manufacture of fabrics, including clothing. Formaldehyde also turns up in wood floor finishes, paint, and wallpaper and in emissions from laser printers, copiers, and personal computers, the U.S. Consumer Product Safety Commission says.[49] And formaldehyde is a product of combustion, so it is also generated from burning tobacco, natural gas, gasoline, and wood.[50]

The U.S. Consumer Product Safety Commission explains that indoor air levels of formaldehyde can change depending on temperature, humidity, ventilation, and ozone level. It notes that both higher temperatures and higher humidity tend to increase formaldehyde emissions, as do higher-pollution or "ozone action" days.[51] So continued global warming signals an even more troublesome forecast for allergies and asthma due to higher formaldehyde exposure in the future.

Allergy and Asthma Linked to Formaldehyde Exposure

"Breathing formaldehyde vapour can result in irritation of nerves in the eyes and nose, which may cause burning, stinging or itching sensations, a sore throat, teary eyes, blocked sinuses, runny nose, and sneezing," explains the Australian Government Department of Health.[52]

Other research focuses on an even more specific link between formaldehyde, respiratory illness, and allergy. "Increased Risk of Allergy in Children Due to Formaldehyde in Homes" is the name of a study from Monash University in Australia that looked at the impact of indoor air pollution from formaldehyde on children's health. The researchers measured formaldehyde levels in 80 homes in Victoria, Australia, and found that glued wood products, such as particleboard, were the main source of emissions of formaldehyde, which was detected in the bedrooms, living rooms, and kitchens at much higher levels than outside.

They discovered that the children's low-level exposure to formaldehyde was linked to increased allergic sensitization to common airborne allergens. What is more, they found that exposure to higher levels of formaldehyde was linked to more severe sensitization.[53] And they noted that the rise in allergies over the past few decades has paralleled the increase in formaldehyde-emitting products used inside homes.

Another study from Australia, published in the *European Respiratory Journal*, focused on asthma and found that exposure to formaldehyde at home "significantly increases the risk of asthma in young children." For the study, parents whose children had asthma as the primary diagnosis were recruited by the accident and emergency department of Princess Margaret Hospital in Perth, Western Australia. The researchers noticed a seasonal variation in formaldehyde levels, with summer bringing greater exposure to the chemical than winter.[54]

This reinforces a troubling trend that I have mentioned earlier: that in a warming world, higher temperatures will likely increase formaldehyde levels. The researchers state that children exposed to formaldehyde at levels of "49 parts per billion (ppb) are

39% more likely to have asthma compared to those who are not exposed to such levels."[55] Comparable results were obtained by researchers at the University of Arizona, who found that children in houses with formaldehyde at levels of 60 to 120 ppb had significantly greater rates of asthma and bronchitis than those with less exposure.[56]

Conclusion

In this chapter I have explored the big-picture reasons behind the allergy epidemic that is sweeping the world. In order to answer the question *Why are we so sick?* I've outlined reasons that are so fundamental to our well-being that they determine in large measure whether or not we can be healthy.

Leading health organizations and medical centers around the world have documented that a multitude of factors—widespread air pollution, global warming, longer pollen seasons, tobacco smoke, toxic chemicals, dust, fast food, processed food such as trans fats and refined carbohydrates and sugar, and an out-of-balance internal ecology of microbes—are all contributing to the rise of allergies.

Is it any wonder that people are getting sick from polluted air when the number of vehicles on earth is nearing two billion, virtually all of them belching toxic chemicals into the air? We'll come back to the subject of toxins later in the book, when I send you on a mission to root them out and reduce their impact in your personal environment.

To address these challenges, a community effort is needed, and that is why I urge you to bring this book with you to see your doctor, so we can all work together to heal ourselves and the planet. In the next chapter I'll take a closer look at how allergy affects our bodies—particularly our immune systems—and why it makes us so sick.

CHAPTER 3

YOU'RE OVERREACTING: IMMUNITY OUT OF BALANCE

Flip is a rock musician, a skilled guitarist who called me in a panic one day, wailing, "I've become allergic to my guitar! This is the end of my career. You've got to help me."

I saw him in my office the same day. He wasn't exaggerating. His fingertips were oozing and weeping, covered with a red, scaly rash where they made contact with the metal strings on his guitar. The diagnosis was immediately obvious: he had developed a condition called allergic contact dermatitis, and the fact that stainless steel guitar strings provoked the reaction made it likely that he was reacting to nickel, which is alloyed to iron in producing stainless steel.

Nickel is one of the most common contact allergens in the world. People with nickel allergy react with a red, scaly, blistering rash when their skin makes contact with the metal, which is found in stainless steel products like costume jewelry, watch casings, and kitchen utensils. The diagnosis can be confirmed by a patch test, in which a small piece of paper containing a nickel solution is applied to the skin. The development of nickel allergy requires skin exposure to nickel and is increased in people with stainless steel earrings that pierce the skin.[1]

Surprisingly, nickel is also found in many foods. It occurs naturally in whole grains and beans and some fruits and vegetables; it's also found in most canned goods, as nickel from the stainless-steel can penetrates the food. People who are nickel sensitive may react to the nickel present in food with skin rashes and with gastrointestinal symptoms such as abdominal pain. This reaction is called systemic nickel allergy syndrome (SNAS).[2] For more information on nickel levels in food, visit www.drgalland.com.

Flip had been playing rock guitar since the age of 10, so I wanted to understand why he had become allergic to nickel suddenly at the age of 30. I noticed that he had a gold earring in his left ear and asked him if that was new; I didn't remember seeing it before. Yes, he told me. He'd had a steel earring inserted a few months earlier, but the puncture site got inflamed, so he had it removed and replaced with a gold stud. I also noticed that he'd lost weight and asked him whether he'd changed his diet. Yes, he said, he'd been trying to get healthy, so he'd cut out refined grains and meat and started eating whole wheat and brown rice and alfalfa sprouts a few weeks earlier.

My analysis indicated a three-step process that had produced Flip's life-altering nickel allergy:

- The steel earring sensitized him to nickel. He had removed the earring because he began reacting to it, but he didn't realize that the rash was an allergy; he thought it was an infection at the site of the piercing.

- The increase in dietary nickel from adopting a healthy, whole-foods diet increased his total nickel exposure and made him more sensitive to nickel in general.

- His skin reacted in the one place where nickel touched it: his fingertips when he played guitar.

The program I suggested had two components: First, Flip was to avoid all skin exposure to nickel for three months. He limited his guitar-playing to acoustic guitar with nylon strings and did not wear a watch or jewelry. Second, he was to follow a low-nickel diet. The skin on his fingertips improved within a few days on this diet, but he maintained it for three months anyway.

Over the next several months, Flip's nickel allergy totally abated. He was able to play rock guitar and eat a whole-foods diet with no skin rash. If he wanted to wear jewelry or an earring, I insisted that it be sterling silver or 14-karat gold, so that he would avoid any undue persistent skin contact with nickel. He's been fine now for six years.

What Is an Allergic Reaction?

An allergic reaction is a self-amplifying chain reaction that begins with a trigger and ends with a series of effects that include the symptoms you experience and the signs a doctor finds on examination. The trigger can be minuscule, and the effects can vary from subtle to catastrophic. If your immune system supplies the amplification, the reaction is considered to be allergy. Whatever the details, the fundamental pattern of allergy is:

Exposure to a trigger → amplification of the signal
by the immune system → effects

The trigger is called an allergen or an antigen. You do not experience an allergic reaction on your first exposure to an allergen. The allergic response requires that a memory of the allergen already be imprinted on your immune system. It's like recognizing a face: you have to have seen the face before. The allergic reaction will show itself only on subsequent exposures—sometimes the second exposure, sometimes not until multiple exposures have occurred.

Allergens come in all shapes and sizes and can be present in anything you breathe, eat, or touch. Allergens initiate the allergic cascade when they attach to a receptor on an immune cell that activates the immune amplification response. Some allergens produce such an overwhelming immune reaction that an amount too small to measure can trigger a life-threatening allergic reaction. This is the case with peanut allergy, which can trigger fatal reactions (see "Peanut Allergy" on page 49).

The Conductors of Your Immune System

Allergic reactions are commonly thought of as misguided or overreactive responses of the immune system, but I believe they are due to a *lack* of function of key immune cells, so they can actually be thought of as resulting from immune deficiency rather than immune excess.

Most people think of immunity as if the immune system were a radio, with the main control over its output being the volume dial: louder or softer, stronger or weaker. But your immune system is much more like an orchestra. There are many sections, and the output from each section must be synchronized with the output from every other section. When you want more from the strings, you have to quiet the horns or the strings will be drowned out. Organizing the synchronicity of immune responses is the job of a group of white blood cells called lymphocytes. They're the conductors of the body's immune system orchestra.

For people with allergies, one particular type of lymphocyte seems to be the weak link. These are the regulatory T-cells, or T-regs, which limit inflammation by turning off unwanted immune responses. Numerous studies have shown that in people with allergies, the T-regs are not functioning properly. This leads to the unwanted immune responses that are the hallmark of allergy.

Scientists in Norway studied immune responses in children with allergy to cow's milk who outgrew their allergy and compared them with the responses of children who remained allergic to milk.[3] All the children in the study followed a totally dairy-free diet for an average of six months. Their prior symptoms, which included diarrhea, vomiting, and eczema, cleared quickly.

Milk was then reintroduced into their diets, slowly and cautiously, building up to 115 millilitres a day. About half the children no longer showed any adverse reaction to milk, but the other half experienced a return of symptoms and milk had to be stopped. A week later, all the children's blood was tested. The major immune difference between the two groups was that the children who had outgrown their allergy had a higher level of T-regs in their blood. Further testing demonstrated that the T-regs were responsible for preventing the allergic response.

The Process of Allergy

The effects of allergy—the symptoms that make you sick—are created by cells called effector cells and by the specialized chemicals they release, which are called mediators. The two major types of allergy effector cells are mast cells and eosinophils, or Eos. Most of the drugs used to treat allergies work by blocking the effects of mast cell mediators; antihistamines are the best-known example. Steroids work in part by killing off Eos. This book offers a different approach: a way to identify and avoid the hidden triggers of allergy and turn down the immune amplification process.

Effector cells produce the effects that we call an allergic reaction. But the first thing to know about these cells is that they do not exist to make you sick; they play an essential role in wound healing and tissue regeneration and also protect your body from infection and toxicity.[4]

Mast cells, for example, are activated by bee venom to produce the swelling and pain associated with bee stings. Eos play an important role in killing parasites. In the current epidemic of allergy sweeping the world, allergy effector cells have been hijacked by allergens and tricked into doing more harm than good.

Mast cells supply most of your body's histamine—one type of chemical mediator—and are the effector cells of the initial, or early phase, allergic response. They are an ancient type of cell, found even in primitive animals like sea squirts, where they function as mainstays of the immune system.[5] In humans they are large cells sparsely distributed throughout all tissues of the body. The chemical mediators that they make, store, and release not only cause the symptoms of allergy, but also attract other cells, especially Eos, that create the late-phase allergic response.

Eos circulate in your blood but readily wander into your tissues, where they release an array of unique mediators of their own. The best studied of these are enzymes that cause considerable damage to cells of all types.[6] Invasion of tissues by Eos is a major feature of chronic allergic diseases including asthma, sinusitis, and gastrointestinal disorders. Eos also shift your immune response pattern in the direction of greater sensitivity. Activation of Eos initiates a vicious cycle, a feed-forward loop in which allergy induces more allergy.

Mast Cell Mediators

Mast cells produce about 200 mediators that create the signs and symptoms of allergic reactions. Most drug treatment of allergy works by suppressing the synthesis or blocking the activity of these mediators.

The best-known mast cell mediators are:

- Histamine: Causes the typical symptoms of acute allergies by dilating blood vessels to produce redness and heat. Histamine makes blood vessels leaky, so that blood plasma seeps out into the surrounding tissues, causing swelling. It also causes many of the symptoms associated with classic allergic reactions, like sneezing and hives. Antihistamines are the standard first-line therapy for symptoms of allergy.

- Serotonin: Constricts blood vessels and increases motility of the gastrointestinal tract. It may cause abdominal cramps and diarrhea. In the brain, serotonin has numerous effects on mood, sleep, and cognitive function. Some drugs used to treat allergic symptoms, especially itching, work by blocking serotonin.

- Prostaglandin D2 (PGD2): Causes constriction of bronchial tubes and plays a key role in the wheezing of asthma. It also dilates blood vessels to cause flushing of the skin or redness of the eyes. Some of the eyedrops used to treat allergic conjunctivitis block the synthesis of PGD2 in the eyes.

- Leukotrienes (LTs): Increase mucus secretion and make bronchial tubes constrict. They contribute to the misery of asthma and hay fever. LT antagonists like monteleukast (Singulair), a prescription drug, may reduce symptoms of allergy.

The Four Types of Allergy

The term *allergy* was coined by a Viennese pediatrician, Claude von Pirquet, in 1906, to explain the sneezing of children exposed to pollen. The clearest translation of its meaning is "altered reactivity," and it soon became clear that allergy involves excessive and abnormal activation of the immune system.

During the 20th century, scientists identified four types of immune activation that lead to allergic reactions.[7] All four types can occur in people with allergic disorders.[8] Each type requires that your immune system recognize a specific allergen because of a previous exposure to it. In the first three types, that previous exposure caused your immune system to make antibodies directed against the allergen. The usual function of antibodies, which are proteins made by cells of your immune system, is to create immunity, helping you resist infection; allergy turns this protective effect into a harmful one. The fourth type of allergy, the type that occurs with nickel dermatitis, does not require antibodies to produce its effects.

Type 1 Allergy

Type 1 allergic reactions, the most common form, result from formation of an antibody called IgE (immunoglobulin E). When IgE attaches to an allergen, it stimulates mast cells to release mediators like histamine into your tissues with explosive force. Standard blood tests for allergies look for the presence of IgE antibodies directed against specific allergens. Skin tests for allergies attempt to measure the swelling produced in your skin when IgE antibodies attach to an allergen that's being injected.

Type 1 is the kind of allergic reaction that occurs with anaphylaxis, eczema, hives, hay fever, and allergic asthma. It has two phases, early and late. Symptoms of the **early phase** allergic response are caused by the release of mast cell mediators. They can occur within seconds of exposure to an allergen and may last for a few hours. Some mast cell mediators also attract Eos to the inflamed tissues.

Activation of Eos creates the **late phase** allergic response. The most potent mediators released by Eos are enzymes that damage cells. They're capable of killing parasites and can inflict the same kind of damage on your own tissues. The late phase reaction may last for days and can cause long-lasting changes to your tissues and your immune system: damaged tissues may heal with scarring, and your immune system may shift so that your lymphocytes further increase their production of IgE antibodies. It's a dangerous cascade that can allow allergies to spin out of control.

If you suffer from allergic eczema, you can see the difference between the early and late phase responses in your own skin. When you eat a food to which you're allergic, your skin becomes red, somewhat swollen, and very itchy. Once this early phase reaction subsides, your skin becomes thickened and scaly, still red and itchy but with less intensity. That's the late phase response, and if it lasts long enough, your skin does not readily return to normal.

Type 2 and Type 3 Allergy

Type 2 and Type 3 allergy depend upon another class of antibody, called IgG (immunoglobulin G), to amplify the allergic signal. IgG is the main class of antibodies circulating in your blood. IgG is essential for a normal immune response, and its deficiency predisposes people to recurrent or chronic bacterial infections.

Type 2 and 3 reactions are the main mechanisms involved in drug allergies and may occur in some people with food allergy, especially when migraine headache, abdominal pain, or arthritis are the allergic symptoms.[9]

Two factors make Type 2 or Type 3 allergy to foods or drugs hard to detect. First, IgE antibodies are not involved, so standard allergy tests, which measure IgE, will not detect this kind of allergy. Second, the onset of the allergic reaction is often delayed, sometimes occurring 24 hours or more after exposure to the triggering allergen. You have to be a really good detective to track down these reactions. The same is true for Type 4 allergy, which is known as delayed hypersensitivity.

Type 4 Allergy

Type 4 allergic reactions do not require antibodies. The triggering allergens directly activate immune cells called helper lymphocytes, which amplify the response themselves, attracting so-called killer lymphocytes to the area where the antigen is found. Killer cells are just as effective as Eos at causing tissue damage.

Type 4 reactions occur in a number of infectious diseases, such as tuberculosis, where they help to control the spread of the infection. They also contribute to the damage that occurs in several autoimmune disorders, including rheumatoid arthritis, Crohn's disease, type 1 diabetes, multiple sclerosis, and Hashimoto's thyroiditis.

The most common allergic disorder employing the Type 4 mechanism is poison ivy, an allergic skin rash caused by exposure to oils from plants in the genus Toxicodendron. Allergic contact dermatitis (like Flip's allergy to nickel, for example) usually involves a Type 4 reaction. For some people, Type 4 reactions may cause asthma. As I describe in Chapter 12, up to 15 percent of asthmatic reactions may occur because of Type 4 allergy. Food allergy may also be caused by Type 4 reactions, especially when the allergic reaction affects the gastrointestinal tract or the skin.

Anaphylaxis: Allergy That Can Kill

The term *anaphylaxis* was coined in 1901 by the French scientist Charles Richet, who received the Nobel Prize for his research in 1913. Richet coined a new word for what he believed to be a new concept: hypersensitization, or, as he expressed it, "the opposite of a protective response."

With an anaphylactic reaction, your body is flooded with chemicals that cause instantaneous, massive swelling of the affected tissues, dilation of blood vessels, contraction of the smooth muscles that line your airways or intestines, and irritation of nerve endings. If the reaction involves your tongue, throat, or respiratory tract, you may be unable to breathe. If it involves your circulatory system, your blood pressure can drop profoundly, producing anaphylactic shock. Swelling of your face, your lips, your eyes, or any part of your skin, as well as wheezing, abdominal cramps, and diarrhea, are other symptoms that may occur with anaphylaxis.

The usual triggers for anaphylaxis are insect stings, specific foods such as peanuts, or medication such as penicillin. Emergency treatment is essential and starts with an injection of adrenaline, which raises blood pressure, constricts blood vessels and dilates bronchial tubes.

Anyone with a history of anaphylactic reactions should carry a device for rapid self-injection of adrenaline at all times and have an emergency action plan worked out with his or her personal physician.

The incidence of anaphylactic reactions has doubled over the past decade, with an estimated 1,500 fatalities a year in the United States, yet most patients receiving emergency treatment for anaphylaxis at U.S. hospitals do not receive an adrenaline auto-injector or an allergist referral when discharged, a missed opportunity for preventing further reactions.[10]

Studies in many different countries have all reached the same conclusion: people prone to anaphylaxis are not adequately armed with adrenaline. As severe as it is, life-threatening anaphylaxis is still underdiagnosed, underreported, and undertreated.[11]

Peanut Allergy

Peanut allergy is one prevalent cause of anaphylaxis. Peanuts contain at least 12 allergenic proteins, two of which can cause anaphylaxis in sensitive individuals.[12] A telephone survey of more than 4,000 U.S. households in 1997 concluded that peanut or tree nut allergies affected 1.1 percent of those surveyed (which translates to about three million people in the U.S. population).[13] A follow-up study five years later found a doubling of peanut allergy among children.[14] By 2007 the prevalence of peanut allergy among schoolchildren in the United States had tripled, and researchers were using the term *epidemic* to describe the increase.[15] A British study documented a tripling in the rate of allergic skin-test reactivity to peanut extract among schoolchildren during the 1990s and a doubling of clinical allergic reactions to peanuts.[16]

The reasons for the increase in peanut allergy are not clear. Most children with peanut allergy get sick immediately on their first known exposure to peanuts. For this to happen, the child must already have been exposed to peanuts, so that his immune system became sensitized to peanut allergens.

Researchers at Imperial College London attempted to identify factors that separated children with proven peanut allergy from children with other allergies or no allergies. The most significant difference was that children who developed peanut allergy had been rubbed with skin care products containing peanut oil (arachis oil) twice as often as children who did not develop peanut allergy.[17] Peanut oil is a common component of skin care and infant care products in the United States as well as the United Kingdom. The list of commonly used topical preparations that contain arachis oil includes Cerumol (for removing earwax), Siopel barrier cream, zinc and castor oil ointment, calamine oily lotion, Dermovate (a potent topical steroid cream used for difficult eczema), and Naseptin cream.[18]

The British researchers also found that peanut allergy was more likely to occur if other family members ate peanuts.[19] Their theory is that exposure to peanut allergens through the skin is the main risk factor for peanut allergy. This theory might explain why children with eczema are at increased risk for developing anaphylaxis from peanuts. The inflamed and broken skin of eczema allows increased absorption of peanut antigens through the skin.

There is at present no specific treatment that can reverse peanut allergy.

The Mystery of Oral Tolerance

How you're exposed to an antigen in infancy can determine whether you react to it as if it is a friend or a foe. When a child eats a food, especially a large dose of the food, his or her immune system usually recognizes the food as safe and responds to it with a reaction called oral tolerance, a reaction that says "friend." If the infant is exposed to the same antigen through the skin, oral tolerance does not occur and allergenic sensitization may result. A study of mice found that exposure to peanut protein on the skin produced an allergic response to peanut allergens followed by an even stronger reaction when the mice were subsequently fed peanuts.[20]

Oral tolerance to food and intestinal bacteria helps to prevent food allergy and intestinal inflammatory disorders like celiac disease, Crohn's disease, and ulcerative colitis. A critical step in oral tolerance is the development of the specialized lymphocytes called T-regs that we discussed earlier in this chapter, which work to prevent dangerous hypersensitivity responses to antigens.[21]

Red Meat Allergy Triggered by Tick Bites

A new phenomenon burst into medical journals in 2009. People who had been eating meat their entire lives suddenly developed hives or anaphylaxis after a meal of beef, pork, or lamb but had no reaction to any other food.[22] In almost every case, the development of red meat allergy had followed bites by hard-bodied ticks. The initial account came from the University of Virginia, but the same strange syndrome was soon reported from places as far-flung as Australia, Scandinavia, Spain, and China.[23]

Although most food allergens are proteins, the Virginia researchers found that in affected people, tick bites caused the development of an IgE Type 1 antibody response to alpha-gal, a sugar that is found in red meat but not in human tissues. Hard-bodied ticks also contain alpha-gal and inject it into the skin of people they bite. Recognizing alpha-gal as a foreign substance, the lymphocytes of some people mount an immune response to destroy it. This disrupts the normal response of the body to potential food allergens, which is oral tolerance. The next time that person eats red meat, the misdirected protective response creates an allergic reaction that can include itching, burning, hives, throat swelling, and even anaphylactic shock. Although it's a Type 1 allergic reaction, which usually starts soon after allergen exposure, the alpha-gal red meat reaction may not occur for several hours after the meat is consumed.[24]

Tick-bite red meat allergy is another example of skin exposure to an allergen creating an allergic reaction that overrides oral tolerance, your natural defense against food allergy.

Conclusion

This chapter kicked off with the case of the rock musician, Flip, who developed a dramatic allergy to his guitar strings. His case helps us answer the question: what is an allergy? Allergy starts with a trigger, followed by amplification of the signal by the immune system that produces the effects, or symptoms. I introduced the concept of the immune system as an orchestra, where white blood cells called T-regs are like conductors who maintain a balance in the music. In upcoming chapters we will look at many ways of supporting the function of these T-regs to help reduce allergic reactivity.

I also outlined the four types of allergy and drilled down to the cellular level of allergy with a look at effector cells and mast cell mediators. Given the medical nature of this material, it is imperative that you bring these pages with you when you see your doctor. Because allergy is complex and carries the potential of a dangerous allergic reaction, you must follow the professional advice of your doctor.

Now that you understand more about what's going on in your body when you have an allergic reaction, let's turn to figuring out what triggers *you*—because knowing what's wrong is the first step toward making it right.

CHAPTER 4

CRACKING THE CODE: UNMASKING HIDDEN ALLERGIES

"Before last year, I never knew the meaning of fatigue. I'd run circles around my husband," Kate said. "I'm a graphic artist. I worked ten-hour days, raised two kids, went for a run before work every morning . . . I'm sorry, I didn't mean to cry," she added, as her eyes filled with tears. "I've lost my life. I can't exercise, I feel like a zombie at work, I'm missing out on my kids' lives. Going to dance recitals or soccer games feels like agony. All I want to do is lie down and rest. My brain feels like glue. Every little thing I do takes so much effort. I'm just not the person I once was."

Like so many other women, Kate had built her life around taking care of other people. Her family and her clients came first. Even with a debilitating illness, her main concern was its effect on others. "I don't even know what to call this disease," she told me. "It's not like I have cancer or heart failure. Sure, I'm depressed, but who wouldn't be?"

Kate's symptoms seemed to come out of nowhere. It's a story I've heard from many of my patients. The inner dialogue escalates like this:

- *I'm working too hard; maybe I need a vacation . . .*
- *Maybe this is what happens when you get older . . .*
- *Maybe I have a virus . . . or I'm anemic . . .*
- *Could my thyroid be underactive?*
- *Could I be depressed?*
- *What's wrong with me?*

Kate stopped making plans to go out on weekends. A pattern emerged. She'd feel worse and worse as the week went on, then spent the weekend resting, trying to recover. She'd feel her best by Sunday night, although never really well. Her internist examined her and ran blood tests. Everything was normal. That was a relief, but also a source of frustration.

When Kate first consulted me, I thought that her weekly symptom pattern was a good place to start. In fact, it quickly led to the most important aspect of her illness: she always felt unwell at her workplace.

The previous August she'd taken two weeks' vacation and traveled upstate with her family. Poison ivy struck on day one, carried on the smoke from a fire in an empty field. A day later her face turned red and began to swell and itch. She found an urgent care center a few miles away, and a doctor gave her a prescription for five days of steroids.

Almost at once a turnaround occurred. Not only did her skin rash clear, but her chronic symptoms greatly improved. Her fatigue vanished; her mood lifted. By the end of the first week she was hiking in the Adirondacks with her kids. Kate was elated.

But when her vacation was over and she returned to work, her world came crashing down all over again. After a few days following her usual routine, the devastating cycle of symptoms returned, but now it was even worse. Her doctor concluded that work stress had to be the culprit and referred her to a psychologist.

Yet after meeting with Kate, the psychologist felt that stress was not the cause, that it had to be something physical, and referred her to me.

I considered various possibilities that might explain Kate's rapid improvement after taking medicine for poison ivy. My leading suspicion was that she was allergic to something in her workplace, which was why two weeks away plus a dose of steroids had restored her almost to normal. If something in her workplace was making her sick, being away on vacation could improve her symptoms. And steroids could temporarily suppress allergic reactions. Putting those two factors together could account for Kate's turnaround on her trip.

I considered that her problem was unlikely to be a simple allergy. If you're allergic to cats, for example, and you visit a friend who has cats, your eyes may itch and water or you may sneeze or wheeze, but the symptoms will usually start soon after you're exposed and will usually clear within hours of leaving your friend's home. Kate's pattern indicated a delayed allergic reaction, one that's more typical of mold allergy.

We needed more information, so I gave Kate two assignments:

- First, find out if there had been any leaks or floods in the building where she worked, and look carefully for signs of water damage or discoloration of walls or ceiling.

- Second, see if she could work from home for a week or two without going into the office.

Kate worked for a major graphic arts company in a midtown office building. As she carefully surveyed the walls and ceilings, she realized that the heating and cooling vents near her desk looked sooty rather than pure white. With a little bit of investigation, she had located a possible source of mold: the ducts that blew air into her work space.

As most of her work was done on a laptop, Kate was able to work from home for a week. The cycle of symptoms began to improve. She wasn't back to normal by the end of the week, the way she'd been on steroids, but she was better on Friday than she'd been on Monday. She'd broken the pattern by avoiding her office, but she wanted to get back to work with the artists on her team.

Through testing at her office, it was discovered that samples taken from within the ducts grew eight species of mold. Fixing the problem required careful cleaning of the ducts and rebalancing of the entire system to prevent moisture from accumulating at junctures in the ductwork. Everyone working in the office noticed how much fresher the air felt, and Kate was able to return to her desk without her debilitating symptoms coming back. But she was still not well.

Finding mold contamination was just the first step. I still needed to address two factors for Kate to regain her normal vitality. Both were factors internal to Kate: allergy and toxicity.

As a result of heavy mold exposure, mold allergy had become a real problem for Kate. We needed to consider other sources of mold, outside her office.

Moreover, two of the mold species found in the air ducts produce toxins that can affect immune function. These toxins don't necessarily leave your body as soon as exposure ends. Your liver discharges them into bile and they're secreted into your small intestine; then they are reabsorbed into your bloodstream, so they keep recycling within your body. Kate would need help with detoxification.

By applying the steps I will share with you in the chapters ahead, I was able to help Kate improve her personal environment. She diminished her mold exposure at home, where excess moisture in her bathroom had permitted mold growth behind the sink. And by following the Immune Balance Diet, she reduced dietary mold and supported detoxification. In order to enhance the detoxification process, I asked Kate to take two dietary supplements:

- NAC (n-acetylcysteine), an amino acid and antioxidant, which I have found to be helpful for detoxification

- Coconut charcoal, because charcoal absorbs toxins; when taken orally, it can trap toxic substances in the intestines so they're excreted from the body rather than absorbed into the bloodstream

Kate's complete recovery took about a month.

To help Kate restore her health, we considered three questions that are essential for anyone who suspects he or she may have hidden allergies:

- Is allergy the cause of your unexplained symptoms?

- Are there dietary or environmental allergens you need to eliminate?

- Why are you allergic? Are there factors creating allergy that you can change?

In this chapter I'll take you through the questions I ask my patients in order to get the answers I need.

The Allergy Solution Process of Discovery

You are about to embark on a fantastic voyage of discovery to an uncharted sphere of new understanding about yourself and your personal environment. It is likely to be a defining event. You will be asking yourself new questions about your symptoms, meant to bring out hidden clues about your health. Some you'll be able to answer right away, like whether your joints ache or whether you have brain fog. Other questions will seem more obscure, like whether you have an abnormal sense of smell or taste. The questions are designed to enable you to gather critically important information about yourself and your personal environment, both around you and inside you.

What may emerge is a whole new way of seeing and thinking about health, with you at the center. Each item can seem like an isolated detail, but even small clues can unlock the mystery of your health journey and get you closer to uncovering what your allergic triggers might be and how they influence your life. There are some thought-provoking questions here, and don't be surprised if the process is emotional. It is often a revelation to stop and think about how your symptoms impact your life.

In the pages ahead, you'll take four steps toward unmasking your allergies.

First, using the Allergy Solution Checklist of Symptoms, you'll identify and record your health issues.

Second, in the Rate Your Symptoms section, you'll use the questions provided to measure the severity, frequency, and duration of your symptoms.

Third, in the Search for Triggers section, you'll find questions designed to help you think about the timing and rhythm of your symptoms, and how these relate to your personal environment. This can help you identify what is triggering your symptoms, bringing you closer to understanding your allergies.

Fourth, in the Search for Origins section, I will highlight key issues that often lead up to allergies.

When you're done, you'll have a lot of new information about yourself and your health. And I want you to bring all of the information you collect here with you when you go to see your doctor. Quite likely it will spark a very productive conversation, stimulating new ideas and new areas for exploration. It is about helping you and your doctor look closer, know more, understand your own health journey more fully, and make significant progress toward uncovering your allergies.

The Allergy Solution Checklist of Symptoms

First step: make a list of the symptoms that bother you. These are the symptoms you're going to rate and evaluate. These are the symptoms you'll be working to eliminate. If you have too many symptoms to remember, this list may jog your memory. For now, just record them. You'll analyze them later.

I've seen each of these symptoms occur as the result of allergies in different patients. If you don't see your symptoms listed here, just fill them in at the end.

List Your Symptoms

- ☐ Fatigue—physical or mental

  - • What have you stopped doing because of fatigue?

    _____

- ☐ General unwellness or malaise

- ☐ Weight problems
  - ☐ Trouble losing weight
  - ☐ Trouble gaining weight
  - ☐ Food cravings
  - ☐ Excessive appetite

- ☐ Pain
  - ☐ Headache
  - ☐ Earache
  - ☐ Sore throat
  - ☐ Sinus pressure

  - ☐ Chest pain

    - • Where in your chest?

      _____

  - ☐ Heartburn
  - ☐ Abdominal pain
    - ☐ Above your belly button?
    - ☐ Below your belly button?
  - ☐ Back or neck pain

☐ Joint pain

- Which joints?

_____

☐ Muscle pain

- Which muscles?

_____

☐ Pain in a different area of your body

- Which area?

_____

☐ Poor sleep
  - ☐ Trouble falling asleep
  - ☐ Trouble staying asleep
  - ☐ Waking up not well rested in the morning
☐ Mood disturbances
  - ☐ Depression
  - ☐ Anxiety
  - ☐ Mood swings
  - ☐ Irritability
☐ Cognitive problems
  - ☐ Brain fog—trouble focusing or concentrating
  - ☐ Poor memory
  - ☐ Confusion
  - ☐ Hyperactivity
☐ Dizziness
  - ☐ Feeling light-headed or off balance
  - ☐ Spinning in your head

- ☐ Itching, swelling, or redness
  - ☐ Face
  - ☐ Eyes
    - ☐ Are they gooey?
  - ☐ Ears
  - ☐ Throat
  - ☐ Hands or feet
  - ☐ Scalp
  - ☐ Butt
  - ☐ Genitals
    - ☐ Is there a discharge?
  - ☐ Different area of your body

    - • Which area?

      _____

  - ☐ All over
- ☐ Runny nose, sneezing
- ☐ Postnasal drip, throat clearing
- ☐ Abnormal sense of smell or taste
  - ☐ Decreased smell or taste
  - ☐ Heightened sensitivity to odors
- ☐ Cough
  - ☐ Dry
  - ☐ Wet—coughing up mucus
- ☐ Difficulty breathing
  - ☐ Wheezing

☐ Palpitation

   ☐ Irregular heartbeat

   ☐ Rapid heartbeat

   ☐ Pounding heartbeat

☐ Gas

   ☐ Abdominal bloating

   ☐ Belching or burping

   ☐ Flatulence

☐ Diarrhea

☐ Constipation

☐ Dry, flaky, or scaly skin

☐ Acne

☐ Hair loss

☐ Other symptoms you are experiencing

_____

_____

Describe Your Symptoms

Allergic symptoms usually fluctuate, depending in part upon your exposure to allergic triggers. Doctors describe these fluctuations using the terms *severity, frequency,* and *duration.* Severity has two parts: how intense the symptom gets at its worst and the overall impact of the symptom on your life. Frequency and duration determine the pattern of your symptoms.

For each symptom you have selected or written down on the above list of symptoms, ask yourself:

Is the symptom always present, or does it come and go?

   ☐ Always present—never completely without it

   ☐ Comes and goes—sometimes it's not present at all

When it's present, does it fluctuate in intensity?

☐ Whenever I have it, it's always the same

☐ Sometimes it's stronger and sometimes it's milder

What percent of time is the symptom at its worst?
10, 20, 30, 40, 50, 60, 70, 80, 90

What percent of time is the symptom at its mildest?
10, 20, 30, 40, 50, 60, 70, 80, 90

What percent of time are you free of the symptom?
0, 10, 20, 30, 40, 50, 60, 70, 80, 90

What percent of the time are you free of all symptoms?
0, 10, 20, 30, 40, 50, 60, 70, 80, 90

Once you understand the pattern of your symptoms, you can rate them. For each symptom on the checklist that you've selected or written down, answer the questions in the section below. This will allow you to keep track of your progress. It's the key to accurate journaling, which will be useful when you start the Power Wash in Chapter 6. Record your answers in the table provided after the questions:

• How much does this symptom impact your life?
(This is Overall Severity.)

1. A little
2. Moderately
3. A lot
4. Can't stand it

• If it fluctuates, how bad is it at its worst?
(This is Peak Severity.)

1. Minor annoyance
2. Somewhat troublesome
3. Very symptomatic
4. Agony

- How often does the symptom occur?

1. Less than once a month
2. About once a month
3. Two or three times a month
4. About once a week
5. Two or three times a week
6. About once a day
7. More than once a day
8. Constantly

- How long does it last each time it occurs?

1. Seconds—a fleeting symptom, however severe it is
2. A few minutes
3. Up to an hour but not longer
4. Up to several hours but less than all day
5. About a whole day
6. Several days
7. A week or longer
8. Too variable to describe this way

Record and Rate Your Symptoms

Use this table to record the symptoms that trouble you and to rate them with regard to:

- Overall Severity (How much this symptom impacts your life)

- Peak Severity (How bad it is at its worst)

- Frequency (How often it occurs)

- Duration (How long it lasts when it occurs)

SYMPTOM	OVERALL SEVERITY (RATE 1 TO 4)	PEAK SEVERITY (RATE 1 TO 4)	FREQUENCY (RATE 1 TO 8)	DURATION (RATE 1 TO 8)

The Search for Triggers

Allergy detective work is the search for triggers. Nothing produces such dramatic and total relief as identifying an allergic trigger and eliminating it. Not all triggers can be eliminated, of course. But knowing what they are is of great benefit in creating an individualized treatment program.

Sometimes the trigger is obvious, because the symptoms are immediate and your exposure is episodic. Allergy to cats or to peanuts usually falls into the "obvious" category. But many of the cases described in this book involve triggers that were not obvious. They had to be ferreted out. The function of the next list is to help you identify the non-obvious triggers for your allergic symptoms.

Please answer the questions below for each symptom on the Checklist of Symptoms that you selected or wrote down. These questions apply to symptoms that fluctuate in severity or that come and go. I've listed the most common types of triggers, but the list is not exhaustive.

☐ Is there a rhythm to the occurrence or severity of the symptom?

☐ Worse during the night or in the morning when you first wake up?

- Could be something you ate the night before.

- Could be something in your bedroom:

  ☐ Dust and dust mites are the most common bedroom allergens. They hide in carpets, drapes, pillows, mattresses, books, and stuffed animals.

  ☐ Laundry detergent or fabric softener used on your sheets might be a problem.

  ☐ Has there been a leak or flood, perhaps in an attached bathroom?

  ☐ Is there a lot of pressed-wood or particleboard furniture? When new or when damp, it can off-gas formaldehyde, an allergen and irritant.

  ☐ Is there a new carpet, new drapes, or fresh paint? These off-gas volatile organic compounds (VOCs), which can provoke allergic or toxic symptoms.

  ☐ Is your mattress brand new or very old? Either way, it may be a source of VOCs.

  ☐ Does your pet sleep with you?

☐ Is the symptom not bad in the morning but worse in the evening or as the day goes on?

- Consider allergy to a food you eat every day.

☐ Worse on weekdays?

- Perhaps there's a trigger at work or school.

☐ Worse on weekends?

  ☐ Do you eat or drink differently on weekends than during the week?

- ☐ What do you do for recreation on weekends? Where do you go?
- ☐ Worse premenstrually?
  - • You may be allergic to progesterone. After ovulation, the level of progesterone in your body rises dramatically. You'll need a skilled allergist to test for that.
  - • You may be allergic to yeast. The level of yeast in your body grows premenstrually, under the influence of increasing progesterone.
- ☐ Worse in spring?
  - • Pollen allergy is likely. Check the pollen levels in your area at the time of peak symptoms.
- ☐ Worse in late summer or early fall?
  - • Pollen allergy is likely. Check the pollen levels in your area at the time of peak symptoms.
- ☐ Worse in mid- to late fall?
  - • Mold allergy is likely. Check the mold spore count in your area.
- ☐ Worse when heat comes on?
  - • Check for contamination in the heating system. Mold, dust, or other pollutants should be considered.
- ☐ Worse when air-conditioning is running?
  - • Check for contamination in the air conditioner or cooling system. Mold is a strong possibility, although some people just react to cold air.
- ☐ Better in deep winter, when there's a freeze?
  - • Mold or pollen is likely.
- ☐ Better in summer, regardless of location?
  - • Food allergy often improves in summer.

☐ Are there any **locations** in which the symptom is more likely to occur or get worse?

   ☐ Indoors: consider indoor mold, dust, dust mites, or some contamination or pollution of your living or working space. There's a long list of possibilities.

   ☐ Outdoors: consider outdoor molds, pollen, or air pollution.

   ☐ In the country: consider mold, local pollen, or agricultural pollution.

   ☐ In the city: consider pollution from car exhaust, diesel fumes, dry cleaners, and other urban sources.

   ☐ In your car?

      • If it's new, high levels of VOCs are likely.

      • If it's old, check for mold or for leaks in the exhaust system.

   ☐ In trains or planes: VOCs from cleaning products are possible culprits.

   ☐ In a hotel:

      • If it's new or newly renovated, VOCs from cleaning products, furnishings, or construction materials are likely.

      • If it's old, mold or dust is likely.

☐ Are there any **locations** in which the symptom is **less likely** to occur or less likely to be severe?

   ☐ On vacation? Maybe there's something in your home or workplace that harbors allergens.

   ☐ In the country, in the mountains, at the beach? Maybe it's a pollutant in city air.

   ☐ In the city? Maybe it's outdoor mold spores.

☐ Are there any **environmental conditions** in which the symptom is more likely to occur or get worse?

    ☐ Damp weather? Might be outdoor mold spores.

    ☐ Before a thunderstorm? Probably outdoor mold spores.

    ☐ On clear, windy days? Probably pollen or dust.

☐ Are there any **activities** during or after which the symptom is more likely to occur or get worse?

    ☐ Housecleaning? Think dust.

    ☐ Gardening? Think mold.

    ☐ Eating or drinking? Think food.

☐ Are there any **medications** you've taken that seem to make the symptom worse?

    ☐ Antibiotics? If you're not allergic to the antibiotic, maybe you're allergic to the yeast that's very likely to be growing in your gut because of the antibiotic. By knocking out bacteria, antibiotics leave your gastrointestinal tract open to a yeast overgrowth.

☐ Are there any **medications** you've taken that seem to make the symptom better?

    ☐ Antihistamines? The symptoms these help are often caused by allergy.

    ☐ Steroids? These usually relieve symptoms of allergy while you're taking them, and they may also help reduce nonallergic inflammation. But steroids have very serious side effects.

    ☐ Antibiotics? These usually help bacterial infections, but some have anti-inflammatory effects that are separate from the antibiotic effects. Consider three possibilities:

        • The symptom that improves with an antibiotic is the result of a bacterial infection stemming from the inflammation caused by an underlying allergic problem.

- The allergic condition is actually the result of a bacterial infection.
- The improvement is unrelated to the antibiotic effect of the medication. There's another explanation.

The Search for Origins

I believe that to identify and reverse your allergies, it helps to understand how they developed. Genetics plays a role, but the galloping allergy epidemic of the last 40 years is due to environmental factors rather than genetic changes. Genes merely create susceptibility. As I explained in Chapter 1, children with a defective gene for creating the detoxifying enzyme GST develop asthma only if they're also exposed to environmental toxins like cigarette smoke or diesel exhaust. That is an excellent reason for eliminating cigarette smoke and diesel exhaust from the environment.

What Leads Up to Your Allergies?

It helps to know which factors tip the balance away from health, because fixing them can enable you to restore health. I call these factors Antecedents. In my clinical experience, the most common Antecedents for developing allergic illness are:

- Exposure to environmental toxins
- Unusually heavy exposure to mold or pollen
- Infection
- Depletion of the body's beneficial microbes
- Nutritional deficiency
- Impaired digestion
- Extreme stress—psychological or physical

I deal with each of these in detail throughout this book. To better understand the origins of your own allergies, ask yourself if your symptoms started during or after the following circumstances:

- Renovation at home or work or moving into a newly constructed or renovated home or work space? Toxic VOCs from construction and finishing materials are likely Antecedents.

- Living in an area with heavy commercial traffic or industry? Particulate air pollution is a likely Antecedent.

- Living or working in a damp or high-humidity building or in a space where leaks or floods have occurred? Exposure to mold or dust mites is a likely Antecedent. The leading dust mite allergen is actually an enzyme produced by the mite that directly damages the lining of the respiratory tract.[1] Exposure to dust mites has a toxic effect on your body, which creates an allergic response to the toxin. The same is true for certain pollens.

- The use of antibiotics? Depletion of beneficial bacteria, and the overgrowth of yeast and opportunistic bacteria, is a likely Antecedent.

- Treatment for indigestion or ulcers? Medical treatment of these conditions usually depends on drugs that suppress production of stomach acid. Just like antibiotics, these drugs have a negative impact on the beneficial bacteria living in your intestinal tract. They are proven to increase development of food allergies.

- Extreme dieting? Rapid weight loss can deplete your body of essential nutrients and disrupt immune function. The Immune Balance Diet in Chapter 8 is designed to provide nutritional support for immunity.

- Stress? Your body's stress response is actually a protective response, designed to help you recognize, confront, or avoid danger. But it comes with a hefty price, and chronic stress can be the main cause of the immune imbalances that underlie allergy.

- Acute illness? If your allergic problems started after an acute illness or became much worse, ask yourself:

  - Did the illness cause you to change your diet or lose or gain weight?

  - What medications did you take for the illness? Could those have provoked the allergies?

  - Are you fully recovered from the illness? Could some aspect of the illness still be making you sick?

Cracking the Case

Now let's look at another case history to see how multiple Antecedents converged to create one woman's personal perfect storm of allergy—and how her detective work cracked the case.

Daphne is a 42-year-old design engineer who has traveled all over the world working on various projects for a number of high-profile clients. Five years ago, when she was asked to be the maid of honor at a friend's wedding in Southeast Asia, Daphne went on a drastic diet. She lost 35 pounds in three months but also developed severe abdominal pain, which improved when she treated herself with over-the-counter antacids.

She went to the wedding, but when she returned, she found that most of the foods she usually ate made her sick with unpleasant gastrointestinal symptoms. With every meal she would suffer nausea, burping, and abdominal bloating. She developed frequent diarrhea, which led to further, unintended weight loss.

She consulted a gastroenterologist who found that she was infected with a stomach bacterium called *H. pylori*, which is a frequent cause of stomach ulcers and inflammation. The doctor suspected she had acquired the infection on her trip to Southeast Asia for the wedding. He treated her successfully with two antibiotics, but curing the infection seemed to do very little to help her symptoms. Daphne continued to have burping, belching, and bloating every day, along with frequent diarrhea, and was beginning to get exasperated.

Then, for the first time in her life, Daphne developed a sinus infection; she went on to develop recurrent sinusitis every few weeks. The sinus symptoms were pressure in her face, swelling of her cheeks, and a postnasal drip. Respiratory symptoms compounded the misery of her digestive symptoms.

Daphne was referred to an allergist who found that she was allergic to dust mites and many types of pollen. A year of allergy shots produced no benefit.

On her own, Daphne realized that drinking milk would cause a runny nose and watery eyes. She decided to totally eliminate all dairy products, and her sinus problems and digestive problems improved for a while.

A year before consulting me, she started a new job in a new building. When the heat went on in November, all her sinus symptoms returned. She decided to investigate the reasons for her illness on her own. She discovered that the building's insulation was made of polyethylene foam, which had been sprayed just before she began working there.

She also learned that isocyanates, a by-product of polyethylene foam spray, are potent allergens and well-known causes of occupational asthma. She obtained a 12-inch chunk of the hardened foam and found that when she held it up to her face her eyes watered, her nose ran, and her face swelled. Once again she thought she had solved her problem.

Daphne took a job in an older building and her sinus problems improved, but only for a short time. She then realized that other environmental chemicals—solvents and cleaning solutions in particular—had the same effect on her as polyethylene foam.

Then, two months before seeing me, she developed intense, burning pain in her legs and debilitating fatigue. She returned to her allergist, who found that she had become allergic to latex as well as to bananas, a fruit that can provoke allergy in people allergic to latex. (Visit www.drgalland.com for more information on latex allergy.) Although she removed possible sources of latex exposure at home and work and avoided foods that cross-react with latex, she got worse instead of better. Now very much unable to perform at her usually high level, she went on medical leave from her job.

When Daphne came to my office, I praised her for her determination to get to the roots of her illness and for her persistent allergy detective work. The key to her illness had been overlooked, and it seemed to me that it was hiding in plain sight.

The complex cascade of increasing allergies had started during her trip to Southeast Asia. Her allergies had been preceded by two significant events: a crash diet for weight loss and the use of antacids. These would produce nutritional deficiency resulting in immune dysfunction and would increase her risk of acquiring a gastrointestinal infection. Her gastroenterologist had identified a bacterial infection, but its treatment had not cleared up her digestive symptoms. Perhaps there was another infection that had slipped beneath the radar.

In fact, there was. I found that Daphne had two parasitic infections: an amoeba called *E. histolytica* and a worm called *Ascaris*. When I treated her with the appropriate antibiotics, there was a remarkable response. For the first few days all her symptoms intensified. She had increased pain in her legs and face, increased facial swelling, and increased mucus drip and runny nose. Then, within two weeks, all her symptoms began to improve. Her energy increased and her food reactions diminished.

Treating Daphne's parasites had the effect of resolving her allergic symptoms, but we still needed to look at her nutrition. She had become quite drained and depleted of nutrients while suffering from gastrointestinal complaints including diarrhea. On the most basic level, whatever she had been eating was not being properly digested, but passing through her digestive system without her getting the full nutritional benefit.

Now that she was able to eat more normally, I had her begin the Immune Balance Diet (which you will read about in Chapter 8) to provide an enhanced level of nutritional support. Her pain, facial swelling, and mucus drip all disappeared. Her sinusitis was gone. Daphne was gratified to have her health back.

Ever the detective, Daphne insisted on visiting her previous office, where she was again confronted with the hardened polyethylene foam and cleaning solvents, just like before. But now Daphne had no adverse reaction to either.

Conclusion

In this chapter we looked at hidden allergies that can cause a bewildering array of unexplained symptoms. We saw how Kate, the graphic artist and mother, went from energetic to exhausted due to an undiscovered allergy. Like a detective tracking down clues, we reviewed a detailed history of her symptoms and learned that these symptoms almost vanished when she was out of the office, which led me to suspect a mold allergy, a common environmental cause of illness that we resolved at Kate's office. Her case illustrates the Allergy Solution Process of Discovery, with the goal of gathering information about yourself and your symptoms to solve the puzzle of your condition.

We met the design engineer Daphne, a world traveler who had developed a mysterious case of abdominal pain and sinusitis. After we cleared up her parasites, we addressed her nutrition with the Immune Balance Diet and resolved her symptoms.

Solving the allergy puzzle involves diligent detective work, and I have provided tools to help you gather the information you need. Now that you've trained a spotlight on your allergic symptoms and the factors most likely to be triggering them, you've taken an important step toward reversing your allergies and regaining your health. I believe this detailed information is so essential to understanding a person's health that you should bring the completed Allergy Solution Checklist of Symptoms—and all the incredibly valuable data about yourself that you gather with the tools here—to your doctor for an in-depth review.

The chapters ahead will provide a way to zero in on aspects of diet that may be contributing to hidden allergies and keeping you from feeling truly well. But first, I'm going to send you on a mission to reduce your exposure to toxins in your personal environment, something all of us should do to remove toxins that may be contributing to our allergies and undermining our health.

CHAPTER 5

MISSION DETOXABLE

Mission: To avoid toxic events that contribute to allergies and undermine your health.

Are you ready to dodge dust mites, crack down on chemicals, and clear the air indoors? Then you have what it takes to stay aware of your surroundings and keep your eyes, ears, and nose alert to major toxic threats. Like freshly painted walls. Diesel fumes. The laundry detergent aisle at the supermarket.

Of course, you can't live in a bubble. That would be no fun. What you can do is minimize your exposure to toxins that increase your risk of allergy and menace your health.

The Toxic Elephant in the Room

Every 2.6 seconds, a new chemical substance is made or isolated. The American Chemical Society has a database of more than 50 million chemicals that are in use somewhere in the world. Many of these can be found in the places where you live, work, study, or shop. Some of them have profoundly negative effects on health, especially for people with allergies or asthma.

Diesel exhaust from trucks and buses, solvents used for cleaning, microparticles and chemicals like styrene and xylene from laser printers and copy machines—these are just a few of the toxins our bodies have to contend with in the modern world. Many of these hitchhike on dust, which is an age-old irritant. Classic symptoms of allergy, like sneezing, coughing, and scratching, are the body's way of trying to keep out or get rid of toxins like these. But with so many toxins, your body's defense mechanisms can easily get overwhelmed.

Environmental toxins are like the giant elephant in the room, up on its tippy toes trying to hide. The amazing thing is that despite its enormous bulk, this toxic elephant is able to hide in plain sight. Most people just take the many toxins around them as a routine part of life and have accustomed themselves not to pay attention to them. How many times have I heard the refrain "The smell doesn't bother me" from people confronted with fresh paint fumes or other toxic hazards?

The fact is that the health of each and every one of us is greatly affected by the toxins we are confronted with in daily life. And they come at us from all sides, from left and right, from up and down. We inhale them into our noses and lungs. We absorb them through our skin, they get in our eyes, and we swallow them in our food and water.

The toxic assault starts from the moment you wake up, before you have even left your house. Pour yourself that first cup of coffee, the one you've been looking forward to since you went to bed. If it's not organic, your cup may very well contain pesticides along with your coffee, because coffee shrubs are among the most heavily sprayed plants in the world.

In the shower you squeeze out some shampoo and lather it into your hair. Most commercial shampoos contain chemicals like the detergent sodium lauryl sulfate, a known skin irritant that can harm skin health and lead to the redness and itch of contact dermatitis.

Or you spray out some shaving cream. Now you probably have a handful of some of the 3,000 potential chemicals that could have been used to create its fragrance, and quite possibly trieth-anolamine, a skin and respiratory irritant, and the same sodium lauryl sulfate that was in your shampoo. They're all in your hand, headed straight for your face. And your day has barely begun.

All this toxicity can take a heavy toll. Many of the mysterious symptoms my patients experience can be traced back to toxic exposures. Often there's more than one source of exposure—cleaning sprays, paint fumes, formaldehyde, fragrances, scented laundry products, or a thousand other things. For many people, it's the total cumulative load of toxins that tips the scales to the breaking point, and they get sick.

So in this chapter I'm sending you on a mission to lighten your load and detox your life, using the strategies that have helped me and my family reduce our exposure to many common toxins.

Employ Evasive Measures

At the core of the Galland strategy is flexibility. When a toxic event happens, you want to be ready to take evasive action. Here's how it works:

- Let's say your favorite gallery just painted its walls in preparation for a big new show. The artwork is up, and everything looks perfect. But it smells terrible, with paint fumes hanging in the air. So what can you do as you walk into the door? Simple—get outta there!

- You approach your favorite coffee shop. But you notice that workers are redoing the sidewalk right in front, with jackhammers breaking up the old concrete and construction vehicles spewing industrial-strength diesel exhaust into the air. What's your move? Try a different coffee shop today, and come back when they're done with the work.

- You're wheeling your shopping cart in the supermarket and come to the aisle with the cleaning products and the heavily scented laundry detergent. I am pretty sure you know what to do by this point. That's right, keep pushing your cart and skip this aisle completely—that's what I do.

This strategy may take some getting used to. If you like, you can think of it as a game. Maybe even an adventure. But it's for real.

Get Allergy Solution Clean

Cleanliness is one foundation of the American dream. The marketing and advertising guys discovered that in the 1950s. You can imagine Don Draper of *Mad Men,* dressed in a suit and tie, pitching his ideas to a client by launching into flights of fancy about the virtues and benefits of a household cleaner. He would make it seem pristine, beautiful, even sensuous. Of course he's just selling a bottle of chemicals, but that is what proves so compelling to the clever minds of the Mad Men: how to bring emotion into something so pedestrian.

True clean, however, doesn't come from a household cleaner in a spray bottle filled with chemicals, or from a floor cleaner loaded with detergent that produces irritating fumes, or from an air freshener that simply covers up odors with something artificial and potentially allergenic. Don't allow an advertising team to determine what products you use and what chemicals you are exposed to. When you are setting out to eliminate allergens in your home (or, for that matter, in your office or school), why bring new chemicals in?

I'm proposing a whole new way of looking at clean—a fresh take on "fresh" that helps you get rid of the dirt, the allergens, and the chemicals all at the same time!

Your mission is to detox your personal space, the Allergy Solution way. I'm going to give you three buckets to use in your cleanup: one for dust and mold, one for indoor air pollution, and one for chemicals like the ones in that spray bottle.

The Dust and Mold Bucket

Dust gets into your home from outside, quietly floating in through doors and windows and silently seeping in through the cracks. Dust and other allergens are generated by many things already inside, too, including your towels, your clothes, your pets, and even your own body. You turn around and there it is again. Dust. It gathers everywhere, like . . . well, like dust. It creates a haven for airborne toxins and for toxic insects like dust mites.

Mold, in turn, grows in damp spaces and can wreak havoc on your health, as we saw in the case of Kate in Chapter 4. Minimizing dust and mold is an excellent first step in detoxifying your personal space and protecting yourself from these major allergens.

Leave Dust and Allergens Outside

As I've just said, dust gets in from outside, so let's not give any more of it a free ride into the house. Kick off your shoes before you come inside. Neon-colored running shoes, dress shoes, flats, loafers, knee-high leather boots, work boots—they can all carry dirt, toxins, and allergens into your home.

And lots of bacteria, according to a research study from the University of Arizona. It found shoes to be contaminated with large amounts of bacteria, including coliforms and *Escherichia coli*, indicating contact with fecal matter, which the study suggests comes from public restrooms or from animal waste outdoors. In the next step of the study, the researchers also discovered that when these outdoor shoes made contact with clean tiles, up to 90 percent of the bacteria they carried could be transferred to the tiles.[1]

Now, depending on your activities outside, you may want to remove more than your shoes. Been digging up the garden? Mowing the lawn? Chances are your clothes are covered in dirt and allergens like tree and grass pollen. You will want to change into fresh clothes and toss the soiled ones into the laundry.

Good Bugs, Bad Bugs: Understanding the "Hygiene Hypothesis"

The Hygiene Hypothesis is a poorly named but currently popular theory of the origins of the allergy epidemic. It's based on a handful of observations: 1) Allergies are very uncommon in the developing world, where sanitation is far less intense than in economically advanced countries. 2) Children living in large families or growing up with pets are less likely to have allergies than those from small families or those who don't grow up with pets. 3) Babies born by caesarean section are more likely to develop allergies than those born through normal vaginal delivery.

The evolving theory behind the Hygiene Hypothesis is that exposure to bacteria and other microbes early in life conditions the immune system to resist the development of allergy, but the overly sanitized modern world deprives us of this protection, allowing allergies to flourish. In my view, this is an incomplete hypothesis, and from a problem-solving perspective it's a dead end. It suggests that the solution to the allergy crisis is less sanitation.

The Hygiene Hypothesis ignores all the data presented in this chapter and throughout *The Allergy Solution*, which show that it's not just the absence of germs that leads to allergies. It's the presence of toxic substances that damage your body's tissues, coupled with nutritional deficiencies that impair your body's ability to protect itself from that damage.

Within this struggle between cellular damage and repair, there is a role for "good bugs": the bacteria that normally live in a healthy body and populate the space in which you live and work. I describe the effects of these bacteria in several chapters that follow. Furthering our understanding of how we can help these beneficial microbes keep us healthy is a fascinating area of my research.

Banish Dust-Catching Clutter from Your Home

Horizontal surfaces, such as a coffee table or kitchen counter, are like magnets for dust. And dust loves clutter, not only because stuffed animals, picture frames, handicrafts, and all sorts of other decorative and household objects are perfect places for dust to hide, but also because clutter makes it harder for dust to get cleaned away. So let's clear the dust, and the air, and get things Allergy Solution clean.

The more stuff you can clear off your kitchen counters, your coffee tables, and your nightstands, the quicker and easier it will be to wipe off the dust and allergens. Later, when they're free of clutter and oh-so-inviting, you will find yourself wiping off those surfaces more often, keeping your home cleaner than ever before.

For dusting, I prefer to use a damp cloth to keep dust from flying around the room. Another trick is to wear a mask while cleaning, to help keep you from inhaling dust. Damp mopping the floor will help keep the dust down as well.

Don't Harbor Dust Mites

Here's another good reason to practice dust control: From that hard-to-reach dusty shelf to the area around your stereo equipment to the space underneath your bed, the dust in your home can contain itty-bitty bugs called, you guessed it, dust mites. You can't see them, and they can't see you. These primitive little creatures have eight legs and no eyes and are related to spiders. They feed on the skin shed by people and their pets. One gram of dust often contains 100 to 500 dust mites.

Dust mites are responsible for most of our allergies to dust. In other words, dust allergy is primarily an allergic reaction to the waste products and bodies of dust mites.[2] What's more, mites contain toxic enzymes that directly damage your respiratory lining, allowing increased penetration of airborne irritants and allergens.[3]

Your body has a protective response, a natural enzyme inhibitor that can limit the damage produced by the toxic mite enzyme, but indoor air pollutants block the effects of the enzyme inhibitor.[4] The combination of dust mites and indoor air pollution can create a perfect storm that leads straight to allergic asthma.

Dust mites are actually misnamed: they don't need dust to survive. They need moisture and a soft place to hide, like stuffed furniture and bedding. To catch the mites most effectively, use a vacuum with a HEPA filter. A regular vacuum could simply blow the dust mites around the room. Use a damp cloth or mop, as noted above, to keep dust down and mop up the dust mites. Using a dry method just spreads them around.

Pull up wall-to-wall carpet or rugs in the bedroom, when possible, and replace with hardwood or tile flooring; this eliminates one of the mites' habitats. Get miteproof covers for your mattress, pillows, and comforter. At least once a week, launder all of your bedding in hot water to kill the dust mites.[5] And keep the relative humidity in your home and workplace low.

A 2014 review article from Harvard Medical School, which looked at the research on minimizing allergens in the home, confirmed this as the most effective strategy for cutting down on house dust mites: cleaning often, using dust-mite-impermeable bedding and washing it in hot water weekly, keeping humidity below 50 percent, and not using carpet or keeping stuffed animals around.[6]

Knock Out Mold

The obvious signs of mold are a musty smell or visible mildew. But mold can be lurking anywhere, especially where it's damp, dark, and warm. Mold, like dust mites, loves high humidity. It thrives in places that are moist, wet, or waterlogged. At a humidity of 70 percent or greater, it grows rapidly. So you'll want to aim for a much lower humidity level—ideally, 30 to 45 percent—throughout your house or apartment.

Think of all the showers you take at home, throwing off all of that steam. That excess moisture has to go somewhere. That's why you don't want your home to be sealed tight like Fort Knox. Instead, you want it to breathe a little, so condensation doesn't build up. Make sure you have adequate ventilation, especially in areas of your home where there's moisture. A clean and well-maintained dehumidifier or air conditioner can also help reduce humidity.

A great hiding place for mold is the refrigerator, so make sure you clean it out regularly. Check all the food in the fridge and throw out any items on which you spot mold. Remember that mold can also grow in food or beverages that are left out of the refrigerator, so place them in the fridge or discard them.

Banish Roaches

Cockroaches can cause big problems when it comes to allergies. The skin, saliva, and waste from these not-so-small critters are all serious allergens. Take steps to banish these bugs from your home:

- Keep your kitchen super-clean, with all food properly stored so roaches cannot get at it. Remember, they have had millions of years of practice at getting meals, so we have to outsmart them and keep everything edible out of their reach.

- Bag your garbage and remove it promptly.

- Use Roach Motel–style traps to catch the bugs and discard them. You can use gloves to do this, latex-free gloves if you're sensitive to latex. (Visit www. drgalland.com for more information on latex allergy.)

The Indoor Air Pollution Bucket

With so much of our time spent inside, understanding the importance of clearing the air indoors is a key goal of *The Allergy Solution*. In addition to banishing dust and mold, you'll want to set your sights on eliminating other challenges to indoor air quality. I highlight some key problems here, but there are many more, so you're going to have to think on your feet and address the particular indoor air pollution challenges that confront you.

Make Your Home a Smoke-Free Zone

Let's end smoking once and for all. Smoking kills people and pollutes the earth. Secondhand smoke does the same. Then there is the problem of thirdhand smoke, the toxic residue from leftover cigarette smoke that clings to carpet, sticks to walls, and infiltrates furniture. A recent study from the University of California shows that thirdhand smoke causes significant damage to the lungs and the liver.[7]

Never allow smoking in your home, and ban smoking anywhere on your property. You don't want any secondhand smoke sneaking in through windows or doors, or cigarette butts or ashes lying around; these can be sources of allergens even after the cigarette has been put out.

Put Out the Fire

Let's clear the air: burning logs, wood pellets, or coal in a stove or fireplace causes both indoor air pollution and outdoor air pollution. Wood smoke is considered a significant source of particulate matter, commonly known as soot, in indoor air. The science shows that this smoke is a risk factor for disease, including asthma.[8]

A study from the remote island of Tasmania, south of Australia, where wood stoves are common, found that exposure to wood smoke is linked to more severe asthma in adults. This was observed for people who burn wood at home, as well as for people who don't but who are exposed to the wood smoke coming from the chimneys of neighbors. The researchers suspect the irritant effect of wood smoke on the respiratory system, along with increased inflammation from the smoke, as factors in aggravating asthma.[9]

Eliminate the use of wood stoves and fireplaces as much as possible to remove this preventable source of both indoor and outdoor air pollution.

Make Your Bedroom a Clean-Air Oasis

You probably spend more hours in your bedroom than in any other room of your home. That means you want your bedroom to be a special place where you can relax and restore yourself and unwind your body and mind after a long day. To make it as tranquil as possible, may I suggest keeping electronic devices to a minimum in your bedroom? All that blaring volume on TVs, all that buzzing and vibrating of phones, is a lot of extra agitation.

Also, you may want to clear the air in your bedroom by putting away any dust-magnet clutter and by leaving newspapers and magazines, with their off-gassing printed pages, outside the room. Did someone mention printers? Keep these out of the bedroom, by all means, because they emit chemicals that you don't want to breathe in. Do not use any type of combustion device, such as a fireplace, a stove, or even candles, in your bedroom.

In your oasis of rest, comfort, and safety, you have removed sources of pollution and allergens. Now you can rest easy.

Park Outside and Keep Your Garage Free of Toxins

Once you go to great lengths to remove toxins from your home and your life, why pull the biggest pollution-generating machine of all, the gas-powered car, into your garage? Pollution from the exhaust and the tires, dust from the brakes and engine, are all sources of toxins and allergens being brought into a confined space. You breathe these toxins into your lungs when you exit the car. And if your garage is connected to your house, these toxins can very well seep into the house itself. If possible, park outside and breathe easier.

The Hidden Air Pollution in Your Backyard

What if there was a hidden source of air pollution in your town? You would want to know about it, right? And what if that air pollution was right in your neighborhood? You would sit up and take notice. But what if it was in your own backyard? You would want to stop it immediately and clean it up.

In a remarkable study, the first of its kind, scientists from the University of Washington revealed a hidden source of air pollution that belches hazardous chemicals into the backyards of millions of homes across America. Not the pollution from a car or truck. Not the smoke from a fireplace or woodstove. No, the scientists identified something that looks quite harmless: the typical clothes dryer. It is not so much the machine itself but what gets vented out of the back of the machine that represents the threat.

The Washington team methodically traced the problem back to its source: fragranced laundry detergents and dryer sheets. These products introduce chemicals into the dryer, where they are heated and then vented outside—into the backyard, for example—creating a toxic cloud of chemicals, including some classified as hazardous by the EPA.

So now you probably want to know what chemicals the laundry products contain. Figuring that out is difficult, because as the University of Washington team noted, just the fragrance alone may contain hundreds of chemicals, and they are not required to be listed on the product label. So the researchers set up a test to identify what exactly was vented out of a typical dryer.

The place: Seattle. The setup: two homes, two days, two dryers in good condition, both venting outdoors. The scientists sampled air from the dryers during the laundry test with 1) no products, 2) fragranced laundry detergent only, and 3) fragranced laundry detergent and dryer sheets.

What they found could knock your clean white socks off.

During the detergent-only test, the two dryers vented out 21 volatile organic compounds (VOCs), including acetaldehyde, acetone, benzaldehyde, butanal, dodecane, hexanal, limonene, nonanal, 1-propanal, and 2 butanone.

As I noted in Chapter 2, VOCs are toxic. They can sting the eyes and irritate the skin and airways. And one of these compounds, acetaldehyde, is classified as a carcinogenic hazardous air pollutant by the EPA, "with no safe exposure level," the Washington researchers explain.[10]

When what is coming out of your dryer is a hazardous air pollutant, it feels like you need to borrow Walter's gas mask from *Breaking Bad* just to run the dryer.

But there is more.

When the use of both fragranced detergent and dryer sheets was tested, the following VOCs were found: acetaldehyde, acetone, benzaldehyde, butanal, dodecane, hexanal, limonene, nonanal, octanal, tetramethylpropylidene cyclopropane. The list goes on, with complex chemistry that it would take a professor to understand fully. The VOCs detected in the above tests were not present in the no-detergent test.

So what is the takeaway from this study? It would be a very good idea to skip the fragranced laundry detergent and dryer sheets.[11] Be part of the solution and help clear the air in your home and neighborhood. Use only unscented products.

The Chemicals Bucket

I'm not going to sugarcoat it. This part of your mission is going to require vigilance. With the thousands of chemicals that already go into the products we use every day, and many more on the way, this bucket keeps getting filled faster than we can empty it. On the bright side, once you make the switch to go natural, there is less for you to spend money on!

Which brings me right to the topic of cleaning products.

With household spray cleaners linked to asthma (see below), steering clear of spray cleaners is a good idea. Fragrances are linked to allergies, so avoiding fragrances is important. What's the solution? It's not as simple as going to the store and picking up a cleaning product whose label says it is "all natural" or "green." I have been disappointed to find the same skin-irritating chemicals show up in "natural" cleaning products. That is why I use water and a little baking soda as my go-to cleaning solution to handle most tasks. I've found that it's effective as an all-purpose cleaner all over the house.

Cleaning Sprays Increase Asthma Risk

In the movie *The Karate Kid*, the main character, Daniel, is being bullied by someone bigger and more powerful. He meets a wise karate master, Mr. Miyagi. With a series of lessons, the master teaches the young student to stand up for himself by thinking for himself. At first it is not easy. It takes some practice for the young student to absorb the lessons of his master. But finally he understands.

Like Daniel in *The Karate Kid*, a big part of *The Allergy Solution* is getting you to think differently about the world around you.

Very differently. Because there are a lot of ordinary, everyday consumer products that are working against your health.

Take household spray cleaners. They are lined up on the shelves of the supermarket. They are a popular product in the United States and also in Europe. Walk into a restaurant, café, or clothing store, and frequently you'll see a staff member holding a bottle of spray cleaner, trying to keep the place spotless. You may notice the smell of the cleaner, or you may not. But one thing is for sure: it's made of chemicals.

Now several recent research studies have shown that these sprays are linked to asthma. In one study, an international team of researchers looked at the relationship between using household cleaning sprays and new onset of adult asthma. Looking at information from the European Community Respiratory Health Survey—from Sweden, Italy, Norway, Switzerland, Germany, Belgium, Estonia, France, United Kingdom, and Spain—they identified 3,503 people who cleaned their own houses and did not have asthma at baseline, and they followed these people for nine years.

The sprays used by the people in the study contained a variety of active ingredients, including alcohols, ammonia, sodium hydroxide, acryl polymers, terpenes, and glycols and glycol ethers. The researchers noted that the mist of chemicals created by the sprays would create chemical exposures to the respiratory tract.

The study found the risk of incident asthma (defined as diagnosis by a doctor and the use of medication for treatment) increased by 30 percent to 50 percent with the use of a spray household product at least once a week. The results suggest that using common household sprays may be an important risk factor for adult asthma. The authors state: "One in seven adult asthma cases could be attributed to common spray use. This indicates a relevant contribution of spray use to the burden of asthma in adults who do the cleaning in their homes."[12]

The researchers also explain that passive exposure to these chemicals in places where the sprays are in use, or have recently been used, could be bad for the people exposed. That is something to think about the next time you see a store employee holding one of these bottles in his or her hand.

Another study looked at data from the Epidemiological Study on the Genetics and Environment of Asthma (EGEA), which gathered data from subjects in five cities in France. The goal of the study was to assess the link between the use of household cleaning sprays and asthma in women. The researchers concluded that use of sprays was associated with increased asthma symptoms and that using the sprays was therefore a risk factor for women.[13]

So what do these studies teach us? The science says that spray cleaners may carry the risk of asthma. Skip the spray cleaners and reduce exposure to the chemicals they contain.

What Lurks Under Your Kitchen Sink?

Your kitchen evokes a feeling of home, of security. This is where the food is. But just below the surface, underneath the counter, danger lurks. A dark, out-of-the-way place contains forgotten bottles that say "WARNING: Harmful if swallowed" or "CAUTION: Avoid breathing vapors. Use protective clothing when working with chemicals." Who knows what toxins and allergens lurk under your sink? If you haven't thought about it lately, check out what's stored down there.

Typical suspects include all types of chemical-laden household products that often creep in one by one. It could start with a spray bottle of all-purpose cleaner, then some detergent for the dishwashing machine. They are joined by other boxes, bottles, and sprays of chemicals that you may have used only once, then shoved out of sight. Pretty soon you have a toxic dump in your home.

These chemicals must be disposed of and handled with extreme caution. The United States Environmental Protection Agency provides information on how to properly dispose of these items to minimize harm to the environment. Visit www.epa.gov/osw/conserve/materials/hhw.htm.

Wash New Clothes Before Wearing Them

"Aww, but I just bought them, and I want them to look new when I put them on." I hear you. But the problem is that new clothes are usually loaded with dyes and formaldehyde, chemicals you don't want next to your skin. Here is what I suggest doing with new clothes you bring home from the store: Remove the price tags, of course, then toss the clothes into the washer. Let them soak overnight in warm water. When you flip open the lid of the washing machine the next day and peer in, see how the dye has colored the water. Now wash them on a regular wash cycle, and see how they smell. You may need to wash them several times. They should not have a chemical odor when you are done washing.

Break Free from Fragrances

Once upon a time, fragrance was much more limited in scope. There was perfume, cologne, and aftershave. Soap and shampoo had some fragrance, but nothing too over-the-top.

Now the whole world has been fragranced. Body wash, body spray, makeup, lip gloss, everything has a not-so-subtle smell.

But fragrances are made from up to 3,000 different chemicals, the toxicity of which is not known. What *is* known is that breathing in these extra chemicals, or absorbing them through your skin, builds up the toxic load in your body.

You know that when you open a fashion magazine you will most likely be hit with the strongly perfumed pages that advertise fragrances. The beautiful models stare out at you, often in a pristine natural setting, looking like they are getting plenty of fresh air even as they provide you with a dose of not-so-fresh chemicals.

Now this advertising method has leapt over the perfume counter right into ads for a wide variety of household products. Scented ads for air fresheners, antiperspirants, body wash, and household cleaners grace the pages of magazines, trying to grab your attention.[14] Though most people don't know this, some publishers are willing to provide scent-free copies of their magazine to readers who request them.[15] So not only do you have the option of choosing products without fragrance added, you can get your glossy magazines scent-free as well.

Air Fresheners—Trouble for Allergies and Asthma

Everyday life is filled with natural odors. Some things are pleasantly fragrant, like freshly brewed coffee or a bouquet of flowers. Others, like the garbage and the bathroom, have always had their unpleasant moments from an olfactory standpoint. But these odors, good or bad, convey information that is important, perhaps requiring our attention.

At some point in time we learned to loathe unpleasant natural odors; they went from being an annoyance to being virtually intolerable. Marketers were only too happy to oblige this new aversion. They had just the thing to cover up offensive odors: a new product, the air freshener. Spray some fragranced freshener into the air, and voilà, the old smell was replaced by a new one. But was the air truly freshened? Whatever was causing the unwanted odor in the first place was still there. Spraying air freshener did not take out the garbage or change the kitty litter. It just introduced chemicals into our environment without any fresh air coming in.

A study from the University of California looked at the health effects of things that cause odors indoors, *including* air fresheners. The researchers explain that air fresheners contain a variety of natural or synthetic perfumes. The most frequently reported health effect of some perfumes is allergies, the study notes. A worsening of asthma is another commonly reported health effect of perfume.

The study further observes that indoor odors are a signal of improper ventilation, and that instead of bringing more fresh air indoors, people look for a quick fix in the form of air fresheners, which bring chemicals into the places we live and work. With more insulation and more airtight buildings, less fresh air gets inside, allowing indoor air pollution to build up. This published research from a leading university highlights the fact that spraying perfumes such as air fresheners is a health risk for allergies and asthma.[16]

Another study looked at the impact of air freshener sprays on the nasal mucosa of rats. After one month of exposure to the sprays, increased congestion was seen. After two months of exposure, mild inflammation was noticed. Following three months of exposure, intense inflammation had begun.[17]

This is science that informs and inspires us to makes changes to protect our health. By bringing to light the little-known risks of fragrances, it challenges us to think and act in a new way. Can we forgo fragrances? Avoid air fresheners? Part ways with perfumes?

Save Your Skin

At this very moment, your skin may be trying to get your attention. Sending you a text, an e-mail, or a message in a bottle. Because your skin is not a happy camper. It is not feeling smooth and comfortable, but dry, red, irritated, and itchy. You may feel like you need to squeeze moisturizer on your skin, but when you do, it barely makes a difference, the skin is still so dry. If that sounds all too familiar, then read on.

Dryness and irritated skin can have many causes, and if you have these symptoms, you should see your doctor to determine the cause. But you can also take steps to make sure you're not making matters worse by the way you treat your skin. Have you noticed that it gets worse the more you shower or bathe? Published research tells us that common, everyday products like shampoo and body wash often contain a chemical that is a known irritant to skin and can cause dermatitis. This is sodium lauryl sulfate, the culprit that I mentioned near the beginning of this chapter. It is used to give the products the foam that we have come to expect.

A long time ago, when people felt the urge to wash, they bathed in a stream or pond. Soap had yet to be invented, so they stuck with what they had: water. Later, as civilization developed, people found new ways of washing themselves. The ancient Greeks applied olive oil to their skin, then scraped it off, hoping to take off any dirt along with it. Luckily for them, pesticides were still unknown, so the olive oil they used was organic.

In our modern times, we can choose from a bewildering array of personal cleaning products. The chemicals in these products can cause irritation with even one use, according to a study from the Indiana University School of Medicine. In fact, sodium lauryl sulfate is so effective at causing irritation that it is used in lab experiments to induce skin irritation when that's the effect researchers require—say, in order to study a remedy for irritation. It has been demonstrated to cause disruption in the skin barrier function, which can lead to allergic (atopic) dermatitis, an inflammatory skin disease that has become much more prevalent over the past few decades. The severe itch that it causes can impact mood and concentration and contribute to poor health.

Think about this for a moment. By using shampoos and cleansers containing a common chemical, you could literally be opening your skin up, making it more vulnerable to the outside world. That sounds like a very bad idea.[18]

Here is one simple way you can help your dry, irritated skin. Give it a vacation from all that soap, body wash, shower gel, bubble bath, and shampoo. Just use a tiny bit where it is needed, and nothing more. Give that whole head-to-toe lathering thing a rest and see how your skin feels after a few days.

And unless you're performing surgery, avoid antiseptic soaps. These are intended to kill bacteria, but they have three undesirable effects.

First, the chemicals they contain are more likely to irritate your skin than ordinary soap.

Second, they deplete your skin of good bacteria that contribute to its health, since the microbes living on healthy skin help to organize a strong protective immune response.[19] Some of them, with names you've never heard of, have actual anti-allergic effects.[20] They're your friends. Don't make them collateral damage.

Third, killing off the friendly bacteria that live on your skin allows the growth of not-so-friendly bacteria that are resistant to the antiseptic agents in the soap. The bacteria that live on your skin do not stay on your skin. They float through the air and become part of the environment in which you live and which you share with others.

The study of bacteria inhabiting homes and workplaces—the "indoor microbiome"—and its effects on health is a rapidly growing area of research. The principal source of these bacteria is you, your skin in particular. So the bacteria growing on your skin determine the bacteria that everyone in your home is exposed to.

You will learn more about this cutting-edge area of science that is transforming our view of health in Chapter 14.

Go Organic and Heal the Planet

This is so basic, so simple, and yet so necessary. It is an excellent way to reduce your exposure to toxins and shrink your toxic load, which is the total amount of toxins you take in through eating, breathing, and contact with the world around you.

You might even say that going organic is heroic. Choosing organic is not just for you; it is for the planet and all the people who live on it. Each time you buy organic lettuce or blueberries, for example, you are reducing the use of pesticides along a vast chain from the chemical factory to the farm to your table. The people who work on organic farms don't have to handle toxic pesticides, so it is healthier for them too. The soil itself, which is really a living thing, can remain pesticide-free. That means less pollution running off into streams, rivers, and lakes.

Back in the day, shopping organic meant traveling across town to a little health food store that stocked a few vegetables and pieces of fruit. Now organic has gone very much more mainstream, with organic frozen fruit and vegetables distributed to many supermarkets. So it is easier than ever before to choose organic. Is it a little more expensive? Yes, but I consider it an investment in health and well-being.

Join the Homemade Coffee Revolution

I invite you to join a little revolution. The good news about this revolution is that coffee will be served.

This is a completely grassroots movement. Anyone can join. No long-winded speeches, no membership, just a win-win-win for you, your pocketbook, and Mother Earth. I am talking about organic coffee, the best way to enjoy your favorite brew.

Years ago, finding organic coffee was a chore. Organic coffee was mostly off the radar, something you had to go looking for. You could walk miles of aisles in your supermarket and it would not be sitting there on the shelf. You had to make a special trip somewhere, or you had to order it from a catalog.

Today that has all changed. Push your cart down the aisle at the supermarket, the big box retailer, or the specialty grocer, and organic coffees will be waiting for you. Recent shopping excursions to big stores have revealed ample supplies of organic coffee from Bolivia, Sumatra, Ethiopia, Nicaragua, Colombia, and Rwanda. I love to break open a bag of one of these coffees, inhale deeply, and have the aroma bring me to far-off lands where lush coffee plants grow. At home, I grind up the beans and make a deeply satisfying and delicious cup.

So that brings us to the critical question: if you are enjoying organic coffee at home, why do you settle for takeout coffee that is not organic when you're not at home? For coffee lovers out there, I have a better plan. Why not brew an extra cup of your favorite organic coffee at home and bring it with you? You know how much better your own coffee can be. Plus, by sticking with organic, you are skipping the pesticides that conventionally grown coffee contains, which could help lower your toxic load.

One of the pleasures of bringing your own coffee with you to work or to school is the independence it gives you. No longer do you need to make that extra stop, wait in line, get a paper cup, and rush on. You can do it yourself, with a sense of pride that you are doing the right thing for your health and for the environment. Think of the millions of paper cups we won't need to manufacture, store, use, and then dispose of in a landfill. Forget that paper cup and join the revolution!

Conclusion

In this episode of *Mission Detoxable* I outlined a mission that is vital to overcoming allergies and improving your health. I assigned you to detox your personal space, clearing out three bucketfuls of dust and mold, indoor air pollution, and toxic chemicals. As we're surrounded in everyday life by toxins such as air pollution, chemicals, and tobacco smoke, I showed you evasive measures to take to safeguard yourself against these threats.

You learned to pay attention to important clues about your surroundings, like a detective, and to jettison air fresheners and cleaning sprays that can lead to asthma and allergies. I briefed you on how to get Allergy Solution clean by banishing dust and knocking out mold. You kicked off your shoes before entering the house, to keep allergens and random bacteria at bay, and enjoyed a cup of organic coffee. You will no doubt encounter new challenges as you go about your mission, should you choose to accept it.

It is an adventure in which you'll be living a little greener and a lot healthier, benefiting yourself and Mother Nature. Remember, this is not an impossible mission, it's Mission Detoxable. You can do it!

This message biodegrades in five seconds . . . Good luck!

CHAPTER 6

THE THREE-DAY POWER WASH

I have seen dramatic, life-changing results when people remove even just one thing—food or beverage—from their routines. Asthma improves. Headaches disappear. Hard-to-lose pounds melt away. Joint pain vanishes. Digestion becomes easy. Skin stops itching. Depression is lifted. Focus, mood, energy all improve. And that is just the beginning of the list of symptoms that can improve when a problem food is taken off the menu.

As we've seen, allergic reactions are self-amplifying chain reactions in which your immune system amplifies the effect of a trigger. One way to think about it is that your body is overreacting to a trigger. With immune system amplification, a tiny trigger can have a big effect. That's why, in my experience, allergy elimination diets that simply remove a trigger can be so powerful and effective in such a short period of time.

But it's not the same triggers for everybody. That's what I've learned while applying the science in *The Allergy Solution* to help so many of my patients with their hidden allergies.

For some people, the problematic food is dairy. For some people it's wheat or corn or soy or peanuts or wine. For other people it could be one (or more than one) of any number of different foods.

That's why it is so important to bring this book with you when you see your doctor before starting the program I'm about to share with you, so your doctor can collaborate with you on this very important journey of discovery.

Clearing the Tracks with the Power Wash

You've already used the tools in Chapter 4 to gain a better understanding of your allergic symptoms. Now comes the next step in the process of reversing allergy and restoring your health: identifying and eliminating your problem foods. As you heal, your need for dietary restriction may diminish. But you can't heal if you ignore the problem food or beverage. I am not saying that once you're well you'll be able to eat the kinds of nutrient-depleted, inflammation-promoting junk foods that are responsible for so much ill health, but that you'll be able eat a wide variety of delicious, nutritious whole foods.

So how can you discover your problem foods? I have developed a method called the Three-Day Power Wash that is based on my clinical experience and research into nutrition science. It's a first step toward discovering hidden intolerance to foods.

The Three-Day Power Wash is not meant to be an ongoing maintenance diet. That's why I call it the Power Wash. It's the first stage of a three-stage process, in which you "clear the tracks" by cleansing your body and reducing the most common allergenic foods. Once cleansed, you'll move on to the second stage, the Re-entry Food Challenge, and reintroduce foods one at a time to determine which ones you need to avoid. In the third stage, you'll discover the Immune Balance Diet: a delicious, diverse eating plan, designed to support your immune system and sustain your well-being, that you can follow for as long as you like.

For most of us, everyday life has become hectic, filled with so many things it can be hard for any one thing to stand out. The same goes for our eating: We grab quick bites on the go and push nutrition to the edges of our busy lives. Eating in something of a random manner, we may have a hard time telling what effect any one food has on us.

The Power Wash is a way for you to cut through the noise of everyday life, the usual eating patterns, to get to a quieter place where you can listen to your body. In that way the Power Wash is like meditation, a program to access the inner stillness and wisdom of the body.

Another way to think about the Power Wash is to compare it to a symphony. When you have a multitude of instruments all playing together, it can be challenging to hear one single instrument. But then there is a dramatic pause in the music, a quiet moment where the audience almost holds its breath. Suddenly you hear the beautiful sound of the violin solo, or the oboe, cutting through the quiet with astonishing clarity. That is what the Power Wash, the quiet, and Re-entry, the solo instrument, are like. The Immune Balance Diet is like the full orchestra coming back in so you can hear the rich, harmonious whole.

How the Power Wash Works

The goal of the Three-Day Power Wash is to enhance intake of nutrients from plants that science has shown can help balance immunity, and to help steer clear of the major allergens. You won't see the following in the Power Wash:

- Milk, milk products, and milk derivatives like yogurt, cheese, ice cream, butter, whey, and any food that contains casein or caseinate, which are major milk allergens
- Eggs
- Fish and other seafood
- Beef and pork
- Wheat, rye, and barley
- Corn
- Soy, other beans, and chocolate
- Nuts and peanuts

- Yeast, which is found in alcoholic beverages, vinegar, fruit juices, dried fruits, grapes, commercial soups and sauces, and anything fermented or pickled

- Mushrooms

- Nightshade vegetables, which include tomatoes, eggplant, potatoes, and bell peppers

- Citrus fruit

- Table sugar, honey, and other sweeteners

- Spices

- Garlic and onion

- Coffee

Don't eat any of the above during the Power Wash. Instead, you will learn to enjoy foods rich in natural substances called flavonoids that may help inhibit allergic responses.[1] You'll also enjoy foods that support the healthy bacteria in your gut—which help reduce inflammation—and concentrated nutrients that aid in detoxification and immune function.

Detoxification is a process that your body performs spontaneously and continuously. It's driven by enzymes in your liver, kidneys, lungs, skin, and intestines. The food you eat affects the natural detox process in three important ways:

- Food supplies the vitamins, minerals, and amino acids that allow detox enzymes to work.

- Certain foods, like broccoli and other cruciferous vegetables, contain chemical components that stimulate your cells to make more detox enzymes.

- Eating foods to which you're allergic produces a leaky gut. Your intestines contain the most toxic environment to which you'll ever be exposed, and a leaky gut can overwhelm your detox pathways to produce systemic inflammation and immune dysfunction.

The Power Wash has three components: The Immune Balance Smoothie is your breakfast and midafternoon snack. The Immune Balance Soup is your lunch and dinner. And you'll enjoy four cups a day of Organic Oolong Tea. I will explain the science of oolong tea in a moment. You'll find the recipes for each component in the next few pages.

During the Power Wash you may eat until you are satisfied, but not too full. In Chapter 9 you will learn about the digestive drawbacks, such as heartburn and GERD, that can come from being too full. Hunger will hinder recovery, not help it. If you want an extra smoothie, go right ahead. If you want an extra bowl of soup, go right ahead.

Important Note

If you've had an allergic reaction to one of the foods included in the Power Wash, don't eat it. There is no food that someone hasn't had an allergic reaction to. Always avoid allergens.

If you are allergic to metals like nickel, you won't be ready for the Power Wash until you overcome your nickel allergy. (Learn more about nickel in food at www.drgalland.com.) If you are allergic to latex or to birch pollen, do not include avocado in your Smoothie. Consult your doctor before starting the Power Wash or acting on any of the information presented in *The Allergy Solution.*

IMMUNE BALANCE SMOOTHIE

Velvety, creamy, and delicious, this smoothie packs a ton of nutrients in one easy-to-sip beverage. The vegetables simply swirl away into the fruit and avocado, and the result is pure heaven, with just a touch of natural sweetness.

450g strawberries, fresh or frozen
1 medium avocado, peeled, with the pit removed
30g chopped rocket
½ head romaine lettuce, chopped (6 leaves)
2 tablespoons freshly ground chia seeds
240ml green tea, brewed for 5 minutes, added hot
1 medium banana, if desired

Place the fruit in a blender and layer the vegetables on top. Add the chia seeds, pour in the green tea, and blend until the mixture is velvety smooth. If you refrigerate it after blending, the smoothie becomes thicker and creamier. Chia seeds are an excellent source of fiber and omega-3 fats.

Note: If you have latex or birch pollen allergy, do not include avocado. Avocados may provoke allergic reactions in people with latex or birch pollen allergy. If you have latex allergy, do not include a banana, as bananas may also cross-react with latex. If you are allergic to strawberries, leave them out. In that case, if you are not allergic to blueberries, you may substitute blueberries. If you are allergic to any ingredient, please leave it out.

IMMUNE BALANCE SOUP

This is a soul-satisfying soup with a delightful aroma, the kind that brings you back to your grandma's kitchen. The flavors of the vegetables blend to create a delicious broth. This soup is so mellow you can enjoy a big mug or bowl any time of day or night, and it's an excellent and tasty way to get the nutrients that support healthy immune function. It gives you an abundance of amazing vegetables in an easy-to-make and easy-to-eat meal—four servings of vegetables per large mug. It's rich in anti-inflammatory carotenoids and flavonoids.

I am excited to share with you one of the Galland family's favorite recipes, a modern classic that combines the art of cooking with the amazing science of nutrition. Once you start making it, everyone will think you took a class at a healthy cooking school.

450g sliced carrots

3 tablespoons extra-virgin olive oil

25g chopped parsley (you can include the stems)

200g chopped green onions (green parts only)

340g broccoli, cut up small (you can include the tender part of the stalks)

85g baby kale, chopped

1 teaspoon turmeric powder

¼ teaspoon freshly ground black pepper (or more to taste; black pepper enhances absorption of the awesome anti-inflammatory flavonoids contained in turmeric)

Salt to taste

1 tablespoon shredded daikon radish, added just before serving

Sauté the carrots in the olive oil for 10 minutes, then add the other vegetables and spices. Heat and stir for 1 minute, then add 2.8 litres of water and bring the mixture to a boil, stirring as needed. Cover and simmer for 20 minutes.

Just before eating, add one tablespoon of freshly shredded daikon radish per serving. Uncooked daikon contains a very special enzyme called myrosinase, which enhances the nutritional value of cooked broccoli. (It's the best-kept secret in nutrition, and a way to make broccoli even healthier, which sounds pretty amazing.) Or, if you like, allow the soup to cool and puree it to a creamy consistency, then reheat it before serving. The daikon should always be added just before eating.

Note: If you are allergic to any ingredient, please leave it out.

If you have any kind of problem with your kidneys, if you have a personal or family history of kidney stones, or if you suffer from chronic vulvar pain or bladder discomfort, check with your doctor before increasing your consumption of kale and parsley, as dietary oxalates may adversely affect some people with those disorders.

ORGANIC OOLONG TEA

Tea has been used as a medicinal beverage for over 3,000 years. Now modern science has discovered that a special type of tea, oolong, may offer unique anti-allergic benefits.

Oolong tea is made from partially fermented tea leaves, giving it a distinctive mellow flavor. Chinese oolong is aged longer than Formosan oolong.

Tea leaves are rich in natural compounds called catechins, which are a family of flavonoids. Fermentation changes the nature of the catechins, which alters the physiological effects of tea drinking.

In laboratory studies, the catechins found in oolong tea were shown to inhibit allergic reactions in rats and were more potent than those found in green tea. In a clinical trial done in Japan, people with allergic eczema that had not improved with medication were given oolong tea to drink for six months. While drinking the oolong tea, the majority of the people in the study experienced a moderate to marked improvement in eczema within one month, with benefits being first noticeable after one to two weeks.

The amount used was 10 grams of tea leaves, equivalent to about three teaspoons of dried leaves or four tea bags, brewed in boiling water for five minutes. According to the Japanese study, the right amount of tea is four cups a day. Do not exceed this amount per day.

To ensure that your tea has a high level of catechins extracted from the leaves, brew the tea in boiling water for five minutes. If the tea is too strong, boil it in a small amount of water and dilute with plain hot water to the desired concentration.

To reduce the amount of caffeine in your tea, first steep the tea leaves in hot water for 30 seconds and discard the water. Then add fresh water and boil for five minutes. Most of the caffeine will be extracted in the initial waste water. Most of the catechins will remain in your tea.

Note: If you are allergic to tea, please do not drink tea. You may have plain hot water, a common beverage in China and Japan.

Getting the Most out of the Power Wash

The Power Wash works well over a three-day weekend. You can start it Friday morning and move on to Stage 2, Re-entry, on Monday. With Re-entry, you begin introducing new foods in a structured sequence so you can identify those that you should avoid.

I want to give you a few key guidelines to help you make this process work.

Track Your Symptoms

As with the Allergy Solution Checklist of Symptoms that you worked through in Chapter 4, tracking your symptoms is essential to understanding the information the Power Wash can give you. Is it headache, itching, rash, wheezing, cough, pain, palpitations, brain fog, diarrhea, bloating, swelling, or any of a hundred other symptoms? Track the symptoms that have been bothering you the most, but also pay attention to minor symptoms that you identified when completing the symptoms checklist. Consult your doctor, who can help you decide which symptoms are most important.

Keep a Journal

For each symptom you're tracking, establish a baseline: how severe is it on a scale of 0 to 10? Then keep a daily record of how you experience this symptom over the course of the Power Wash, along with a record of what you're eating. Your symptoms may not improve at first during the Power Wash. In fact, some of them may get worse before they get better. That's usually a good sign. Improvement may take a week or more and only occur during Re-entry.

Watch Out for a Withdrawal Reaction

People with food allergies are sometimes physically addicted to those foods and may experience a withdrawal reaction. They may feel better when they eat the allergic food and start to feel worse when they avoid it. The most substantial withdrawal reactions I've encountered came early on, long before I developed the Power Wash, when I first started exploring the role of food allergy in chronic illness. These are extreme stories, but they illustrate the effects of the addiction/withdrawal phenomenon in hidden food allergy. You should consult your doctor if you experience a withdrawal reaction.

A Withdrawal Reaction

Emily, a schoolteacher in her 50s, had an arthritis flare-up so severe she needed hospitalization. Her hands, feet, elbows, and knees were so swollen and painful that she could barely move. I strongly suspected food allergy as the underlying cause, because her flare-up occurred during Christmas break after she had visited family in different nearby towns and eaten far more food than she normally did.

Because Emily was in the hospital, I placed her on a prescription elemental diet for the Power Wash elimination phase. An elemental diet is a liquid formula made up of amino acids, vitamins, and minerals. There are no food proteins. On the third day of elimination, Emily's pain got worse than ever and she developed a fever of 101 degrees. I treated her symptoms to get her through the night, and the next day all her pain and joint swelling disappeared. When she left the hospital the day after, she was symptom-free on no medication.

Emily's case is a dramatic example of a withdrawal reaction. This is what can happen with an elimination diet like the Power Wash that removes allergic triggers.

Staying Stable for Two Weeks

Try to maintain a stable environment for two weeks while you're doing the Power Wash and Re-entry. This may be challenging because you don't live in a research laboratory; you live in a world where there are variables you can't control. If possible try to eat out as little as possible, if at all. Don't decide to clean out your attic or take a trip or start a new job while you're doing this. Make sure your kitchen is well stocked with the right foods, which you'll learn more about as I take you through the Re-entry phase and the Immune Balance Diet in the next two chapters.

Support Your Power Wash Detox

Since you are making the effort to detox and clean your body, I encourage you strongly not to smoke or use tobacco products during this period. In fact, if you smoke, this would be the perfect time for you to quit for good, which would be the best thing.

Alcohol is a toxin, so please avoid alcohol during the Power Wash to help minimize toxins in your body.

Beyond Allergy—Foods That You May Need to Avoid

Now that we've drilled down into food allergy, I would like to look at the broader issue of why you may need to avoid certain foods. In addition to allergy, there are a few different ways in which foods and beverages can make you feel worse. For example, you may have an adverse metabolic reaction to a food or beverage. Another reason could be the way food interacts with the microbes in your gut.

Adverse Metabolic Reactions to Sugar or Coffee

There are foods that, for some people, lead to an adverse metabolic reaction, and for that reason they need to be avoided. Two very common examples are 1) sugar and sweets and 2) the caffeine in coffee.

Sugar and Sweets

Many people can't tolerate sugar or sweets. When they consume these, their blood sugar rises too quickly and then crashes, leaving them fatigued, shaky, and sweaty. This is called hypoglycemia, or low blood sugar, and it's caused by insulin, a hormone that is secreted when people consume a meal that's high in sugar. This is not an allergic reaction, it's a hormonal reaction.

Coffee

Lattes, cappuccinos, espressos. It seems that the whole world is walking around with a cup of coffee. But not everyone. There are many people who just can't tolerate coffee. For some people the caffeine in coffee can make them feel uncomfortably sped up and anxious and interfere with sleep. Sometimes they are able to drink tea without issues, but others need to avoid caffeine in any form. As important as they are, however, metabolic responses to diet change are different from food allergy.

What's Going On in Your Gut Can Make Some Foods a Problem

From the moment you start chewing and swallowing, your body begins to process and interact with what you are eating. As the food you consume continues along your lengthy digestive tract, it enters into an incredibly crowded new world where a variety of gut microbes play a major role, one that is sometimes helpful but other times causes problems. Common foods and beverages like milk, fruit, juice, vegetables, and wheat may interact with the microbes in your gut, leading to a variety of symptoms.

Milk

If you suffer from a condition called lactose intolerance, drinking milk may cause abdominal cramps, bloating, gas, and diarrhea. The reason: to be absorbed from your intestinal tract, milk sugar, or lactose, must first be digested to its component parts, which are simpler sugars called glucose and galactose.

Your intestines quickly absorb glucose and galactose but cannot absorb lactose. If you lack the enzyme needed for breaking lactose down into glucose and galactose, the undigested lactose reaches your large intestine, where it is fermented by intestinal bacteria to produce acids that irritate your gut. This fermentation can lead to the abdominal symptoms I noted above.

Fruit and Juice

With another common condition called fructose malabsorption, some people get fermentation in the gut if they eat fruits that are high in fructose, which is often called "fruit sugar." Humans have a limited ability to absorb fructose, and it varies greatly from person to person. Once you exceed your body's quota, any fructose you eat will quite likely be fermented in your large intestine. If you have fructose malabsorption, fruit juices and dried fruit of any kind can rapidly overload your gut's ability to handle fructose. Apples and pears tend to be the most problematic whole fruits.

Vegetables and Wheat

Wheat and some vegetables contain polymers of fructose called fructans. For some people, eating high-fructan foods can contribute to the symptoms of fructose malabsorption.

Most of the patients I see who have digestive complaints when they eat wheat actually suffer from fructose malabsorption. In their cases, we have determined that they are not allergic to wheat and are not sensitive to gluten, which is a major wheat protein. For them the problem is not with the proteins found in wheat but with fructans, which are carbohydrates.

The profound interaction between your diet and your gut microbes is at the cutting edge of nutrition research. During my medical career I have been a leading pioneer in applying this new knowledge of the gut microbiome to clinical practice and teaching other doctors about this in my writing and lecturing. I'm delighted to see mainstream medicine finally recognize its importance.

These interactions are not allergic. But because diet can change the nature of your gut microbes, which in turn influence your immune system, I've applied the profound insights of this cutting-edge research on gut microbes and health to the Allergy Solution program. You'll read more about what's going on in your gut—and how it can affect you—in Chapter 14.

Conclusion

This chapter served up a special tea, smoothie, and soup that I created to help detoxify the body and supply it with plant-based nutrients that help support the balance of the immune system. I enjoy preparing these recipes in my kitchen, getting all the wonderful vegetables out on the counter and ready for the soup pot and blender! It is a great way to put that kale, broccoli, carrots, green onion, parsley, and other nutrient-rich ingredients to use.

I explained that detox enzymes in your digestive system, liver, and other organs help rid the body of toxins and that vitamins, minerals, and amino acids from food support the work of these enzymes.

I also outlined some non-allergy reasons why you might need to avoid certain foods. For a variety of reasons that I touched upon in this chapter, things like sugar, coffee, wheat, milk, fruit, juice, or vegetables may need to be avoided because they don't work in harmony with your body.

Before starting on the Three-Day Power Wash, have your doctor take a look at the recipes and instructions and get his or her professional advice on whether or not this program is appropriate for you.

CHAPTER 7

THE RE-ENTRY FOOD CHALLENGE

Jennie, a college field hockey player, suffered from chronic sinusitis that would flare up during hockey season in the fall. The sinusitis made her miserable and interfered with her game. She had seen an allergist, who found allergies to mold and dust. Jennie had been prescribed antihistamines, but even the "non-drowsy" type made her feel drowsy. Nasal steroids gave her nosebleeds. A prescription anti-allergy medication caused profound mood swings. Clearly Jennie needed a different approach.

Jennie was a cheese-aholic. Sharp cheddar was her daily fix. This was an important clue. So when she came to my office I applied two principles: First, if there's a food you crave, you are probably both addicted to, and sensitive to, that food. A Re-entry trial may be worthwhile. Second, people who are allergic to airborne mold often have issues with molds found in food. Aged cheese is a mold-based food, and fall is a time for environmental mold, especially in Connecticut, where Jennie lives. I suspected mold might have an additive effect in creating her nasal congestion.

I recommended that Jennie stop eating cheese and milk-derived foods. The look on her face told me that I was right: Jennie was seriously addicted to cheese. I asked her to avoid it for five days and to call me after she had reintroduced her favorite cheeses on Days Six and Seven.

The call came early on Day Six. Fifteen minutes after eating 55 grams of her beloved cheddar cheese, Jennie felt very bloated and congested. She felt gas and had to relieve the pressure by passing gas numerous times. Bloating, burping, gas, diarrhea, and other digestive symptoms are one of the not-so-subtle ways the body tells us that it is not happy with a food or beverage. For Jennie, the digestive disturbances were probably her body's response to avoiding her favorite food for five days and then eating it again. The bloating, gas, and congestion were enough to convince Jennie that healing her allergies had to start with the elimination of cheese. I assured her that this was not forever. There were ways to eventually overcome her problem with dairy, but they wouldn't work if she kept taking her daily dose of cheddar.

Learning What Foods Make Your Body Happy

After the Three-Day Power Wash, the next step is the Re-entry Food Challenge. Re-entry follows a standard medical procedure of structured food challenges, used in medical centers and universities around the world, to uncover hidden food sensitivities. Jennie's story is one example of how reintroducing foods may produce unexpectedly strong responses, which is why you should always consult your doctor before and during Re-entry. If you have a known food allergy, you should not consume that food. People with asthma must not follow the Re-entry Food Challenge: asthmatics *must* avoid foods to which they may be allergic.

If you want to continue the Power Wash for another few days, you're free to do so. Just remember that the Power Wash is not designed to be an ongoing maintenance diet, so don't continue for more than seven days total.

During Re-entry you continue drinking the Immune Balance Smoothie and Organic Oolong Tea and continue eating Immune Balance Soup. You also begin expanding your diet step by step. Continue keeping your journal of symptoms, and keep a record of every food and beverage you add each day. If you experience symptoms, you'll need this record to bring with you to your doctor for evaluation in order to understand which foods, if any, may contribute to symptoms.

Re-entry is based on science. Its purpose is to help you connect with the wisdom of your body. Once you've completed the Power Wash, your body can tell you which foods you need to avoid for healing to occur.

During Re-entry, you will expand your diet in three stages. You are likely to notice changes in your body during each of them. Sometimes the changes will be immediate responses to a specific food you've just added. It may be a food you consumed regularly and had no idea you had an issue with, like Jennie and cheese. Other Re-entry responses may be delayed: a response may require more than one exposure to the food or may not occur for a day or two after eating the food. A delayed response is fairly common.

If you experience an adverse response after starting a new Re-entry stage, stop and proceed to the section on page 124 called "Zeroing In." If you experience no symptoms, continue to follow the Re-entry schedule until you've gone through all three stages.

Re-entry at a Leading Medical Center

In the 1980s, a famous British immunologist, Professor J. F. Soothill, teamed up with German neurologist Josef Egger— whose research on food allergy and ADHD you read about in Chapter 1—to investigate the role of food allergy in epilepsy and migraine among children. They conducted their research at the leading pediatric hospital in Britain, the Hospital for Sick Children in London, among patients who had epilepsy that was not responding to medication.[1] Since this was a research study with very sick children, they used an extended and rigorous protocol that should not be attempted outside a medical center, but their findings prove the importance of delayed food reactions.

They gave the children an elimination diet with a very limited range of foods for two weeks. This diet consisted of one or two starchy foods like rice or yams, chicken or lamb for protein, one vegetable, and one fruit. They found that 80 percent of the children who had epilepsy combined with headache, abdominal pain, or hyperactivity responded to the elimination diet with fewer seizures or complete cessation of seizures, along with improvement in their other symptoms. Children who only had epilepsy did not get better with the diet. They then had the children undergo a food challenge phase, in which each child received one new food a week, to see if specific foods would provoke symptoms. Symptoms were provoked by 31 different foods, with most of the children being reactive to several foods.

When the researchers confirmed these results with a double-blind, placebo-controlled food challenge, they observed that the reactions could take several days to occur. Using this technique, Soothill, Egger, and their colleagues enabled 60 percent of these children to remain completely free of epilepsy without drugs.

Important Notes

ALWAYS consult your doctor before attempting the Re-entry Food Challenge.

If you suffer from anaphylaxis or asthma, you should NOT attempt the Re-entry Food Challenge.

If you have ever experienced an adverse reaction from eating one of the foods mentioned in this chapter, do not eat it during Re-entry. Reintroduce only those foods that you believe are safe for you to eat.

Re-entry Stage One

This stage will last for a minimum of two days. After completing the Power Wash, you can add brown rice and poultry (chicken or turkey) to your diet. You can mix these into the Immune Balance Soup or eat them together as a separate dish. The poultry should be oven roasted and flavored with salt and pepper but no other spices except turmeric, if desired. Eat as much food as you need to prevent hunger.

- If you prefer to not eat poultry because you are a vegetarian, you may skip the poultry and have green peas in addition to rice. If you would rather have lamb than poultry, you can eat lamb as a substitute. Poultry and lamb are the meats included in the classic elimination and challenge programs.

- Rice allergy is rare in Europe and the Americas but common in Asia. If you suspect you have a rice allergy, choose oats or oatmeal instead of rice. Oatmeal can be eaten with blueberries for flavor, but with no milk added.

- If you prefer to avoid starches or grains, skip the rice and eat cauliflower or green peas in addition to chicken or turkey.

- Continue the Immune Balance Smoothie, the Immune Balance Soup, and the Organic Oolong Tea. When you include all the components, Stage One can be followed for up to a week, and you can enter Stage Two on your own timing.

If you experience any type of symptoms during Stage One, stop and follow the instructions under "Zeroing In" on page 124. If you've had no symptoms after two days of Stage One, you can proceed to Stage Two.

Re-entry Stage Two

This stage usually lasts for five days. It's designed to allow you to expand your diet, so that you're eating a variety of nutritious and flavorful foods. You can continue the Immune Balance Smoothie and Organic Oolong Tea for the unique nutrients they supply. The Immune Balance Soup is optional. Foods you may add are:

- Any vegetables you like, except those in the nightshade family, such as tomatoes, peppers, and eggplant. Use fresh or frozen vegetables, but not canned. Also avoid corn, which is a grain. You may enjoy your vegetables cooked or raw. I recommend trying squash, sweet potatoes, cabbage, and cauliflower. Do not eat any type of hot pepper.

- Beans, peas, lentils, and other legumes. But no nuts or peanuts, and no cocoa beans or chocolate.

- Beef, pork, and lamb. These are optional and should not be consumed more often than twice a week. Beef should be free-range and grass-fed.

- Organically grown coffee, if desired, but it must not be sweetened and should be taken black or with rice milk or coconut milk. At this point you do not yet know whether you can tolerate soy, almond, or cow's milk well. Why organic? Because coffee is one of the plants most heavily sprayed with pesticides on the planet.

- Fruit (with the exception of citrus fruit), fresh or frozen, but not canned. No dried fruit, no juices, and no syrup. Limit fruit to no more than three servings a day. If there are fruits to which you've previously had an allergic reaction, such as an itchy mouth or throat, continue to avoid them.

- Your choice of herbs and spices, fresh or dried, with the exception of cayenne, habañeros, jalapeños, and paprika. These spices are members of the troublesome nightshade family.

If you experience any type of symptoms during Stage Two, stop and follow the instructions under "Zeroing In" on page 124. The foods in Stage Two are diverse and nutritious enough that you can remain in Stage Two for as long as you like, although five days is the minimum. If you've had no adverse reaction after five days of Stage Two, you can proceed to Stage Three.

Re-entry Stage Three

This is where you test more foods and expand your menu further so that you have many delicious choices on your menu. I recommend that you test each food or food group separately for two days. During the two-day test, you may eat the food twice a day. Remember that a response may not occur on your first exposure to the food and that it may be delayed. If at any point you experience symptoms, stop adding new foods and move to Zeroing In. If at any time you want to stop testing new foods and maintain the diet you've been following, go ahead and do so. By now you've reached the point where there are enough foods available to you that you should be able to sustain the diet for as long as you like.

This is the order in which you may add foods in Stage Three. You do not have to eat any of these foods if you don't want them. Just skip what you dislike and move on to the next choice.

- Eggs: boiled, poached, fried, or as omelets. If you use oil in preparing eggs, use a little extra-virgin olive oil. Extra-virgin olive oil contains anti-inflammatory and antioxidant flavonoids that play an important role in the Allergy Solution.

- Fish. Choose low-mercury organic or wild fish: salmon, sardines, sole, flounder, and tilapia. Shellfish and high-mercury seafood such as tuna, sea bass, or swordfish should not be among your staple foods and are not included in the Immune Balance Diet.

- Nuts and seeds: dry roasted or fresh and raw, unsalted. Walnuts and almonds have the greatest nutritional benefit. Brazil nuts are rich in selenium but should be limited to no more than two per day, for a total of fourteen in a week. Peanuts are not really nuts; they are legumes. They are naturally contaminated with mold, which grows *inside* the peanut shell. Some of the healthiest seeds to chew on are pumpkin seeds, which are an excellent source of zinc, and sunflower seeds. Flaxseed should be freshly ground to convey its health benefits. Careful with sesame, though. It's a major allergen.

- Nightshade vegetables. The most nutritious members of this family are tomatoes and bell peppers, especially the orange and red varieties. All peppers except black pepper (peppercorns) are members of the nightshade family. Skip jalapeños, habañeros, cayenne, and paprika because they can mimic allergy and aggravate pain, inflammation, and asthma through a nonallergic biochemical reaction. Spicy peppers cause nerve endings to release a chemical called Substance P, which can increase inflammation in your tissues. That is why I recommend that you not consume hot peppers during Re-entry.

  - Some berries come from plants in the nightshade family. The most common of these are goji berries, also known as wolfberries. They are native to Asia and are now popular as health foods in North America and Europe. They can be eaten raw or dried or made into a juice. You can test unsweetened goji berries as part of the nightshade family.

  - Other common nightshade foods are potatoes and eggplant. They do not play an important role in the Immune Balance Diet because they lack the anti-inflammatory benefits of tomatoes, peppers, and goji berries.

- Citrus fruit: lemon, lime, grapefruit, tangerine, and all varieties of oranges. They can be eaten fresh or taken as juice, but limit the quantity of juice to no more than 230 millilitres a day. Organic fruit is recommended, because citrus can be heavily treated with pesticides.

The Final Four: Milk, Wheat, Corn, and Soy

These four foods are staples of the Western industrial diet, which makes them part of the problem. There are many reasons why they should not be staple foods, including genetic modification and contamination. They are not mainstays of the Immune Balance Diet, and you can easily live without them.

If you are happy avoiding milk, wheat, corn, and soy, go ahead and keep them off the menu. However, if you decide to try these, to know if any of them may be an issue, test each group separately, following the same protocol I've just described for other foods in Stage Three:

- Soy can be eaten as tofu or as whole soybeans (edamame) or drunk as unsweetened soy milk.

- Corn can be eaten as corn tortillas or grits or as whole kernels or corn on the cob.

- Wheat can be eaten as pasta, matzo, or wheat cereal. Bread, crackers, and baked goods contain too many other ingredients to allow a "wheat only" challenge.

- Milk can come from cows, sheep, or goats. Milk products include milk, yogurt, and cheese.

  - Casein, an allergenic milk protein, is concentrated in milk curd, so it's at its highest in cheeses. It is also a common food additive, listed on labels as sodium caseinate or calcium caseinate. When testing cow's milk, you can include foods with added caseinate.

  - Whey protein is also isolated from milk. You may remember the nursery rhyme about Little Miss Muffet eating her curds and whey. Whey is more soluble than casein. It comes as a powder, and at this point you can mix it into your Immune Balance Smoothie.

Re-Entry will only work if you've already cleared the tracks with the Power Wash and brought down the level of allergic inflammation in your body. Otherwise there will be too much noise for you to be able to listen to your body.

Zeroing In

If you experience symptoms during Re-entry, you might want to determine which food may have been a problem and whether the effect was just a chance association. Take the following steps:

- Stop testing new foods.

- Avoid any foods you've added to your diet in the past three or four days. Remember that Re-entry responses may be delayed, so how you feel can be due to a food you started eating two or three days ago rather than a food you ate today. Rolling your diet back a few days will help eliminate any foods that may have been part of delayed responses and leave you with a better diet.

- Maintain your improved diet until the reaction clears, which may take one to four days.

- Begin testing individual foods, starting with what you ate most recently before the symptoms occurred. The journal you've been keeping will really come in handy now. Let's say that on Saturday you added green peas and lentils, on Sunday you added beef, and on Monday you had scrambled eggs for the first time. Then Monday afternoon you broke out in a rash. Eggs would be the most likely culprit, so you'll retest them first, but only after cutting out beef, peas, and lentils and allowing the rash to subside. If eating eggs once more does not provoke a rash, then challenge yourself with beef, peas, and lentils, one food at a time. If the second round of challenges does not provoke a rash, the symptom may have been a coincidence, the result of an environmental exposure or stress or some factor other than food allergy. If you do experience a rash, you'll have a better theory about which food may be an issue.

Conclusion

Here I introduced the concept of Re-entry, which is based on the standard medical procedure of structured food challenges, used in medical centers and universities all over the world. For Jennie, the field hockey player with sinusitis, the issue was with milk-derived foods such as cheese. After cutting out all dairy for five days, she experienced bloating and gas after reintroducing her favorite cheese into her diet. Eliminating cheese from her diet was the next step.

Food allergy carries the risk of a dangerous allergic reaction. Re-entry must be supervised by a doctor. If you suffer from anaphylaxis or asthma, you must not attempt Re-entry.

Once you've used Re-entry to identify and remove the foods that may be an issue, you are ready to create long-lasting immune balance by learning about the research on nutrition science in the next chapter.

CHAPTER 8

THE IMMUNE BALANCE DIET

Snow-white peaks jut up into the clear blue sky. It's 9:30 A.M. and I am standing at the top of a mountain in Colorado. I take a deep breath of the crisp morning air, point my skis downhill, lean forward, and leap into the deep powder. My skis bank within the snow, cutting arcs to the right and then the left as I turn. It is an act of balance, feeling the snow, the air, and the steepness of the slope as I descend rapidly down the mountain. I reach the bottom of the run and feel exhilarated.

Balance is everything. It doesn't matter how strong you are; if your balance is off, you're likely to fall. The simple act of walking shows you how balance works in your body: it's the coordination of opposites. Right and left. You use both legs to walk. When one foot steps forward, the other stays on the ground, supporting your weight. When you're walking, your arms move in synchrony with your legs. Alternating right arm, left leg. Left arm, right leg.

Your immune system also depends on balance for its proper function—and I have discovered that nutrition plays a key role in balancing immunity. Our modern diet, high in sugar and refined carbs and filled with fast food, has knocked us off balance and thrown us off our skis.

In this chapter I will reveal breakthroughs in the science of allergy-fighting with nutrients from delicious, natural foods and beverages. These breakthroughs in nutrition inspired me to create the Immune Balance Diet, to help support the body against allergies by feeding the lymphocytes called T-reg cells that I talked about in Chapter 3.

Science teaches us that T-regs love vitamins and phytonutrients from fruit, vegetables, and tea, so the Immune Balance Diet is full of these delicious, natural sources of nutrients. I will be explaining the exciting nutrition research from around the world, and I'll also be introducing some incredible natural foods that you can find right in your local supermarket or farmer's market.

The full list comes later in this chapter, but here is a quick preview. Red, ripe strawberries, fresh parsley, and mellow green tea and oolong tea are just three of the nutrition rock stars that I want to talk about.

You will also learn why I'm so enthusiastic about the special nutrients in vegetables such as spinach, asparagus, and brussels sprouts, and why I am a big fan of legumes such as lentils, black beans, and garbanzo beans. Sweet potato is at the top of the list as a source of one key nutrient I will explore, and it's joined by carrots, sweet bell peppers, and mangoes. All of these satisfying foods will help restore balance and get us back on our skis. It is going to be a delicious, exciting ride. Are you ready?

Fighting Allergy Naturally—with Food

Do you believe that there is something fresh and vital in natural foods like fruits and vegetables that you can't get from a bottle of pills? Of course there is. Mother Nature provides us with the unique gifts of fiber, vitamins, minerals, and other important nutrients directly from whole, natural foods, which form the foundation of nutrition.

The goal of the Immune Balance Diet is to help you feed your T-regs and support their function. When T-regs are working well, they help us overcome allergies. The Immune Balance Diet is a healthy way of eating that can provide nutritional support to help fight allergies over time. Following it for 6 to 12 months may lead to a gradual subsiding of allergies.

Dietary factors found to enhance T-regs include folates from food, vitamin A, and various plant-derived nutrients called flavonoids, especially one found in tea.[1] Some flavonoids also inhibit the activity of cells that cause inflammation, so they can knock out allergies in two ways.[2]

Having gone through Power Wash and Re-entry, you have already begun to balance your immunity by enriching your diet with some nutrients that boost T-regs. The Immune Balance Diet is designed to help you further nourish your T-regs and also to combat allergies in four other important ways. The Immune Balance Diet:

- Helps to avoid your problem foods, which you have discovered through Re-entry

- Supplies optimal nourishment for the cells of your body

- Supports the growth and maintenance of healthy gut microbes that aid your efforts to reverse allergy

- Helps you steer away from inflammation-promoting junk food, which has played such a major role in creating the allergy epidemic

Balance Immunity on the Immune Balance Diet

So what foods do you eat to balance immunity? Science provides the answer. To begin with, at least nine servings of brightly colored vegetables and fruits every day, choosing those that are rich in natural folates, vitamin A, and fiber. Folates from food are needed for cell growth and repair, immune function, and brain function. Their deficiency can cause anemia, fatigue, depression, cognitive disturbances, and immune impairment. Brightly colored vegetables and fruits are also rich sources of flavonoids.

On the Immune Balance Diet, the Immune Balance Soup and the Immune Balance Smoothie can still be staples of your menu.

The Smoothie is rich in folates, flavonoids, and vitamin A; the Soup is packed with nutrients, and one bowl supplies four servings of vegetables. You can add other ingredients of your choice to the soup, such as whole scallions, beans, chicken or fish, and additional spices like garlic or ginger. Keep the original ingredients and add to them to make this soup your own.

In addition to the Soup and the Smoothie, you can eat any of the foods that tested well during the Re-entry process described in the last chapter: meat, fish, poultry, eggs, nuts, seeds, beans, fruits, vegetables, herbs and spices, even dairy products and whole grains. Re-entry allows you to experience the ways in which different food groups affect you as a unique individual. Know your body and listen to it.

If you're not allergic to them, nuts and seeds are an excellent source of vitamins, minerals, protein, and fiber, and they make a great snack food. I make my own trail mix, using almonds, walnuts, sunflower seeds, pumpkin seeds, and a few Brazil nuts. Almonds are high in magnesium. Walnuts supply healthy fats. Sunflower seeds are an excellent source of vitamin B6 and folates. Pumpkin seeds are the highest plant source of zinc. Brazil nuts are rich in selenium. But the benefits of eating nuts and seeds can't be reduced to the individual nutrients they contain. People who eat nuts and seeds regularly may be less likely to suffer from obesity, diabetes, and heart disease, according to research.

Let's take a closer look at the nutrients that form the backbone of the Immune Balance Diet.

Natural Folates from Food

It is necessary to get natural folates from foods. Dark-green, leafy vegetables and legumes like lentils and beans are among the best sources. In the box on page 131, I've listed the best food sources of natural folates and the amount you'll get in a common portion of each. Choose those you like and eat them regularly as part of the Immune Balance Diet. You can add beans, peas, lentils, and asparagus as desired to the Immune Balance Soup. Asparagus can be added fresh, but the legumes need to be precooked, because the soup is boiled for just 20 minutes, which is not enough time to cook the legumes.

I designed the Immune Balance Smoothie to provide ample folates from food. One 340-millilitre glass a day can supply abundant natural folates for optimal T-reg function. It's so fresh, creamy, and delicious that I look forward to drinking mine every day. In addition, the Smoothie can provide ample amounts of vitamin A from vegetarian sources and carefully chosen flavonoids.

Excellent Food Sources of Folates

Food	Folates
Lentils	358 mcg
Black-eyed peas	356 mcg
Pinto beans	294 mcg
Garbanzo beans	282 mcg
Spinach	263 mcg
Asparagus	262 mcg
Black beans	256 mcg
Navy beans	254 mcg
Kidney beans	229 mcg
Lima beans	156 mcg
Beets	136 mcg
Split peas	127 mcg
Papaya (one medium)	115 mcg
Green peas	101 mcg
Brussels sprouts	100 mcg
Broccoli	96 mcg
Avocado	90 mcg
Romaine lettuce	76 mcg
Winter squash	57 mcg
Cauliflower	55 mcg
Green beans	42 mcg

Oranges (one medium)	40 mcg
Summer squash	36 mcg
Grapefruit (one medium)	30 mcg
Strawberries	25 mcg

Nutrient measurements are based on one cup, unless otherwise specified.

Vitamin A from Food Sources

Vitamin A is a critical nutrient for cell repair, vision, healthy skin, and proper immune function. Vitamin A deficiency can cause blindness, slow wound healing, and poor resistance to infection. Whole-food sources of the building blocks of vitamin A are the best way to obtain this important nutrient.

Vitamin A is a general term used to identify families of naturally occurring molecules called *retinoids* and *pro-vitamin A carotenoids*. Retinoids come mostly from animals, and carotenoids come mostly from plants. You can make all the retinoids you need from the pro-vitamin A carotenoids found in plants, which means that vegetarians may enjoy a better vitamin A status than omnivores if their diets are rich in vegetables and fruits.[3] The names of the pro-vitamin A carotenoids are beta-carotene, alpha-carotene, and beta-cryptoxanthin.

I recommend that you get your vitamin A from foods that are rich sources of these, like carrots, spinach, and sweet potato, because these contain not only natural vitamin A but also many phytonutrients that come only from whole food sources.

Carotene gets its name from carrots, and it's their high concentration of beta-carotene that makes carrots look orange. Carotenoids and retinoids are both absorbed better if you consume fat along with them. That's why the recipe for Immune Balance Soup begins by having you sauté carrots in olive oil.

I believe the best way to meet your need for vitamin A is from food, especially carotenoid-rich vegetables that also give you flavonoids, fiber, and phytonutrients at the same time. A list of plant foods high in vitamin A is shown in the box on page 133. These foods also give you related carotenoids, like lycopene, lutein, and zeaxanthin. Although your body does not convert them into vitamin A, they may yield health benefits through important mechanisms of their own. The Immune Balance Soup and the Immune Balance Smoothie are designed to supply ample vitamin A from plant foods.

Excellent Food Sources of Vitamin A

Food	Vitamin A
Sweet potato, one medium	1,403 RE (retinol equivalents)
Spinach, 15g	573 RE
Carrots, 75g	459 RE
Cantaloupe, 75g	135 RE
Pepper, sweet red, 85g	117 RE
Mango, raw, 1 whole	112 RE
Black-eyed peas, boiled, 60g	66 RE
Broccoli, boiled, 85g	60 RE

Fabulous Flavonoids: The Best-Kept Secret in Nutrition

You won't see flavonoids listed on any food label. That's because flavonoid deficiency has not been described in the way that vitamin and mineral deficiencies have been, so flavonoids are not treated as essential nutrients. But flavonoids are every bit as important as vitamins and minerals.

It's my belief that the chronic inflammatory disorders that result from a Western diet and lifestyle are in part caused by flavonoid deficiencies. High intake of dietary flavonoids has been associated with a reduced risk of heart disease, diabetes, cancer, and asthma in research studies. The modern Western diet contains about 1,000 milligrams of flavonoids per day. A traditional

Asian diet contains about four times that amount, much of it from herbs, spices, and teas.

Tea Flavonoid Helps Reduce Inflammation and Fight Allergies

There are more than 400 flavonoids in the human diet. As a group, flavonoids have potent anti-inflammatory and antioxidant effects. I'd like to focus on two flavonoids that are important for T-regs and that play a key role in the Immune Balance Diet.

The first is found in tea; let's call it tea flavonoid. Although green tea is a well-known source of this flavonoid, the levels in oolong tea are just as high.[4]

The ability of tea flavonoid to combat inflammation has been studied for more than 25 years. Its effect on T-regs was first studied at the University of California and reported in 2010. Here's a quick look at the research:

- University of California researchers measured the function and the number of T-regs in the blood of overweight and lean people. Both function and number were impaired by obesity and restored by exposing blood cells to tea flavonoid.[5]

- Researchers at Tufts University demonstrated similar effects when they fed low doses of tea flavonoid to mice.[6]

- Further laboratory research has shown that the increase in T-regs produced by tea flavonoid causes a reduction in blood levels of the IgE antibody, indicating a functional anti-allergic effect.[7]

- Low doses of tea flavonoid appear to work better at reducing inflammation than very high doses.[8] That is why I prefer to get tea flavonoid from drinking tea, four cups a day, and not from dietary supplements.

Enjoy Your Own Little Tea Ceremony

You just need a quiet moment all to yourself, away from the pressures of everyday life. I understand. You need a moment to gather your thoughts. Or maybe to let your mind empty and let all your cares and worries flow away. To leave behind the ever present pull of the present and give yourself a little quiet time.

Escape with a tranquil tea ceremony of your own.

Put your cell phone out of reach with the volume turned down. Get ready to settle into your favorite comfy chair or sofa.

But first, about that cup of tea. The kitchen. Your favorite mug. Be aware of the simple and satisfying rhythm of brewing the tea, how you move around the kitchen, the sound of water coming to a boil, the color and texture of the tea itself. As you brew the tea, notice how the tea infuses the water and how the inviting aroma wafts into the air.

With the cup in your hand, settle carefully into your seat. Feel the heat of the cup warming your hands, and watch a faint whisper of steam rise into the air. You are going on an imaginary journey to a faraway place where you can let your mind be still.

Achieving a peaceful mind through meditation or prayer, even for just a short time each day, provides real benefits for your health. While the idea of mind-body medicine was once considered esoteric, a recent study from Harvard University found it moving into the mainstream, with health care providers giving patients "prescriptions" for meditation and yoga.[9]

I'll talk more about mind-body well-being in Chapter 10. For now, sip your tea and enjoy knowing that you're not only getting valuable flavonoids, you're giving yourself an invaluable moment of peace.

The Super-Antioxidant in Strawberries

One of the best-kept secrets in nutrition is the flavonoid fisetin, and the richest dietary source of fisetin is strawberries. Fisetin is a potent antioxidant that increases the concentration of glutathione in your cells, according to research from the Salk Institute for Biological Studies.[10] (You read about glutathione in Chapter 1, and we'll discuss it in more detail in Chapter 13.) Glutathione helps to protect your T-regs from damage; a lack of it makes T-regs susceptible to destruction induced by environmental and food toxins,[11] which is one factor contributing to the epidemic of allergy.

Although the first effect of fisetin is to protect T-regs from damage by enhancing glutathione levels, laboratory experiments have demonstrated other important benefits. For instance, administration of fisetin decreases several aspects of the allergic response and protects laboratory animals from allergic asthma.[12] And at the Salk Institute for Biological Research, scientists have demonstrated numerous protective effects of fisetin on the aging nervous system.[13]

I designed the Immune Balance Smoothie to supply you with fisetin, tea flavonoid, folates from food, and vitamin A. Make it fresh every day. One 340-millilitre glass supplies four servings of fruits and vegetables, almost half of what you need every day. To enhance the amount of tea flavonoid in the green tea used in the Smoothie, I recommend that you boil the tea leaves for five minutes instead of just steeping the tea bag in hot water.

Strawberries, a Delicious Way to Help Fight Allergies

With a delightfully distinctive aroma, flavor, and color, naturally sweet and luscious strawberries deliver nutrition the way nature intended. Two hundred grams of these beautiful berries is only 49 calories and provides you with 98 milligrams of vitamin C as well as the minerals potassium, calcium, and magnesium and 3 grams of fiber.

And that is just the beginning. In research labs around the world, science is unlocking the amazing nutritional power of the simple strawberry. It turns out that strawberries are a delicious source of the anti-allergy nutrient called fisetin, a flavonoid that can fight allergic reactions by supporting the health of T-regs. That is why I made strawberries a star ingredient in my Immune Balance Smoothie.

At the peak of strawberry season, nothing compares to finding beautiful, ripe berries, which are a perfect snack or natural dessert. I always buy organic berries. When fresh berries are out of season, I enjoy using frozen organic berries, which are now easier to find than ever. They give my smoothies the delightful aroma and mild sweetness of strawberries year-round.

A study from Washington State University discovered that organically grown strawberries had higher levels of vitamin C and total antioxidants than conventionally grown strawberries. What is more, the study found that in consumer comparison testing, organic berries were judged to be sweeter and have better flavor and appearance than conventional berries. The study also tested the quality of the soil where the berries were grown and found that the soil on organic strawberry farms was healthier and supported more life than the soil on conventional farms.

So is it worth it to go organic? When it comes to strawberries, the science has spoken. More nutrition, fewer pesticides, better taste, and farming practices that are better for the environment— all this makes buying organic something we can really feel good about.[14]

Enjoying the Wonderful Freshness of Parsley

Bright green, aromatic parsley brings an unmistakable freshness to an amazing variety of dishes. I have added parsley to soups, tossed it onto salads, sprinkled it over pasta, and stir-fried it into rice and vegetables. I love placing a big bunch of fresh parsley on the kitchen counter to make the Immune Balance Soup. The leaves are lovely, but don't forget the stems, which provide a satisfying crunch. I have found that once you get started using parsley, it becomes an easy-to-use favorite that adds great flavor to your cooking.

But the culinary delights of parsley are just the beginning. In addition to enhancing eating pleasure, parsley is an excellent source of nutrients. It is high in carotenoids; it has even more of this nutrient than carrots. Parsley is also a great source of the flavonoid apigenin. Like many other flavonoids, apigenin has anti-allergic and anti-inflammatory effects, but it also activates a switch in the immune response.

Exciting research on apigenin from the Nanjing Medical University in China found that the apigenin switch decreases the activity of allergy-inducing lymphocytes and reduces IgE levels.[15]

This is another reason to continue eating the Immune Balance Soup, which is packed with parsley.

So what do you look for when shopping for this herb? Fresh parsley can be found at the supermarket, the farmer's market, and the natural food store. Freshness is key. The parsley should look like a beautiful bunch of fresh-cut flowers.

Just like flowers, parsley likes water, so when you are ready to use it, toss the parsley into a bowl of water to soak off any dirt. Give it a good rinse and then pat it dry with a paper towel. Now it is ready to use in your kitchen creations!

What Not to Eat

To begin with, you should avoid eating any food or group of foods that you were intolerant of during Re-entry and Zeroing In. Avoid them carefully for at least six months. By the end of six months, you may be able to eat some of those foods again, if you've followed all aspects of the Allergy Solution program and you find that those foods do not cause you any symptoms.

You probably noticed that Re-entry did not include candies, pastries, processed foods, artificial colors and flavors, high-fructose corn syrup, most vegetable oils, or any of the foods commonly thought of as junk food. Once you have gone through the Power Wash, you have cleansed yourself of these foods. There is no Re-entry for donuts, cakes, pies, muffins, or fries. These foods are all part of the problem and cannot be part of the solution. These things are roadblocks to healing. Brian's story is a good example.

Brian was a 35-year-old software designer who had had eczema since childhood. At its worst it covered his arms, face, and legs, with a special predilection for his eyelids and the folds inside his elbows and behind his knees. It was a scaly, itchy rash that would usually clear in summer. The rest of the year he'd control it by applying cortisone cream. Stress always made it worse. One summer the rash wouldn't clear and his skin burned every time he took a bath or shower. That's when he came to my office.

Brian had already started eating what I call a pseudo-healthy diet. He ate lots of salad; he had gone gluten-free, cut out red meat, and started using alternative grains like amaranth and quinoa; and he was mixing hemp seeds into his fat-free Greek yogurt. But then he'd pour two tablespoons of agave nectar into the yogurt, add two teaspoons of honey to his organic green tea, and stay up till two in the morning surfing the Internet while munching gluten-free cookies and eating all-natural chocolate.

Break Free from Sugar Cravings

If you have sugar cravings, you know how compelling, how insistent, how gripping, and how real they can be. It's like having Darth Vader enticing you to come over to the dark side, forcing you against your own will to devour that chocolate cake or pint of ice cream. The dark side of sugar cravings makes you eat things that you don't want to eat.

So how do you escape the forceful grasp of these cravings? You know that, like the bad guy in a movie, cravings don't just disappear on their own. Keep indulging in sugar and the cravings stick with you, not going anywhere, because each time you have sugar you are actually feeding and encouraging your desire for more. No, it is going to take a heroic leap on your part.

The magic happens when you take that brave step and walk away from sugar, leaving it cold. Something quite extraordinary occurs: the cravings go away. In as little as two or three days, they vanish. That constant pull of sugar, the need to munch on a cookie or candy bar, is gone. You can literally sense the weight coming off of your shoulders. You are free.

When setting out to eliminate sugar from their routine, many people are surprised to find it hiding in their favorite products. Sugar has a talent for showing up in places it shouldn't. You expect sugar to star in decadent desserts like red velvet cake or frosted cupcakes. But sugar has a way of sneaking into savory items such as soup, spaghetti sauce, and crackers, just to name a few. Sugar blends in almost everywhere and can go unseen until you read the label. Make it a habit to look closely at the ingredient list on food labels—where sugar may be listed as cane sugar, cane juice, sucrose, dextrose, fructose, corn syrup, beet sugar, and malt—and you will be able to eliminate a lot of it.

It's difficult enough to stay vigilant against hidden sugar in your own kitchen, where you're in control. When you're on the go, it's even tougher. So you don't get stuck trying to improvise or ad-lib this effort, I'm going to provide you with a plan. You don't want to be at the mercy of what you can grab from a vending machine when you are out—and sugary snacks are everywhere, while healthy choices take a little bit of planning. Remember you are doing something heroic, and give yourself plenty of credit.

Plan Your Escape from Sugar

- Pack plenty of healthy snacks and beverages in your bag when you go out. Cut some veggies and eat them by the handful. Carrots and celery sticks give you plenty to crunch on and will help you avoid sugary temptations.

- If you are not allergic to nuts, then almonds, cashews, walnuts, and pecans make a crunchy, satisfying snack.

- Pack your favorite fresh fruit, such as apples, oranges, pears, blueberries, and strawberries. Whole fruit has fiber, antioxidants, and other nutrients that come with natural sweetness.

- Bring an unsweetened yogurt with you, and add some unsweetened fruit juice concentrate to give it more flavor and color.

- Pack a small container of guacamole or hummus, and have that with some baked chips.

- Carry a sandwich bag of seeds like pumpkin seeds, pignoli nuts, or sunflower seeds.

- Opt for healthy beverages like tea, water, and organic coffee that will keep you from gulping down sugar. Skip the sodas, sports drinks, lemonades, and sweetened iced teas.

Listen to Your Body

Brian's road to healing was like a roller-coaster ride. He stayed on the Power Wash for five days and remained in Stage One of Re-entry for a week. Even though it was the middle of winter, his skin became clearer than it had been in years.

Then he stopped using cortisone cream and his skin began to itch again. I explained to Brian that his skin had become dependent on cortisone and he was experiencing a withdrawal reaction. I gave him a two-week schedule for tapering off the cream, which diminished the rebound effect of steroid withdrawal, and the healing of his skin continued. That's when things got more interesting.

First, he began losing weight. When I first saw him he was about 30 pounds overweight and had not been able to lose weight even when he cut back on sweets. I explained to him that steroids interfere with weight loss, so as long as he relied on steroid creams to control his eczema, he'd have a hard time with weight control no matter how few calories he ate or how much he exercised. Off the steroids and following the Immune Balance Diet, weight loss would come naturally.

Then came the holidays and celebrations: Memorial Day, his nephew's high school graduation, his cousin's wedding, Independence Day. Each of these was an occasion to chow down on cake or candy, sometimes with a beer or two, and each time Brian's eczema would flare up, typically a day or two later. Each time it took a week to heal.

With each flare-up he'd gain a few pounds, his hands would feel puffy, and his face would swell just enough for his girlfriend to notice the difference. These changes were not due to food allergies; we'd established that through the Re-entry process. Brian's body was very sensitive to the inflammatory effects of sugar, which I discuss in more detail in my weight-loss book, *The Fat Resistance Diet*. For Brian, itching of his skin was like a barometer of his sugar intake.

Each time Brian's eczema flared, he'd call me up and say, "Doc, I can't believe I'm so sensitive to sugar. Could that really be true?"

And each time, I'd say, "You know the answer, Brian. Listen to your body."

Optimal immune function depends on optimal nutrition. The food you eat nourishes the cells that prevent allergy, help fight infection, and work to control inflammation. The best diet is not the same for everybody. Optimal nutrition is individualized nutrition. It must take into account your own specific food allergies and sensitivities, your tastes, and your culture. I've designed the Allergy Solution program to help you find the nutritious foods that fit your needs and then enhance that diet with foods that ensure optimal T-reg function.

Conclusion

This chapter highlighted exciting research from around the world on nutrition and allergy, with a focus on dietary factors that can help balance the immune system and reduce allergies. Breakthroughs in nutrition science have revealed that we can support the function of the special T-reg cells that are the conductors of the immune system. With T-regs functioning well, allergic reactions can be prevented.

I created the Immune Balance Diet as a natural source of vitamins and phytonutrients, based on nutrition research from around the world. We explored natural food sources of vitamin A and folates. We learned about the special nutrients in strawberries, parsley, and tea that may help fight allergies.

The case of Brian, the software designer, demonstrated how a taste for sugar and sweets could contribute to eczema: his roller-coaster ride of cleaning up his diet, seeing an improvement in his skin, then succumbing to sugar cravings leading to skin flare-ups convinced him just how sensitive his body is to the inflammatory impact of sugar. Luckily, sugar cravings can be overcome, as I explained in the section "Break Free from Sugar Cravings."

I am confident that when you share this chapter with your doctor and discuss what you have learned, she or he will be able to decide on your nutrition program and guide your journey of healing.

CHAPTER 9

ARE ALLERGIES MAKING YOU FAT?

"I don't understand it," cried Madeline. "My body changed when I became pregnant, and it's never been the same since."

Madeline had gained 50 pounds with her first pregnancy and had been struggling to lose it for the past ten years. With intensive exercise and dieting, she'd lost 10 pounds, but she was still 40 pounds away from her goal.

When Madeline came in to see me, she cited recurrent chest infections and fatigue as the reasons for the consultation. Once we started talking, her frustration with her weight quickly made weight loss the main topic.

Growing up in Minneapolis, she'd been lean and physically fit, although she suffered from lifelong allergies to pollen and dust and had frequent colds. In her teens she developed constipation and abdominal pain and was told she had an irritable bowel. She was advised to stop eating meat and increase dietary fiber from whole grains. Her constipation improved.

In her mid-twenties she married her high-school sweetheart, Brad, who had just gotten a new job in Atlanta. Giving up her own job for the move and cooking for her husband every day, Madeline gained the first ten pounds. She had always been a runner, which was one way she stayed lean, but the long pollen season in Atlanta caused her nose to water and itch any time she went for a run between March and November. A strong antihistamine overcame that problem.

Two pregnancies gave her two healthy children but left her 50 pounds overweight and suffering from daily heartburn. Despite her switch to a vegetarian diet, her weight refused to budge.

Once she'd finished nursing her children, Madeline was back on a prescription antihistamine for eight months of the year. Her doctor added a second drug, this one for heartburn. The drug was a proton pump inhibitor, or PPI, which relieves heartburn by suppressing the production of stomach acid. It created a new symptom, abdominal bloating, which made Madeleine feel even worse about the weight she'd gained.

The illness that led her to my office was pneumonia. She'd had two episodes in two years, each time following a cold and each time responding promptly to antibiotics. I'd helped a friend of hers recover from pneumonia, so when Brad came to New York on a business trip, she joined him and they both came to see me for her consultation.

"There's not just one cause for your weight problem," I explained. "There's a vicious cycle in which weight gain increases allergies and allergy increases body weight, and the drugs you've been given actually make it worse. Your problem isn't unusual. I've seen it many times."

Brad worked for a biotech firm and had a degree in chemistry. "I wondered about something like that," he said. "But no other doctor has ever thought about it that way." He asked me for the evidence.

Obesity and Allergy: A Vicious Cycle

"There's a direct connection between allergy and weight gain," I explained. "It results from the interaction between fat cells and the cells that create allergic responses, which are called mast cells and eosinophils."

As I explained in Chapter 3, mast cells store dozens of chemicals that create inflammation. Whenever there's an allergic reaction, mast cells dump these chemicals into your tissues, where they produce most of the common symptoms of allergy, like itching, swelling, redness, sneezing, and wheezing. A little-known fact is that some of these chemicals also promote the growth of fat cells.[1]

Fat cells, for their part, also store many chemicals. As you gain weight, these chemicals are released by the fat cells and circulate in your blood. Most of them provoke more inflammation.

There's something in your fat cells that does the opposite: a hormone that reduces inflammation. It is called adiponectin. Adiponectin has direct anti-allergic effects.[2] It calms down eosinophils (Eos), cells that release enzymes that can damage tissues and harm your immune system.[3]

Here's the problem: the larger your fat cells, the less adiponectin they make. So as your fat cells get fatter, the Eos get restless and produce more allergic inflammation, which increases activation of mast cells, which promotes the growth of fat.[4]

I believe that this vicious cycle explains the powerful link between having allergies and being overweight, a connection that has been documented in medical research. The science shows us:

- Increased body fat is associated with increased prevalence of asthma, allergic rhinitis, and eczema.[5]

- People with chronic allergic sinusitis are two and a half times more likely to be overweight than a control population without allergies.[6]

- Use of prescription antihistamines, a sign of clinical allergy, is associated with increased body weight, according to a study done at Yale University utilizing data from the U.S. government's National Health and Nutrition Examination Survey.[7]

- For children and adolescents, being overweight or obese increases blood levels of allergic IgE antibodies, especially to food.[8]

- Even for women of normal weight, an increase in waist size increases the risk and severity of asthma. The implications of this are very serious, because the rate of abdominal obesity among women in the United States is almost twice the rate of general obesity and reflects a heightened state of inflammation in the body. The inflammatory effect of excess abdominal fat may explain why weight loss by itself improves asthma control in people who are overweight.[9]

I explained the vicious cycle of allergy and weight gain to Madeline, then reminded her that the medication she was taking might actually be making the situation worse. For people who have allergies or are overweight, the development of heartburn and its treatment with PPIs accelerates the turning of this vicious cycle.

The Heartburn Connection

The epidemic of allergy over the past 30 years has been accompanied by the obesity epidemic and an epidemic of GERD, which stands for gastroesophageal reflux disease, or simply reflux. Scientists have made the case that these three epidemics are closely interrelated. Being overweight not only increases your risk of allergy, it also increases your risk of developing GERD, which can increase allergic respiratory symptoms.

If you suffer from heartburn, reflux, asthma, cough, or chronic rhinosinusitis, or if you habitually use drugs for heartburn, you need to read this section carefully, because the conventional treatment of heartburn may actually make your allergies worse.

Heartburn is the chief symptom of GERD and occurs when stomach juices travel backward up the esophagus, where they may produce pain and inflammation. This reverse flow is called reflux, and the inflammation is called esophagitis. Sometimes the feeling of heartburn is called acid indigestion because the burning feels acidic.

Drug ads attempt to separate ordinary heartburn from GERD; however, they're essentially the same condition, differing only in the degree of inflammation they cause.

Here's how GERD can intensify your allergy symptoms:

- Esophagitis can stimulate an increase in mucus production in your nose and sinuses through a reflex involving your vagus nerve, aggravating the symptoms of nasal or sinus allergies.[10]

- Medical research from Emory University in Atlanta determined that GERD is very common among people who have undergone sinus surgery and are still suffering from recurrent rhinosinusitis.[11] The researchers believe that GERD is the main reason for nasal and sinus inflammation in this group of people.

- If stomach juices reach the throat, they may cause a sore throat, a hoarse voice, or a sour taste in your mouth. This condition, called LPR (laryngopharyngeal reflux), is essentially an extension of GERD.

- Stomach juice can also be inhaled into the bronchial tubes, where it produces coughing or aggravates asthma. Numerous studies have found that asthmatics have a much higher rate of GERD and LPR than people without asthma. Studies indicate that GERD prevents good asthma control.[12]

If you suffer from chronic asthma or relapsing rhinosinusitis, it's important to consider GERD as a factor. But here's where things get challenging, because the standard treatment of GERD may make your allergies worse.

The Trouble with Heartburn Drugs

Drugs that suppress production of stomach acid are the standard treatment for GERD and LPR. These drugs fall into two categories. The stronger ones are called proton pump inhibitors (PPIs); this is the type of drug that Madeline's doctor prescribed for her. The weaker ones are called H2 blockers. The best-known PPI is omeprazole (Prilosec); the best known H2 blocker is ranitidine (Zantac). Here is a list of commonly used acid suppressors.

Acid-Suppressing Drugs

Proton pump inhibitors suppress enzymes that transport hydrochloric acid from acid-secreting cells to the surface of the stomach lining. Some common examples of PPIs include:

- Prilosec, Zegerid (omeprazole)
- Prevacid, Dexilant (lansoprazole and dexlansoprazole)
- Nexium (esomeprazole)
- Aciphex (rabeprazole)
- Protonix (pantoprazole)

H2 blockers prevent histamine from performing one of its normal functions, which is to increase the output of stomach acid. Some common examples of H2 blockers include:

- Zantac (ranitidine)
- Tagamet (cimetidine)
- Pepcid AC (famotidine)
- Axid (nizatidine)

Antacids are drugs that neutralize stomach acid without suppressing its release. There are many brands, all available without a prescription. They all contain highly alkaline mineral salts like magnesium hydroxide (milk of magnesia) and aluminum hydroxide. Examples include Maalox, Mylanta, and Gelusil.

Although acid-suppressing drugs are among the most widely used drugs in the United States, there are four reasons why you should not rely on them for treating your heartburn:

1. Acid-suppressing drugs do not prevent reflux. They merely convert acid reflux into non-acid reflux, which can still be irritating and damaging. Much of the damage done by GERD is due to bile and to the enzyme pepsin, both of which are present in stomach juice even when acid production is suppressed.

2. Acid-suppressing drugs, especially the PPIs, may have serious side effects. With long-term use they increase the risk of bone loss, fractures, and nutritional deficiencies. With any use they increase the risk of pneumonia, food-borne infection, and *Clostridium difficile* colitis, a life-threatening infection of the large intestine.[13]

3. A major study of the effects of PPIs on asthma done in 19 U.S. academic centers and conducted by the American Lung Association found an increase in the frequency of respiratory infections in subjects receiving a PPI, but no improvement in asthma control.[14] I believe that Madeline's recurrent pneumonia was directly linked to her use of PPIs.

4. Three-quarters of the people who use PPIs for longer than a year have undesirable increases in body weight.[15]

The Risk of Suppressing Stomach Acid

There's another important reason why you should not rely on acid-suppressing drugs for treating heartburn: suppressing stomach acid increases the risk of allergy to foods and medications. Here's the research:

- Scientists at the Medical University of Vienna studied 152 adults who received acid-suppressing drugs for three months. These patients had no previous history of food allergy. After taking PPIs, 15 percent of them developed IgE antibodies to foods like milk, wheat, potatoes, celery, carrots, apples, oranges, and rye flour. A third of those still showed food allergic antibodies five months after the drugs were discontinued.[16]

- A study at Emory University in Atlanta found that the use of acid-suppressing medication by children with allergies was associated with a 500 percent increase in levels of IgE antibodies to peanuts and a 70 percent increase in clinically diagnosed food allergy.[17] Laboratory studies confirm that the food allergy induced by acid suppression can produce an anaphylactic skin reaction.[18]

- Hospitalized patients receiving PPIs have four times more allergic reactions to orally administered drugs than similar patients not receiving PPIs.[19] Lack of stomach acid is believed to be the cause.

- The use of acid-suppressing drugs in pregnancy is associated with a 70 percent increased risk of asthma in the child born of that pregnancy.[20]

Why does suppression of stomach acid increase the risk of food allergy? It's largely because a major effect of stomach acid is to initiate the digestion of protein. Digestion reduces the ability of protein to elicit allergic responses by a factor of 10,000! Thus, suppressing stomach acid allows food proteins that reach the small intestine to maintain a much higher than normal degree of allergic potential.[21]

The bottom line: if you suffer from heartburn or have evidence of GERD or LPR, reflux may be aggravating your allergic respiratory symptoms, but you need a strategy other than acid suppression to reverse it. Fortunately, there is one, and I've used it to help many people with chronic GERD or LPR overcome their reliance on PPIs or H2 blockers.

Breaking the Cycle: Controlling GERD Without Drugs

My program for alleviating respiratory allergies that are aggravated by reflux—*without* using acid-suppressing drugs—is based on a clear understanding that GERD is not caused by excess acid. It is caused by a malfunction of the lower esophageal sphincter (LES) valve separating the esophagus from the stomach, which allows stomach contents to flow back into the esophagus, and by poor esophageal motility, which keeps the reflux from being quickly expelled.

The main trigger for GERD is a full, distended stomach. The proper treatment for GERD, then, is not acid suppression but avoidance of stomach distension, improvement of esophageal motility, and tightening of the LES valve.

I explained to Madeline and Brad that controlling her reflux without the use of acid-suppressing drugs was an essential first step in helping her lose weight. I gave them my simple program for controlling GERD without drugs. This program has allowed 90 percent of the patients I've treated to discontinue their use of drugs for heartburn. Here's what it consists of.

The Right Way to Eat

The way you take your meals can make a significant difference in how you experience reflux:

- Eat relatively small meals, stop eating before you are full, and be careful not to overeat. This can prevent distension of your stomach, which is the main trigger for GERD.

- Relax while eating. Make mealtime a quiet time to focus on your food, and chew your food well. This enhances normal esophageal motility.

- Don't lie down within two hours of eating. Give your stomach a chance to empty while gravity is helping prevent reflux.

Alkaline Water

Use alkaline water, with a pH of 8.5 to 9.0, as your main source of drinking water. Alkaline water is available from several natural sources.

Drinking alkaline water is very different from suppressing stomach acid: alkaline water is not strong enough to reverse acidity in your stomach, but it can help to neutralize the acidity of stomach contents outside your stomach, in your throat and esophagus.

Much of the damage done by GERD results from activity of the enzyme pepsin, which requires a highly acidic environment to be active; alkaline water can inactivate pepsin in your throat and esophagus. Note: Do not use liquid or chewable aluminum-containing antacids in an attempt to inactivate pepsin. Aluminum alters immune function in the direction of allergy promotion, and aluminum-containing antacids may be as bad for your allergies as PPIs.[22]

Calcium Citrate Powder

Calcium citrate powder, about 150 mg, dissolved in a small amount of alkaline water, may be taken after each meal and at bedtime. Calcium citrate powder is readily available from several sources.

Calcium is required for normal esophageal motility and for closing of the LES. When your esophagus is healthy, there is enough calcium stored inside the cells of the esophagus to properly regulate motility. Laboratory studies have shown, however, that when the esophagus is inflamed, esophageal motility becomes dependent upon external sources of calcium. Calcium supplements can help improve esophageal motility and reduce or prevent GERD.

Most people misunderstand the role of calcium in preventing GERD. They think of calcium as an antacid. Calcium aids in the prevention of reflux through two mechanisms that have nothing to do with neutralizing stomach acid. It speeds up esophageal motility, moving whatever has refluxed into the esophagus back into the stomach, and it can also tighten the lower esophageal sphincter (LES). In my clinical experience, I have found that calcium citrate, which is a mildly acidic form of calcium, works better than calcium carbonate. The reason: calcium citrate is more soluble than calcium carbonate, so the calcium gets into the cells of the esophagus faster.

Here's a key point: calcium tablets do not work for this purpose. The calcium must be chewed or swallowed as a powder or liquid, because it must be available in solution in the lower esophagus and upper stomach. There, unlike acid-lowering drugs, it prevents reflux without decreasing stomach acid.[23]

Power Wash

Follow the Power Wash and Re-entry program to help you determine which of the foods you're eating may contribute to heartburn, sore throat, stuffed nose, cough, wheezing, or weight gain. Once you've gone through Power Wash, these foods usually show their effects pretty quickly. Avoiding them can greatly relieve symptoms of GERD or LPR.

Note: if you have been using a PPI or H2 blocker for several weeks or longer, it may be inadvisable for you to stop the medication suddenly, because long-term use of acid-lowering drugs can lead to a condition known as acid rebound. When the secretion of stomach acid is turned off through a drug's action, your stomach responds by increasing the number of acid-producing cells. Then, when you stop the drug, you will have true hyperacidity. Most people do better if they taper down the drug dose gradually. Ask your doctor how to do this.

Because these drugs may affect the way your body responds to other drugs you are taking, always ask your doctor's advice before changing them or stopping them.

Food Allergies and Heartburn

So far, you've learned that GERD can aggravate the symptoms of respiratory allergy, worsening asthma and sinusitis, and that acid-suppressing drugs, which are the standard treatment for heartburn, can make your allergies worse.

Here's the third part of the heartburn/allergy cycle: *food allergies can be the cause of heartburn.*

The name of this condition is eosinophilic esophagitis (EoE). You'll remember from Chapter 3 that eosinophils (Eos) are allergy effector cells. When there's an allergic reaction, Eos are activated to cause inflammation of tissues. They play a major role in the permanent lung damage that occurs with chronic asthma.

Invasion of the esophagus by Eos was first described more than 30 years ago; initially it was thought to be a rare disorder producing chest pain and difficulty swallowing. During the past 20 years, EoE has received increasing attention. It may affect as many as 150,000 people in the United States. Extensive research has made it clear that EoE is caused by food allergy and that eliminating the food triggers can produce complete, sustained remission of this disease in many people who suffer from it.[24]

About 90 percent of adults with EoE respond well to a six-food elimination diet, avoiding cow's milk, soy, wheat, egg, peanuts/tree nuts, and seafood. About 40 percent of people with EoE are allergic to the yeast *Candida albicans*, which can colonize the mouth and esophagus.[25] Reduction of *Candida* levels requires a low-sugar diet, so you don't feed the yeast the sugar it thrives on.

The healing of EoE is a slow process that takes several months. If you have received a diagnosis of EoE, you should modify the Re-entry process after you do the Power Wash. You should delay reintroducing the six food groups mentioned above for several months and consult your doctor about being retested for esophagitis before returning them to your diet.

Madeline's Weight-Loss Solution

Using my program for controlling GERD without drugs, Madeline was able to discontinue her use of heartburn medication fairly quickly. She'd been on acid suppressors for so long that I had her taper down the dose according to a schedule I devised, rather than abruptly stop. Then she followed the Power Wash and Re-entry protocols.

She lost five pounds during the Power Wash and five more pounds during the first ten days of Re-entry. When she challenged herself with tofu and whole soybeans (edamame) during the second week of Re-entry, she gained four pounds in 24 hours and experienced heartburn and nasal congestion.

For Madeline, the main problem food was soy, a food she'd greatly increased in her diet since becoming a vegetarian. Once she fully removed soy from her diet, she was able to lose weight normally by following the Immune Balance Diet and staying mindful of portion size.

I've seen this pattern over and over again among people unable to lose weight despite a healthy, calorie-controlled diet. There's a specific staple food that needs to be eliminated, because the allergic reaction it provokes interferes with weight loss. People who are overweight because of food allergies usually lose several pounds during the Power Wash, just as Madeline did. Much of what they lose initially is not fat. It's allergic bloating and swelling. If this is your problem, you'll find that you look as if you've lost even more weight than you actually have, and your friends will comment on how good you look even before you've shed many pounds. The reason: before you lose actual fat, you shed that allergic bloat that makes you look and feel swollen.

Foods That Can Prevent Weight Loss

The foods most likely to prevent weight loss because of allergy are:

- Wheat and products made from wheat. Remember that white flour is just refined wheat flour. Wheat is the main ingredient in most breads, crackers, pastries, pasta, and noodles. It's also used to thicken sauces, soups, jams, and jellies.

- Milk and milk products, which include cheese, yogurt, cream, ice cream, and butter. Milk solids or milk proteins like casein or whey are often added to prepared foods, so check ingredient lists to be sure you're avoiding milk products in all forms.

- Yeast, which is added to breads and other baked goods as well as to beer and commercial soups and sauces. It also occurs naturally on the surfaces of many fruits and vegetables. Vinegar, wine, sauerkraut, and other fermented foods often contain yeast proteins. So do dried fruits and commercial fruit juices and ciders.

- Soy, which is often added to foods as soy protein or soybean oil or lecithin. Soy as an ingredient is often listed under an alias, such as textured or hydrolyzed vegetable protein, vegetable oil, or mono- and diglycerides. Soy may be a hidden ingredient in foods such as sausage, doughnuts, and bouillon cubes.[26] It's used in many canned foods, fast foods, baked goods, luncheon meats, ice creams, and chocolates.

- Corn, which is widely distributed in our food supply as corn syrup, cornstarch, corn sweetener, and corn oil or hidden under an alias as dextrose or maltodextrin. When xanthan gum, acetic acid, ethyl acetate, ascorbic acid (vitamin C), or vanilla extract appears on a food label, corn was probably the source from which it was made. Corn is the foundation of U.S. agribusiness.

The Science of Weight-Loss Nutrition

I tailored the Immune Balance Diet to boost adiponectin, the anti-allergic hormone that increases when you lose weight. Scientific studies have shown that specific foods or food components can increase production of adiponectin by fat cells in a direct fashion, independent of body weight. These include:

- Oolong tea. Scientists in Japan gave four cups of oolong tea a day to overweight diabetics. After 30 days, the group receiving oolong tea showed a significant increase in blood levels of adiponectin. The control group, given water, showed no change.[27] In another study, Chinese scientists gave four cups of oolong tea a day to overweight men and women for six weeks and found significant reductions in body weight and waist size, despite no change in diet.[28]

- Fisetin, found in strawberries (an ingredient of the Immune Balance Smoothie). Laboratory research shows that fisetin stimulates the production of adiponectin.[29] Fisetin has also been shown to prevent obesity in mice fed a high-fat diet.[30]

- Apigenin, found in parsley. In most recipes, parsley is just a garnish. That has always seemed like a real waste of parsley's potential! It's not only a delicious herb, it's packed with nutrients, including the fabulous flavonoid apigenin. So I packed the Immune Balance Soup with loads of parsley. When your fat cells are subjected to the stress of inflammation, their production of adiponectin drops dramatically. Apigenin can prevent that decline.[31] Higher intake of apigenin among women in particular is associated with higher blood levels of adiponectin.[32]

Adiponectin is such an important anti-inflammatory hormone that several studies in humans have looked at dietary influences on adiponectin levels, independent of body weight. The science tells us the foods consistently associated with higher adiponectin levels are nuts, seeds, and berries.[33] That's one reason I encourage their inclusion in the Immune Balance Diet.

As we have seen, allergies to foods you eat every day may interfere with attempts at weight loss. Madeline's case showed us how controlling your allergies through careful analysis of foods that you may be allergic to can help you shed the pounds that you've been unable to lose from diet alone and overcome the food-craving/food addiction cycle that is so closely linked to hidden food allergies.

If you pay attention to fluctuations in body weight and feelings like swelling and bloating when you go through Power Wash and Re-entry, you should be able to determine whether the allergy-weight connection applies to you. You can then identify and eliminate the foods that are keeping you from losing weight. You'll probably notice other benefits from avoiding those foods too, including improvement in energy and mental clarity.

Advanced Strategies for Controlling Heartburn without Drugs

If your weight problem is associated with heartburn, GERD, or LPR, don't fall into the routine of taking drugs that suppress stomach acid every day to control symptoms. Those drugs can increase the severity of your allergies and contribute to weight gain. If you require more than the simple steps I've outlined in this chapter to overcome your reliance on acid-suppressing drugs, advanced strategies may be called for. Consult your doctor about taking one or more of the steps below.

- Take digestive enzymes, in pill or powder form, with each meal to decrease distension of the stomach.

- Try melatonin, especially if you suffer from nocturnal reflux or cough. Most people think of melatonin as a sleep aid, but melatonin has two other important effects. It is the only product, aside from calcium, that directly tightens the LES. The dose needed is 3 to 6 mg, which should be taken at bedtime.[34] Second, melatonin shifts immune function in a direction that opposes allergy. Caution: some people cannot take melatonin because they feel hung over the next day. This sensitivity does not improve with time, so if you feel drugged by melatonin, stop right away.

- Reduce your intake of sugar and starch. People who have used acid-lowering drugs for an extended period of time are susceptible to bacterial or yeast overgrowth in the stomach. These microbes readily ferment dietary starches and sugars, producing gases that can distend your stomach. Stomach distension, as I said before, is often the main trigger for GERD. If your symptoms improve when you eliminate dietary sources of starch and sugar, you may have developed bacterial or yeast overgrowth caused by lack of stomach acid. Discuss this possibility with your doctor.

- Ask your doctor to check you for celiac disease. Celiac disease is a common genetic disorder in which symptoms are triggered by eating gluten, a protein found in wheat, oats, and barley. For people with celiac disease, a gluten-free diet can help alleviate GERD. Ask your doctor for a blood test.

Conclusion

In this chapter I revealed the powerful science that connects allergies and your weight. I explained how allergic reactions contribute to inflammation and the growth of fat cells and discussed the vicious cycle in which weight gain increases allergies and allergy increases body weight. I also looked at the relationship between esophageal reflux, allergies, and weight gain and discussed the research on how drugs for heartburn can increase allergic reactivity.

We met Madeline, a mother of two who had pollen allergy and heartburn and was struggling to lose the 50 pounds she had gained since her pregnancies; I taught her how to control her heartburn without relying on the acid-suppressing drugs that can make allergies worse. I explored how food allergies can prevent weight loss and looked at exciting nutrition science that shows how oolong tea, strawberries, and parsley can help with weight loss.

Since evaluations concerning health care and medications need to be made with a health care professional, bring this chapter with you next time you see your doctor, and work together with him or her on every aspect of your health.

CHAPTER 10

MIND-BODY HEALING

Laura had suffered from food allergies her entire life. If she deviated from a restricted diet, she would feel the consequences: abdominal pain, diarrhea, and headaches. Eating out at restaurants was especially hard on her, because there would often be some hidden ingredient in a meal that would make her sick. She had read my book *Superimmunity for Kids* during her first pregnancy and had applied its concepts to feeding her family over the next two decades.

"I know exactly what I'm supposed to do," she told me. "But I just don't have the time."

Between raising a family and managing a retail business, Laura had little time for taking care of herself. Once her kids were out of the house, her father became ill and moved in with her. Like so many women, she'd gone from caring for her children to caring for a parent. "Maybe I just need a pep talk," she said.

I considered Laura's lifestyle—a never-ending cycle of responsibilities, spinning at a hectic pace. I'd been there myself; I'm sure you've been there, too. When life's responsibilities become overwhelming, laying down more rules to follow is not the solution. We needed a different approach. If Laura couldn't stick to a diet that would improve her health and daily quality of life, if she couldn't regulate what was going into her body despite everything she'd learned and even put into practice for her family, we needed to tackle the problem closer to its inception—not in a physical way, but in a mental one.

The Stress-Allergy Connection

Much like the evil mastermind in a James Bond film, stress may be found at the heart of many illnesses and physical ailments. Allergic symptoms are no exception. The association between stress and allergies reaches back to the the dawn of Western medicine in ancient Greece. Asthma was referred to as "asthma nervosa" in early medical texts, and 2,500 years ago Hippocrates theorized a link between an angry mind and shortness of breath.

Medical research continues to explore the stress-allergy connection. A study done at Ohio State University revealed that in allergy sufferers the frequency of allergy flare-ups is directly linked to the persistence of mental stress and that less stress can lead to fewer flare-ups.[1] Some people in the study reported allergy flares within days of increased stress. The research suggests a disturbing snowball effect: symptoms such as sneezing, runny nose, and watery eyes can add stress to sufferers and, for some, may even become the main cause of stress. While alleviating stress may not reverse allergies, it can help decrease episodes of intense symptoms.

The Ohio State researchers also demonstrated that psychological stress and mood can directly impact allergic reactivity. They did skin tests on people with nasal allergies before and after having the subjects perform mental arithmetic in front of a small audience. Greater anxiety increased the size of the itchy red wheal that formed in response to the skin test. This increase in allergic reactivity persisted for more than 24 hours, and it did not occur in people who were not given the stressful task but just sat in the same room.[2]

In an article from the University of Mississippi Medical Center, researchers reviewed numerous studies on stress and allergy and summarized the data, finding that stress was linked to:

- The development of asthma
- An increased rate of admissions to the hospital for asthma
- A higher rate of allergic reactions on skin tests[3]

The Mississippi scientists recommended stress reduction coupled with training to improve coping skills in the face of adverse situations. They noted that psychological interventions such as expressive writing and relaxation therapy had been found helpful in improving asthma. They also noted that psychotherapy reduced emergency room visits and asthma exacerbations for patients who were depressed.

A study of university students from Finland concluded that stressful events such as personal conflict or the illness of a family member increased the risk of developing asthma and allergic rhinoconjunctivitis.[4]

Mind over Allergies

Stress not only provokes allergy symptoms, it is also a well-documented factor in promoting inflammation. The confluence of stress and inflammation led scientists from the University of Wisconsin to state: "Psychological stress is a major provocative factor of symptoms in chronic inflammatory conditions."[5] The role of inflammation in asthma (described in Chapter 12) makes stress management an important modality of treatment for people with asthma.

The Wisconsin researchers compared an eight-week meditation course with another healthy-practices intervention to see how each modality might reduce stress and thereby inflammation. The healthy-practices intervention, called the Health Enhancement Program, consisted of exercise such as walking; strength, balance, and agility training; education in nutrition; and music therapy.

The meditation program was mindfulness-based stress reduction, developed at the Center for Mindfulness at the University of

Massachusetts Medical Center. Considered the primary form of meditation in health care settings, mindfulness-based meditation seeks to cultivate an awareness of the present moment through focused attention on the body and mind while sitting, walking, or practicing forms of movement such as yoga.

In the Wisconsin study, the participants were given a stress test that consisted of public speaking for five minutes followed by five minutes of mental arithmetic. Both the meditation and the healthy-practices program helped their participants cope better with the mental stress of the test. Mindfulness-based stress reduction, however, also produced a decrease in inflammation that was not seen with the healthy-practices program. The researchers noted that the ability of meditation to reduce inflammation might make it particularly helpful as a therapeutic tool for inflammatory conditions.

Doing Less Helps You Do More

One of the great paradoxes of our shared experience on this earth is that *not doing* can actually make you more productive. I'm talking about creating stillness, which is not to be confused with mindless inactivity. This truth has not only been grasped by all religions of the world, it has been studied by modern scientists as well. Medical research has proved that just a few hours of training in meditation can increase the efficiency of connections in your brain and enhance your ability to focus your thoughts.[6]

The regular practice of meditation increases the efficiency with which you make decisions, improves the depth and speed with which you process new information, and helps you preserve brain function as you age.[7]

I described the benefits of "creating stillness" to Laura and told her about a study done at Duke University a few years ago in which researchers developed a workplace stress reduction program consisting of meditation or yoga for highly stressed employees. Both relaxation techniques lowered the participants' mental distress and improved the quality of their sleep.[8]

I recommended that Laura take some time each day for meditation, yoga, or focused relaxation, because finding stillness on a daily basis would help her manage a busy schedule with less pressure and greater efficiency. In this way, she would soon find the time and energy to manage her dietary needs with less effort. I gave her several simple methods that I describe later in this chapter. There's no evidence that one technique is superior to another. Choose those that are most appealing to you. It's the method you actually use that will help you the most.

Mental Stillness Leads to Mental Toughness

At a glance, the advice I gave Laura that day seems simple enough: find time for meditation and focused relaxation. But if you try this and find that it's not as easy as it first appears, that's okay. It's the repetition of trying it that's important. If you can't find ten minutes a day to meditate or relax in some way, do it for five. If five minutes is too long, try doing it for two. Once the practice is part of your life, you'll be able to bring your mind to a place of deep relaxation in under 30 seconds, so that you're never very far from stillness, no matter how busy you are.

This practice is also a way to develop the quality that often sets top athletes apart from others—the factor that puts one on the podium with a medal or gets another one the big trophy. This quality is known as mental toughness. It's what gives athletes the ability to withstand the tremendous pressure of competition and do their best when it matters. It's the result of cultivating calm and focus and practicing how to maintain it on a daily basis.

If you're like my patient Laura, seeking balance and calm in order to maintain a healthy lifestyle amid the storm of modern life, you're an Olympic athlete in your own right. The principle of creating stillness, and in the process developing mental toughness, in order to work more efficiently and with a greater capacity is not only reserved for events like the World Cup. Each day of juggling our responsibilities in the workplace and at home can feel like a tennis championship, and we must remember to calm our minds for the sake of our overall health.

Calming the Mind Heals the Body

Before Laura left my office, I told her that there could be another, deeper benefit of creating stillness: it was likely to reduce the severity of her symptoms, essentially making her less allergic. I told her about one study in which a single 20-minute meditation was able to significantly reduce pain in people suffering from migraine headaches, and another demonstrating that regular meditation and focused relaxation could decrease abdominal pain and diarrhea in people with irritable bowel syndrome.[9]

There are other examples. Progressive muscle relaxation (described on the next page) decreases the amount of itching experienced by people with eczema, improving their sleep quality.[10] Progressive muscle relaxation also decreases asthmatic symptoms in pregnant women and teenage girls.[11] Both yoga and meditation have been found to improve quality of life in asthmatics.[12]

In particular, meditation with visualization was shown to improve lung function as well as respiratory symptoms in a group of people with asthma.[13] A study of subjects with migraine headaches and abdominal pain done at Case Western Reserve University in Cleveland found that focused meditation and visualization not only reduced pain but also reduced laboratory signs of allergic inflammation.[14]

Getting Started with Meditation

You don't need to sit quietly to meditate, and I'll describe some types of moving meditation and active relaxation later in this chapter. However, sitting quietly is a good way to start. Find a quiet place and a comfortable spot to sit, perhaps sitting up in bed or on your sofa. Before you start, turn off the TV, the radio, and your phone and enjoy the stillness.

Head-to-Toe Relaxation

Let your arms rest gently by your side. Close your eyes. Become aware of your breath, just noticing how you are breathing, not changing anything. You may find your belly rising as you breathe in and falling as you breathe out. That's good—you have just achieved a level of awareness of your body.

Let your attention drift down to your toes. See how your toes feel, just becoming aware of your toes. Flex your toes, and then let them relax. Wiggle your toes around. Let your toes enjoy their freedom.

Now bring your focus to the bottoms of your feet. Perhaps your feet feel tight or tired. Gently flex your feet, curling your toes toward your heels a little bit, and then let go. Let the tension go out of your feet and feel your body relax. Perhaps you let out a little sigh as you do this, which is perfectly all right. You may want to take a moment to appreciate your feet for all the effort they make to support your whole body throughout the day.

Next, let your awareness come to your ankles. Gently pull your toes up until you feel a slight flex, then release them, letting your ankles and shins relax. From there, let your focus turn to the backs of your legs, to your calf muscles. Point your toes as you would when doing toe raises, and feel the muscles in your calves contract. Let go and feel the heaviness of the calf muscles as they relax.

Now move up to your thighs, among the most powerful muscles in your body. Without moving your legs, simply squeeze your quadriceps and feel the muscles bulge a little bit, then let them go. You may feel a slight sensation of warmth coming into your legs from the contracting.

Now feel the backs of your legs, from the hamstrings up to the buttocks. Squeeze this area and then let it go, letting it relax and soften.

Coming back around to the front of your body, notice your belly. Ever so gently flex your stomach muscles, then let them go. Continuing on up, flex your chest muscles by squeezing your elbows into your sides gently, then release.

Now flex your biceps in the classic "make a muscle" pose, then let go. Feel your arms relax. Gently draw your fingers in to make a fist, then let them go. Give your shoulders a little shake and let your arms and your hands hang loose.

Your face is waiting to let go of tension as well. Gently scrunch your face up for a moment, then let go. You might feel your entire head relax.

Now notice how your whole body feels, from your head down to your toes. Feel the stillness, the quiet, the calm. Relax and enjoy the moment. Remember this feeling throughout the day, and return to it in your mind when you feel like you need to de-stress.

Detox Your Thoughts Meditation

Do you ever feel like your thoughts are going around and around in your head? Maybe you feel irritated by some of the thoughts that go through your mind. Maybe you feel they're distracting you from focusing on something more important. Cutting through that static, turning down the noise, is one of the main goals of meditation.

So here is a short practice to help you detoxify those troubling thoughts and gain greater peace of mind right away. I have used this method many times, and I've found that it can provide a unique sense of calm in a very short amount of time.

Sit in a comfortable place, much as you would for the Head-to-Toe Relaxation described above. Imagine that a hand is resting on your forehead. It is there to give comfort to your mind, to soothe your thoughts. Give this imaginary hand the ability to absorb any irritating thoughts. Let those thoughts float out of your mind into the hand. Notice the unique sense of spaciousness and calm that you can have without those extra thoughts.

Now imagine that the hand is cradling the back of your head, just above your neck. Again let your thoughts get absorbed by the hand, and let your mind become still.

You might be wondering what you will do with all the extra brainpower you can access with meditation. The answer is: plenty. All the positive steps you want to take for your health and your life require a lot of focus and energy, and that is exactly what meditation can give you.

Yoga-Based Meditation for Asthma

There are many types of yoga. Some seem more like a competitive sport than personal meditation. Strenuous yoga seems to be the fashion at certain gyms: either poses held forever that put agility and strength to the test, or the instructor running through a series of difficult maneuvers while making it all look easy. But the type of practice I want to talk about now is about quieting the mind, which lies at the heart of yoga.

Indian researchers wanted to find out if a type of meditative yoga called Sahaja yoga could help improve symptoms and lung function in people with asthma. They recruited people for the study from newspaper ads, primary care practitioners, and asthma clinics. All participants were 18 or over and had suffered from mild to moderate asthma for at least six months. They formed two groups, one that received the Sahaja yoga intervention for two weeks and a control group that received conventional medical treatment.

The Sahaja yoga group was counseled in achieving mental stillness through the use of silent affirmations of health and well-being. They also viewed instructional videos and had the opportunity to discuss any issues with the instructor. In addition, this group was encouraged to practice at home for 10 to 20 minutes each day to achieve a state of mental tranquility. The meditation was done while sitting.

The group receiving yoga training showed a progressive improvement in lung function that was first measured at two weeks and continued for another six weeks after the instruction was completed. Both groups showed an improvement in asthma-related quality of life and a decreased use of medication, but the benefits were more pronounced and occurred faster in the group practicing yoga.

The study highlights the benefits of mind-body relaxation techniques and yoga meditation as a complementary approach to asthma. What made the yoga meditation helpful in the study? As one potential explanation, the authors point to how meditation seeks to create a positive or benevolent view of the self and others. They emphasize that both mind-body relaxation and yoga should be considered as an addition to conventional drug therapy, not as a replacement.[15]

Relax Your Mind by Moving Your Body and Feeding Your Spirit

There are times when I am not inclined to sit still for meditation, when I need to move to shake off the stress. Many kinds of movement can be stress releasing, particularly those that help you clear your mind, enjoy deep breathing, or even enter profound silence, be it walking, yoga, or tai chi. These practices encourage you to focus entirely on body and breath and allow the mind's chatter to subside. For those of you who prefer more physical ways to de-stress, here are a few ideas to help you chill out.

Walk Your Stress Away

Sometimes when you are feeling stressed, just getting the body moving—even taking a leisurely stroll for as little as five minutes—can help you burn off that stress right away. It makes perfect sense, when you think about the connection between the mind and the body, that releasing pent-up physical tension can lead to a new state of peacefulness. If you're feeling stressed by a problem at work, getting away from that problem for a few minutes can be an effective way to de-stress and maybe even find a new way to a solution. You can consider the rhythmic swinging of your arms and the repetitive motion of putting one foot in front of the other as a form of meditation that can reconnect you with your body and refresh your mind.

Get Back to Nature

We are all profoundly linked to our natural environment, so reconnecting with nature from time to time can bring us back to our roots. According to a review article from the University of Illinois, our contact with natural environments has many benefits for our physical and mental health. Nature can help reduce stress and relieve sadness and depression. Access to nature is also linked to enhanced brainpower, more self-discipline, and improved mental health.

And getting in touch with nature can improve functioning of the immune system, enable greater physical fitness, and help diabetics better control blood glucose levels.[16] The Illinois researchers point out that the experience of nature can range from being in a forest to enjoying an urban park to looking out the window at a view of nature. Any contact with nature is preferable to no contact with nature.

Take a Relaxing Mineral Bath

Stress can reduce our levels of magnesium.[17] In Chapter 13 I explain some consequences of magnesium depletion and suggest excellent dietary sources of this essential mineral. Here's another way to overcome the magnesium-depleting effects of stress. Set aside a half hour for a hot bath. Get out a fluffy towel and a favorite bathrobe. The only other thing you will need is a box of Epsom salts, which are composed of magnesium sulfate. Pour 380g of Epsom salts into the tub while you are running the bathwater.

The magnesium in Epsom salts is a natural muscle relaxant that can help you unwind as you soak. In a study from the University of Birmingham in Great Britain, people who soaked in an Epsom salts bath 12 minutes each day for seven days raised their magnesium levels measurably.[18] Giving yourself a wonderful treat like this might be just what you need to shift gears from "doing" to "being." With your cares and worries floating away in the water, you could emerge from the bath feeling relaxed and reinvigorated.

Bathe Your Feet

If you don't have time for a soothing bath, try soaking your feet for about five minutes in a tub or basin of warm water. Find a comfortable sitting or reclining posture, immerse your feet, and close your eyes. If it's a hot day, you might prefer to soak in cool or room-temperature water, which will help bring down your body temperature. For maximum benefit, breathe slowly and focus entirely on your breath and your bodily sensations, letting go of all your chores and obligations.

Music to Your Ears

Listening to beautiful music is one of life's great pleasures. When you are immersed in the music you love, you are easily carried away by the emotions that the music induces, and you let your worries float away. Music is a great source of inspiration that can help us gather our strength and rouse us to action. It can also help us relax and find inner peace.

A team of researchers from the United States, Canada, and France have noted that listening to music can influence people to be happier and more positive. Even more important, in their study they demonstrated that relaxing music can reduce levels of the stress hormone cortisol, which may account for the stress-reducing effect of music.[19]

For relaxation purposes, I like classical music. It could even be chanting, or the sounds of nature, such as birds chirping, waves breaking, or the patter of raindrops. The important thing is that you select something that you find truly, deeply relaxing. As a relaxation exercise, lie down on your bed or a comfortable sofa and play the music at a low to medium volume. Let your mind drift away on the sounds, almost as if they were the sweet murmurs of your loved ones or a lullaby caressing your soul. Immerse yourself in the beauty of the music. Follow your imagination and let the enchanting tune take you to a faraway place. Like meditation, this can bring you to a state of peace and deep relaxation.

Dance Your Ills Away

Music and dance have been a source of joy and expression from the earliest moments of our existence. We've used dance for celebration, entertainment, communication, and expressing spiritual rapture. The rhythm of dance can lighten the burden of work. Dance may be personal or communal, but it always transforms experience.

Modern researchers have demonstrated the benefits of dance therapy for fibromyalgia, depression, high blood pressure, heart failure, cancer-related fatigue and quality of life, Parkinson's disease, rheumatoid arthritis, and asthma.[20]

Dance improves balance, mood, and fitness in people of all ages. When researchers at New York's Albert Einstein College of Medicine followed 469 healthy elderly adults for five years, they found that those who danced socially enjoyed a 76 percent decrease in the risk of developing cognitive impairment.[21]

Dance to music you love as often as you can. Neither the type of dance nor the type of music matters. The pleasure you derive from dance is all that counts. In her delightful book *Goddesses Never Age,* Dr. Christiane Northrup recounts the exhilaration she felt dancing the tango in Buenos Aires. She describes it as an epic event that truly spoke to her soul. With profound insight, she explains, "Movement that is in tune with our core being is movement that is sustainable—and it's the type of 'exercise' we all need."[22]

Reconnect with People

So many people are spending so much time staring at little screens . . . and big screens . . . that it seems there just isn't time to talk to other people. But this dependence on technology can end up isolating us. You have heard it said that humans are social animals. Connecting with others is a deep part of who we are.

Scientists reason that over our years of evolution, being part of a group that worked together increased our chances of survival.[23] Today medical research tells us that loneliness is linked to poor health, impaired immunity, more chronic diseases, increased inflammation, and *lower* odds of survival.

Relationships are so important that I named them the first Pillar of Healing in my book *Power Healing.* A sense of community, of belonging, can help buffer the effects of stress and contribute to our overall health. So find ways to reconnect with people you care about, and see how doing so supports your well-being.

A study from Carnegie Mellon University and the University of California looked at the impact of an eight-week meditation course on the link between loneliness and inflammation in senior citizens. They were particularly interested in finding out how participating in group instruction in Mindfulness-Based Stress Reduction (MBSR) would affect perceptions of loneliness and the raised levels of inflammation that often accompany loneliness.

At baseline, before training in MBSR, the seniors had elevated levels of C-reactive protein (CRP) in their blood. CRP is so strongly linked to adverse health outcomes that it has become the most commonly used marker of inflammation in clinical trials. A critical gene involved in producing inflammation was also found to be more active, or up-regulated.[24]

The training in MBSR consisted of a two-hour group session each week, a daylong retreat in the sixth or seventh week, and 30 minutes a day of home mindfulness practice. The control group was studied while on a waiting list to receive the MBSR training, which they did after the end of the trial. At the end of eight weeks, the participants who had done the training were understandably less lonely, while those on the waiting list felt more lonely. MBSR produced a reduction in upregulation of the pro-inflammatory gene and tended to reduce CRP.

What is most significant about this study is that participation in a meditation group decreased systemic inflammation at its roots by decreasing the activity of a gene that promotes inflammation. Although you cannot change your genes, you *can* change what your genes do.

Flex Your Green Thumb

If you have a patch of vegetables or flowers in your own back-yard, just looking at them can fill your heart with pleasure. Notice how plants grow, mature, and wither. This is the cycle of life. Rudolf Steiner, the Austrian mystic and philosopher, believed that understanding this cycle was the first step in spiritual enlightenment. Raking the soil from time to time, harvesting the veggies for your kitchen or simply standing quietly with a hose can be terrifically therapeutic. Even five minutes spent gardening can relax your mind and refresh your spirit.

If you don't have a yard, try growing herbs indoors. Italian parsley is my favorite. It's easy to grow in pots, thrives in window light, and doesn't need much water. The leaves are joyfully green and great to chew with a wonderful, fresh aroma. They're a key ingredient in the Immune Balance Soup.

Enjoy Creative Time in the Kitchen

For many people, the quiet, peaceful act of working with food can be a meditative experience—rinsing veggies, choosing ingredients for a beautiful salad, carefully arranging fruits and vegetables on a plate—can bring immense joy. When everything is done and food brought to the table, just seeing your friends or loved ones enjoy the food you've created can be therapeutic and relaxing, releasing the stress from a day's work.

Morning Coffee Meditation

For those of you who cherish that glorious first cup of coffee in the morning, I have some very good news. I propose a meditation that blends perfectly with your routine. While these two might not seem to go together, a closer look reveals that both coffee and meditation can help you to sit quietly, fill your senses, and contemplate nature. In this way they complement each other surprisingly well.

As you'll see, this practice works best with organic coffee, decaf or regular, from small farms or plantations. The magic starts right when you begin to brew the coffee, when that amazing aroma wafts up into the air, signaling that your day has begun. Warm your mug by pouring a touch of hot water into it, waiting a moment, then pouring it out. Slowly fill your mug with freshly brewed coffee, then bring it with you as you settle into your favorite seat. Cup the mug in your hands and feel the warmth, taking a moment to savor the aroma again. Wait with expectation as it cools off enough to drink, then enjoy that first sip with deep appreciation.

Carefully holding on to the mug so you don't spill en route, let your mind travel to lush, green, subtropical coffee-growing mountains. Picture in your mind's eye row upon row of green-leafed coffee bushes, adorned with bright red coffee beans. This is farm country, timeless, with just a couple of traditional clay-roofed farmhouses and a dirt road.

Now picture the gently sloping sides of a majestic mountain rising in the distance. As you breathe in, imagine that you can embody the mountain, absorbing its strength and solid mass. The mountain helps you feel grounded to the earth, and it is an image you can carry with you throughout the day.

As you sip your coffee, take a moment to appreciate the organic farmers who tended the coffee plants with care and the roasters who skillfully brought out the flavor of the beans. Allow yourself to feel content that you are supporting organic farming, helping to protect the farms and the farmers. As you continue to drink your coffee, take satisfaction from connecting with the people who create it and the places where it originates, right down to the fertile soil.

As your thoughts return to where you are, you may find that the inviting aroma of coffee has spread throughout the house. If there are other people around, you may have a moment to connect with them over coffee and spread the feeling of contentment from your meditation. If you work at home, this meditation is a nice way to feel a sense of connection with the outside world right from the start of your day.

What if you don't make coffee at home, but grab a coffee on the way to work instead? Even if you are in a rush, you can still do this meditation on the train, bus, or subway, making sure to keep a good grip on your coffee container. Notice how you feel at the end of your journey, maybe a little more calm and relaxed.

Sleep Your Stress Away

Sleep is essential to our well-being. Nothing helps us to beat stress and restore our energy more than a good night's sleep. Our natural immune system counts on sufficient hours of sleep to shore up our defense against any physical or mental threat.

There is scientific evidence on the interaction between chronic stress and sleep problems. The American Academy of Sleep Medicine found that people with chronic stress report shorter sleep duration, worse sleep quality, and more daytime functioning impairments. This is also true the other way around: the study indicates that poor sleep may be a cause of stress. And people who report more fatigue and less total sleep are more likely to report more stress. The simplest, and likely best, advice given by the researchers for individuals with high stress and poor sleep is to look at some of the lifestyle choices they are making and ensure that sufficient sleep is at the core of those choices.[25]

Sleep is a healing process, an active time when your body melts away the stresses of the day and restores itself, preparing you to face new challenges. Sleep deprivation in animal experiments has been found to increase susceptibility to viral and bacterial infection. In humans, insomnia reduces natural killer cell activity. Healthy young men awakened from sleep between 3 and 7 A.M. show a 30 percent dip in natural killer cell activity the next morning.

Sleep is a key health marker, too. A National Sleep Foundation survey revealed that stress and poor health are linked to less sleep and disrupted sleep. Those who report they are in very good or excellent health sleep 18 to 23 minutes more than those who say their health is not as good. If you take control of your sleep with a positive approach, you are on your way to less stress and better health.

The natural sleep requirement for adults varies from six to ten hours per day, with most people needing seven to nine hours, preferably without interruption. Daytime relaxation is also crucial. Quiet meditation each day may lower blood pressure, relieve anxiety, improve nighttime sleep, and reduce the discomfort of chronic headache and other painful conditions.

However, environmental factors such as noise, light, temperature, and the mattress you lie on can make it more difficult for you to get a good night's sleep, so you need to take care of your bedroom environment, too.

Here are some healthy tips to help you sleep better:

- Get some exercise during your day. It could be your regular fitness routine or a half-hour walk.

- Avoid caffeinated tea and coffee in the evening. Also avoid alcohol in the evening. All of these can disrupt your sleep. Eat light for dinner. Try not to eat less than two or three hours before bedtime. Never smoke.

- Choose a comfortable mattress and pillows. If your bedding is inviting and relaxing, it can have a wonderfully restful effect on you. Also, of course, make sure your bedroom is free of dust and other allergens.

- Keep your bedroom at the right temperature. It should be cool—between 60 and 67 degrees.

- Enjoy a relaxing bedtime ritual. It could be drinking a warm cup of chamomile tea, placing lavender close to your bed, or using calming lavender oil as aromatherapy.

- Wind yourself down to a calming mode about an hour before bedtime. You may read a book, but avoid television and other screens such as computers and smartphones, as these can affect the quality of your sleep. Exposure to light during the evening and early nighttime hours suppresses release of the sleep-facilitating hormone melatonin and shifts the circadian clock, making it harder to fall asleep at bedtime.

- Have two glasses of tart cherry juice a day as a sleep aid. Researchers from England's Northumbria University discovered that cherry juice gives adults longer sleep time on average, reduces daytime napping, and increases overall sleep efficiency. The secret is in the melatonin content of cherries—a powerful antioxidant critical for sleep-wake cycle regulation.[26]

According to the Centers for Disease Control and Prevention, about one-third of all Americans suffer from sleep disturbances. If you improve your sleep, you can reduce your stress level and make a big difference in your quality of life—including your symptoms of allergy.

Conclusion

In this chapter, we looked inward to see how our inner lives and our responses to stress could reflect on our well-being. We brought to light important medical research that is unraveling the secrets of how stress, inflammation, and allergy are intertwined.

You met Laura, a working mom with food allergies, stomach-aches, digestive trouble, and headaches who was unable to stick to her diet while overwhelmed with stress and responsibilities. I recommended she try meditation or other relaxation methods. She enrolled in a beginning yoga class and found she really enjoyed it; it was a positive step that gave her a sense of stillness and at the same time energy and focus. We were able to build on that so she was able to eat the way she'd always wanted. Her headaches vanished and her stomach distress gradually improved.

We explored the stress-allergy connection and learned about the science that teaches us that stress can lead to increased inflammation, higher rates of hospital admissions for asthma, and greater allergic reactivity. We learned how, by using simple mind-body techniques such as meditation and yoga, we can take an active and powerful role in reducing stress and nourishing our own well-being. Getting back to nature, listening to soothing music, dancing, and taking a mineral bath are other methods we reviewed for beating stress. Try one and you just may discover a new, more harmonious relationship with yourself and the world around you.

CHAPTER 11

MORE THAN JUST A RUNNY NOSE: NASAL AND SINUS ALLERGIES

Grace worked as a buyer for a luxury retailer. She loved her job because she loved to shop, but it required frequent air travel, which was really hard on her sinuses. As a clothing buyer, she frequently entered showrooms filled with the latest fashions. She found that the air in many showrooms and clothing warehouses would irritate her nose and make her sneeze. The reason: new fabric is usually treated with formaldehyde, an irritating chemical that evaporates and fills the air in fabric shops, showrooms, warehouses, and clothing stores.

She came to see me because she was sick of being sick, and because she wanted to save her job, which was in jeopardy because she missed so much work due to illness.

Grace had suffered from nasal allergies since childhood and had first seen an allergist when she was ten years old. Skin tests done by the allergist showed allergic reactions to house dust, dust mites, and several types of mold. Allergy shots were not helpful.

As a teenager Grace began to experience frequent colds, which occasionally caused sinus infections. In college she underwent surgery, first to correct a deviated nasal septum, then to clean and drain her sinuses. Nasal polyps were found and removed at the time of surgery, and she was advised to use a steroid nasal spray every day to prevent them from returning.

Following surgery, Grace had some relief of her chronic nasal and sinus congestion and mucus drip, but she still caught every cold that came around and each cold led to a new sinus infection, which was treated with antibiotics and steroid pills.

When she first came to see me she had been ill for about four years with continuous nasal and sinus congestion despite daily use of antihistamines and nasal sprays. She was getting steadily worse and had reached the point where almost every airplane ride caused a sinus infection requiring antibiotic therapy. Her doctors recommended further surgery, but Grace doubted it would be of much help, because the first one had not prevented her health from deteriorating.

One doctor thought that her sinus problems were the result of acid reflux. This is a common problem that may affect up to 40 percent of people with chronic rhinosinusitis (CRS), the term for the combined nasal and sinus disorder that afflicted Grace.[1] With acid reflux, as we saw in Chapter 9, your stomach's contents travel backward up your esophagus and into your throat. The most common symptom of reflux is heartburn, but throat and nose irritation may occur and can contribute to the development of CRS.

The standard treatment of acid reflux is the use of drugs that suppress production of stomach acid, but as I noted in Chapter 9, there are many reasons to avoid the use of acid-suppressing drugs. In Grace's case, they simply didn't work. She had used them for two years without benefit.

In an effort to get relief, Grace had changed her diet, eliminating dairy foods like milk, yogurt, cheese, and ice cream and also gluten-containing foods like wheat, rye, and barley. Her daily congestion improved somewhat, but her energy plummeted and she continued to get sick every time she traveled.

When I first saw her, her nose and sinuses were clearly inflamed and she had a thick, yellow postnasal drip. I suspected that the extreme drop in energy she'd experienced on a gluten-free diet might have been due to the dramatic decrease in carbohydrate consumption when she eliminated wheat. Some of my patients feel more energetic on a low-carb diet, but some feel more fatigued. It's an example of the differing ways in which diet change can affect different individuals that I described in Chapter 6.

I thought that Grace needed an additional change to her diet. She was about to leave on another trip, so Power Wash and Re-entry would have to wait until she returned. In the meantime, she needed immediate help. My solution had three components:

- As with many of my mold-allergic patients, the dietary change she most needed to make, after eliminating sugar and junk food, was to eliminate dietary yeast and mold. She'd already stopped eating bread and cheese, because of her milk- and gluten-free regimen, and she rarely drank alcohol. When I reviewed her diet, I realized that the main foods to target were vinegar and dried fruits. She ate salad twice a day and loved to smother it with dressing, and she constantly snacked on raisins. I recommended that she use only olive oil and lemon on her salads and snack on nuts instead of raisins.

- In eliminating wheat, she had drastically reduced her dietary carb intake, and the raisins she grazed on all day just supplied a quick sugar fix that did not really make up the deficit. I recommended that she eat more high-carbohydrate vegetables like sweet potatoes and squash and order rice or potatoes when eating out.

- I thought Grace could also benefit from a few nutritional supplements. These included:

  - NAC and bromelain for their demonstrated effects in acute and chronic sinusitis (I discuss these more on page 201)

- An extract of *Lactobacillus* that I've found helpful in preventing respiratory infections among people who get sick when flying

- Vitamin D and zinc, because her blood levels of both were low

What Are Nasal and Sinus Allergies?

Nasal allergy, or allergic rhinitis, is the most common allergic illness in the United States, affecting almost 60 million people.[2] Around the world, it affects a total of 500 million people.[3] It can make you feel pretty miserable. Stuffed nose. Runny nose. Sneezing. In addition to its relentless symptoms, it causes a great deal of time lost from work or school and wreaks havoc with quality of life.[4] It can easily ruin a night's sleep, producing additional symptoms like fatigue, irritability, and depression and damaging memory and concentration.

Scientific research has identified a little-known but troubling fact: nasal allergy can impair reaction time and driving performance, increasing the risk of motor vehicle accidents. In a controlled experiment conducted in Holland, people with pollen allergies were tested on a closed driving course out of season before and after being exposed to the pollen to which they were allergic.[5] The impairment produced by pollen exposure was equivalent to that seen at a blood alcohol level of 0.05 percent, the legal limit in many countries. Treatment of symptoms with antihistamines or nasal sprays partially—but not completely—blocked the impairment.

In a similar experiment conducted at the Veterans Affairs Medical Center in Washington, D.C., pollen exposure had a major adverse impact on vigilance and response times and decreased the efficiency of working memory and the speed of reasoning and computation.[6] The effect was comparable to taking a sedative drug. But this was not a drug effect. It was a direct effect of the allergy itself. From the perspective of public health and safety, nasal allergy is a serious disease that needs to be taken seriously.

Having allergic rhinitis increases your susceptibility to asthma, colds, and sinusitis, the medical research observes.[7] Proper treatment of allergic rhinitis has also been found to improve school performance.[8] However, research has shown that treatment of allergic rhinitis is often inadequate.[9]

The usual treatments for allergic rhinitis are antihistamines taken either as pills or as nasal sprays, steroid nasal sprays, and drugs like monteleukast that block the activity of allergic mediators called leukotrienes. All these drugs work best when used continuously and daily, but side effects like fatigue, nosebleeds, and excessive dryness can limit their usefulness.

Nasal Allergies and the Common Cold

The interaction between allergic rhinitis and rhinovirus, the group of viruses that cause the common cold, creates a vicious cycle. Rhinovirus enters your cells by attaching to a molecule called ICAM-1, which is a mediator of inflammation. Having nasal allergies increases the levels of ICAM-1 in the cells that line your nose, increasing the opportunity for rhinovirus to cause infection.

Rhinovirus infection then further increases the levels of ICAM-1, which aggravates nasal allergies.[10] Laboratory research has shown that zinc, an essential mineral often lacking in modern diets, can bind to ICAM-1 and prevent rhinovirus from attaching to it.[11] This effect of zinc probably explains the benefits of zinc treatment in decreasing severity and duration of the common cold, which has been demonstrated in numerous controlled clinical trials.[12] Maintaining optimal zinc status is one component of the Allergy Solution program that can help build your antiviral defenses.

Types of Rhinitis and Sinusitis

Allergic rhinitis predisposes you to developing allergic sinusitis. The combined disorder, chronic rhinosinusitis (CRS), affects 12.5 percent of the U.S. population.[13] In addition to nasal symptoms,

CRS causes postnasal drip, sore throat, cough, facial pain, head-ache, and fatigue. Like simple rhinitis, CRS may interfere with sleep and mental concentration and plays a major role in causing or aggravating asthma.[14]

There are two major types of allergic rhinitis and two major types of CRS. Allergic rhinitis may be seasonal (SAR) or year-round (perennial rhinitis); CRS may occur with or without nasal polyps, which are soft, painless growths in the lining of the nose. Understanding these distinctions may help you in applying the Allergy Solution program to heal your own allergies. Nasal polyps, for example, are strongly associated with food allergy, and dietary treatment may greatly enhance the effect of conventional treatment.

Seasonal rhinitis is usually triggered by pollens or outdoor mold spores. If you suffer from SAR, the timing and severity of your symptoms will depend upon what's in the air. Unfortunately, the pollen count is going up almost every year, a result of the increased carbon dioxide content of the earth's atmosphere due to industrial emissions.

Perennial rhinitis is triggered by allergens to which you are continuously exposed, like food, dust, pet dander, or indoor mold, and may also be caused by allergic reactions to bacterial or fungal microbes growing in your nose or sinuses.

Air pollution aggravates all types of allergic rhinitis and sinus-itis by irritating the lining of the respiratory tract.

Out-of-Control Ragweed Now Growing in Your City?

In many action films the future is a barren wasteland where few green plants grow. But what if the real future looks different, with nature somehow hijacked by greenhouse gases and plants growing in unnatural ways?

That scenario is previewing in a city near you. Ragweed plants are growing more quickly, flowering sooner, and getting bigger. The reason? Higher temperatures and higher levels of carbon dioxide in the city than in the countryside. It turns out that more pollution and higher temperatures create a greenhouse effect that makes ragweed thrive. But more ragweed spells big trouble for millions of allergy sufferers, because ragweed is the main allergen triggering seasonal allergic rhinitis.

Scientists at the U.S. Department of Agriculture sought to discover the impact of global climate change on ragweed pollen. Unable to travel into the future, they instead went to the inner city of Baltimore, where pollution had already generated elevated carbon dioxide levels and higher temperatures, just like global warming will produce worldwide. They planted ragweed seeds in aluminum bins, using the same soil, and placed the bins in the city, a nearby suburb, and a country field 40 miles away. Urban ragweed grew to be twice the size of rural ragweed and released five times as many pollen grains.[15]

Allergic Fungal Sinusitis

Fungi are plantlike organisms that lack chlorophyll and feed on organic matter. They include yeasts, molds, mildew, rusts, and mushrooms. A form of sinus allergy called allergic fungal sinusitis (AFS) occurs when common environmental fungi growing in the nose and sinus tract provoke allergic reactions. The chronic sinusitis resulting from AFS resists conventional treatments, which are aimed largely at bacterial sinusitis. AFS tends to occur in young adults and causes thick, highly viscous nasal secretions. People with AFS may have several types of allergic reactions to fungi. Type 1, 3, and 4 allergic reactions have been found in people with AFS.[16]

The biggest mystery of AFS is why fungal colonization of the nose and sinuses stimulates a severe inflammatory response in people with AFS and no response in people without chronic sinusitis. Medical research sought answers:

- Scientists at the University of Texas tackled that mystery with a laboratory test. They exposed blood cells from people with AFS to fungal extracts and compared the response with that of healthy controls.

In healthy people, fungal exposure stimulated increased activity of T-reg cells. This protective response failed to occur in people with AFS.[17] AFS, like most allergic disorders, develops because of impaired function of T-regs.

- Deficiency of vitamin D also contributes to the development of AFS and can be corrected with supplementation.[18]

In addition, an Atlanta physician observed that the degree of nasal inflammation among patients with chronic sinusitis correlated directly with the level of mold in their homes.[19] This suggests that exposure to environmental mold may impact how allergic you are to the fungi that normally grow in your nasal passages.

AFS is a complex and difficult disorder that should be treated by a physician with experience in that condition. You can support proper medical treatment by controlling environmental mold exposure (see Chapter 5), maintaining a healthy level of vitamin D, and using the Immune Balance Diet to enhance T-reg function.

Diet, Environment, and Nasal Allergy

The role of environmental allergens in producing allergic rhinitis is well recognized. However, the role of food in either provoking or soothing nasal allergy is underappreciated. In perennial rhinitis, food alone may be the trigger. In SAR, specific foods have been shown to aggravate the allergic reactions to specific pollens. This aggravation is called cross-reactivity. It's especially strong for ragweed and birch pollens (see "The Pollen-Food Connection," below). In my clinical practice, I've found that people who are allergic to environmental mold are often sensitive to mold in food and can improve their symptoms by avoiding dietary mold and yeast. This was the case for Kate, whose story I told in Chapter 4.

Chronic Sinusitis and Food Allergy: The Staph Connection

Several studies from Europe have demonstrated a very high frequency of food allergies in people who have CRS with nasal polyps. In one study, 81 percent of people with nasal polyps had positive allergic skin tests to specific foods.[20] In another study, food allergy occurred in 70 percent of people with nasal polyps and was twice as common as inhalant allergy.[21]

Researchers have linked this phenomenon to the heavy growth of staphylococcal bacteria (staph) in the noses and sinuses of people who develop nasal polyps. Staph bacteria produce toxins called superantigens that are swallowed when mucus drips into your throat. These toxins travel along the intestinal tract, where they induce allergic reactions to food that you've eaten.[22] Staph toxins stimulate inflammatory reactions and inactivate T-reg cells or even change their functions, making them promote rather than reduce inflammation.[23] The standard medical treatment for nasal polyps is a steroid nasal spray, which causes polyps to shrink. Having allergies, however, causes people with nasal polyps to respond less well to steroid sprays than do people with nasal polyps who do not have allergies.[24] This is surprising, because symptoms of allergic diseases are usually well controlled by steroids. Staph may be the reason. Staph toxins induce resistance to the effects of steroids[25] and at the same time induce food allergy, both of which are critical components of chronic sinusitis for many people.

Nutritional research has observed that dietary flavonoids are able to bind to and inactivate staph toxins,[26] and this is one of the many mechanisms by which the Immune Balance Diet helps in the fight against CRS.

Antibacterial Soap Linked to Staph

Environmental toxins can increase the growth of staph in your nose. Triclosan is an unregulated synthetic chemical increasingly used over the past 40 years as an antibacterial ingredient in soaps, gels, and toothpaste. It's also applied to clothing, kitchen counters, and medical equipment as a disinfectant. Once in contact with your skin or mouth, triclosan is absorbed into your body.

Researchers at the University of Michigan found triclosan in the nasal secretions of almost half the people they tested. Higher levels of triclosan were associated with greater colonization by the most dangerous species of staph. Looking further, the researchers found that triclosan increased the ability of staph to attach itself to human cells and exposure to triclosan made laboratory animals more susceptible to staph infection.[27]

Triclosan also pollutes the outdoor environment. Triclosan contamination of streams increases with urbanization and can dramatically alter the ecology of fresh water, reducing the diversity of normal bacteria and increasing the abundance of potentially toxic cyanobacteria, a major ecological and human health problem worldwide.[28]

The triclosan story demonstrates a fundamental theme of *The Allergy Solution*: environmental toxins can alter the microbial ecology of your body, creating changes that increase your susceptibility to allergy. Read labels and avoid products made with triclosan. Steering clear of toxins is good for you and good for the planet.

Yeast and Mold in Foods

Yeasts and molds are common food additives, used to preserve food, to induce fermentation, and to enhance flavor. They also occur naturally in some foods. Beer, for example, is produced by the addition of brewer's yeast to a mash of malted barley. Wine is created when crushed grapes are fermented by yeasts that naturally live on their skin. Mold is likely to be found growing on any food that is fermented, aged, or spoiled.

With all of this fermenting of yeast and growth of mold, it is no wonder that such a profusion of allergens confronts us. Indeed, scientific studies have identified more than 150 human allergens in various yeasts and molds.[29] Researchers at the world-renowned National Jewish Hospital in Denver have demonstrated that people allergic to inhaled molds commonly show allergic reactions to oral challenge with mold extracts.[30] I often recommend that people who are allergic to airborne molds try eliminating food sources of yeast and mold to test their reactivity.

Here are some typical foods and beverages that often contain yeast or mold. Please note that mold and yeast can be found in a wide range of foods and beverages.

- Bread and crackers
- Beer, wine, and other fermented beverages
- Vinegar and pickled vegetables
- Dried fruit and commercial fruit juices
- Many cheeses and other aged foods
- Commercial tomato sauce
- Black tea
- Yeast extract, a common component of commercial soups and sauces
- Mushrooms
- Anything malted
- Smoked foods, including meat and fish
- Grapes and cranberries, even when fresh
- Melons, which contain antigens that may cross-react with mold

The Pollen-Food Connection

People with pollen allergy may experience allergic symptoms when they eat food that contains proteins similar to those found in the pollen to which they are allergic. This cross-reactivity has been most widely studied with ragweed, grass, and birch pollens. I was able to help Vivian, whom you met in the Introduction, control her acute mystery illness by using the birch pollen–food connection.

Ragweed, Grass, and Pan-Allergies

Ragweed pollen is the major trigger for late-summer hay fever throughout much of the United States. Scientists estimate that a single ragweed plant can release one billion grains of pollen over the course of a single ragweed season. The grains are so light that they float easily on gentle breezes and can travel incredible distances. Ragweed pollen has been detected as far as 400 miles out to sea and as high as 2 miles up in the atmosphere.[31] People with ragweed allergy are often sensitive to melons or bananas and may develop symptoms that range from an itchy mouth or swollen lips to aggravation of hay fever.

The cross-reactive allergens between ragweed and food appear to be proteins called pan-allergens, which are found in many plants and pollens, including ragweed and grass pollen. Pan-allergens are the allergic triggers for about a third of all pollen allergies and are the likely triggers if a person with pollen allergy is also allergic to melon, watermelon, bananas, citrus fruits, tomatoes, or latex.

Pan-allergens may also provoke symptoms outside the respiratory tract, including hives, diarrhea, abdominal cramps, anaphylaxis, and itching or swelling of the throat or lips, which is called oral allergy syndrome.[32] Sometimes pan-allergens require an additional factor, such as exercise or the use of painkillers (aspirin, ibuprofen, or naproxen), to provoke symptoms.

If you have late-summer rhinitis due to ragweed pollen (hay fever), or late-spring rhinitis due to grass pollen (spring fever), your symptoms may be aggravated by eating foods containing pan-allergens, especially during the allergy season.

Birch Trees

Birch pollinates in the early spring and may cause sneezing, coughing, and itchy eyes. Researchers in northern Europe, where birch trees abound, have determined that almost three-quarters of people with birch pollen allergy are allergic to plants that contain proteins similar to the main birch pollen allergens, which are called Bet v 1 and Bet v 6.

Apples, celery, carrots, hazelnuts, soybeans, peaches and other stone fruits, oranges, lychee fruit, strawberries, persimmons, and zucchini may all cross-react with birch pollen and can cause allergic symptoms in people with birch pollen allergy, especially in springtime.

In a study at Germany's Paul Ehrlich Institute, about 70 percent of patients allergic to birch pollen were found to experience symptoms when exposed to birch pollen–related foods.[33] And although pollen-related food allergens are often destroyed by cooking, recent studies have shown that hazelnuts and celery may provoke symptoms even after being thoroughly cooked.[34]

In a creative clinical experiment done in Finland, people with birch pollen allergy ate birch pollen in honey daily from November through March. During the subsequent birch pollen season in April and May, they reported a 60 percent reduction in symptoms of allergy, had twice as many days with no symptoms, and decreased their use of antihistamines by 50 percent, compared with a control group.[35] The mechanism for the protective effects of oral birch pollen was presumed to be the phenomenon called oral tolerance, which I discussed in Chapter 3.

Air Pollution and the Pollen-Food Connection

Most of the allergens responsible for the pollen-food syndrome are defense proteins made by plants to protect themselves. Science has uncovered a troubling fact: environmental stresses like air pollution or climate change can stimulate the expression of these proteins, making both pollens and foods more likely to provoke allergic reactions.[36] Research indicates that increasing global air pollution and climate change are not only increasing the amount of pollen to which we're exposed, but making the pollen grains themselves more allergenic.

Probiotics for Nasal Allergies

Probiotics are cultures of living bacteria with possible health benefits. Most probiotic cultures contain species of *Lactobacillus* or *Bifidobacterium* or combinations of different species. Several have been shown to help people with nasal allergies by relieving symptoms and by improving immune balance, according to double-blind, placebo-controlled clinical trials.[37]

The species with the best track record for allergic rhinitis is *Lactobacillus paracasei*. Different strains of *Lactobacillus paracasei* have been used with those suffering from seasonal or perennial rhinitis. All seem to produce similar effects and may improve symptoms and quality of life; they may also stimulate the immune system in ways that counteract Type 1 allergy. In a head-to-head contest with a mixture of *Bifidobacterium lactis* and *Lactobacillus acidophilus*, *L. paracasei* came out on top.[38] Here's the science on probiotics for allergic rhinitis:

- *Lactobacillus paracasei* strain ST-11 (LP-11), given for four weeks as a fermented milk product, was shown to decrease the allergic response to grass pollen in people with grass pollen allergy.[39]

- When given as a powder supplying ten billion bacteria per day, LP-11 significantly reduced nasal itching during the grass pollen season.[40]

- Another strain of the same species, *Lactobacillus paracasei* strain 33 (LP-33), reduced symptoms of people suffering from dust mite allergy and improved their quality of life.[41]

- When given to people with grass pollen allergy who experienced incomplete relief on antihistamines, LP-33 enhanced the treatment response by decreasing itchiness of the eyes and improving quality of life.[42]

- When *Lactobacillus paracasei* strain HF A00232 was given to subjects who relied on daily antihistamines to control their chronic nasal symptoms, it allowed them to discontinue antihistamines after eight weeks without experiencing an increase in symptoms. Allergy-related quality of life actually improved when antihistamines were discontinued.[43]

- *Lactobacillus johnsonii* strain EM1 was added for twelve weeks to antihistamine treatment of subjects with perennial rhinitis. Benefits of the probiotic became evident at four weeks, progressively increased over the next eight weeks, and were still evident three months after the probiotic was stopped.[44]

Other probiotics shown to help relieve symptoms of nasal allergies in controlled clinical trials include:

- *Lactobacillus salivarius* strain PM-A0006, given as a powder, four billion units a day for 12 weeks, to subjects with dust allergy. It produced a significant improvement in nasal and eye symptoms that started between four and eight weeks of supplementation.[45]

- *Lactobacillus acidophilus* strain L-92, given as a fermented milk product. It relieved symptoms of people with perennial rhinitis due to dust mite allergy.[46]

- *Bifidobacterium lactis* strain NCC2818, given during the height of grass pollen season in Switzerland. It reduced nasal allergies and diminished the allergic inflammatory response, with benefits noticeable after three weeks.[47]

- *Lactobacillus acidophilus* strain NCFM (ATCC 700396) and *Bifidobacterium lactis* strain Bl-04 (ATCC SD5219), given as capsules supplying five billion bacteria per day to subjects with birch pollen allergy, administered for four months, starting two months before the birch pollen season in Finland. Those who received the probiotics showed a decrease in allergic inflammation on nasal swabs and some decrease in symptoms.[48]

- *Bifidobacterium longum* strain BBS36, given in yogurt for 14 weeks. This reduced symptoms associated with allergy to Japanese cedar pollen and significantly reduced the use of medication.[49]

This fascinating research indicates that probiotics of *Lactobacillus* bacteria or *Bifidobacteria* may improve symptoms of allergic rhinitis. They seem to work by shifting immune balance in a direction that resists allergic responses. *Lactobacilli* may be more potent in this effect than *Bifidobacteria*. The benefits of probiotics for nasal allergies may take between three and eight weeks to become evident and may last for many weeks after the probiotics are stopped.

Products containing multiple types of bacteria may not be better than those with just one species. The bacteria may not even need to be living to have an effect. My clinical experience has taught me over and over again that no single probiotic is best for everyone. If your main symptom of allergy is rhinitis, there are many types of probiotics from which you can choose.

In addition, probiotics have been shown to help reduce the incidence and the duration of colds.[50] Reducing the incidence of colds is important for reducing nasal allergy, because the severity of both depends on the inflammatory mediator ICAM-1, as mentioned earlier in this chapter. Colds are also a major factor in the development of CRS.

Grace Finds Balance

So what happened to Grace, whom you met at the beginning of this chapter? She made it through her trip without getting sick. When she returned, we had to work on keeping her well. There was a lot more to do:

- First, I advised her to stop humidifying her apartment. Excess moisture encourages the growth of mold and dust mites, both significant allergens. Humidifying her apartment was hurting her sinus problems, not helping them. I also recommended the use of protective covers on her bedding to limit exposure to dust mites, which live comfortably in mattresses.

- Second, I guided her through Power Wash and Re-entry to help her find her ideal diet. Vinegar quickly provoked nasal congestion and headache. It turned out to be Grace's major food allergen, followed closely by dairy products. Gluten was free of blame in Grace's case, but yeast was not. Along with vinegar, she avoided all the significant yeast- and mold-containing foods I listed earlier in this chapter.

- Third, I evaluated the impact on her body of years of antibiotics, which had depleted her body's beneficial bacteria and encouraged the overgrowth of yeast in her own tissues, along with undesirable bacteria that provoked inflammation rather than immune balance. That healing process, which I call reflorastation, is described in Chapter 14.

- Finally, I helped her realize that creating immune balance required that she create some balance in her whole life, not just her diet. She rarely exercised. There were close friends she rarely saw. Her leisure time was spent mostly watching TV. She needed a life outside of work.

For many people, balancing life is the final part of the Allergy Solution program, as it was for Grace. In order to control her life she needed to break out of the vicious cycle of illness that resulted from her allergies and escalated her allergies. By establishing control in one vital area, improving her health through her own efforts, she gained the confidence that allowed her to make other changes. She even wound up changing her job to become a designer instead of a buyer. Paradoxically, she'd come to me to keep from losing her job because she was sick all the time. Once she became healthy, she decided to leave her job for one she liked more.

The Allergy Solution Program for Nasal and Sinus Allergies

Nasal and sinus allergies are never just problems involving your nose and sinuses, but involve your entire body. They are systemic ailments that require systemic solutions. That being said, there are some local treatments that can provide relief, especially if nasal staph or fungi are helping to create the T-reg dysfunction that underlies allergy.

Here are some steps that may help improve the health of your nose, sinuses, and upper respiratory tract:

- Create an oasis in your home and workplace. Despite increasing environmental pollution, you can decrease your own exposure to toxins and molds by following the steps in Chapter 5.

- Follow the dietary protocols in Chapters 6, 7, and 8 to eliminate allergen-provoking foods, improve resistance to air pollution, and enhance the function of your anti-inflammatory T-reg cells.

- If you are allergic to pollens, try avoiding foods that cross-react with them during the pollen season but eating these foods liberally before the season begins to help induce oral tolerance. NOTE: If you experience itching or swelling of your face, mouth, or throat; wheezing, sneezing, or trouble breathing; or dizziness or trouble standing when you eat any cross-reactive food, you should not attempt to establish oral tolerance. Discuss the reaction with your doctor.

- Correct nutritional deficiencies and imbalances that impact immune function.

- Vitamin D deficiency is common among people with CRS, and lower levels of vitamin D in blood correlate with more severe sinus disease.[51] Vitamin D has unique effects on immunity: it stimulates defense against several types of infection and at the same time acts to suppress inflammation.[52] Ask your doctor if you should be taking a supplement of vitamin D and if testing your blood level would be useful.

- If you're prone to frequent respiratory infections, ask your doctor to check the level of plasma or serum zinc in your blood, to see whether zinc supplementation may be worthwhile.

- Raise your level of glutathione, the most potent detoxifier and antioxidant made in your cells, following the guidelines you'll find in Chapter 13.

- NAC (N-acetylcysteine) is an amino acid and an antioxidant that raises levels of glutathione and also has respiratory benefits of its own. A major problem in CRS is the stickiness of mucus secretions, which are hard to clear and encourage infection. NAC decreases the stickiness of respiratory secretions and enhances the ability of respiratory cells to eliminate mucus.[53] I frequently recommend NAC to my patients with CRS, at a dose of 600 to 900 milligrams two to three times a day.

- Bromelain is a complex of enzymes derived from pineapple stems and available without a doctor's prescription. It has been used in the treatment of sinusitis since the 1960s.[54] Bromelain is generally given as an add-on to conventional therapy. Double-blind, placebo-controlled trials have found that bromelain speeds recovery of acute sinusitis significantly better than a placebo.[55] For people with CRS, bromelain improves symptom scores, quality of life scores, and tissue inflammation.[56] Like NAC, bromelain decreases the stickiness of nasal secretions.[57] It also has direct anti-inflammatory effects. The typical dose is 500 to 1,000 milligrams per day.

Conclusion

This chapter looked at the most common allergy in the United States, allergic rhinitis, with symptoms such as congestion, a runny or stuffed nose, and frequent interference with sleep. Quality of life suffers, and irritability and fatigue often occur.

I told you about research done in the United States and Europe that showed a direct impairment of mental focus and performance resulting from nasal allergies. I reviewed the types of sinusitis and the critical role of nutrition and environment in this condition. I explored how what you eat can increase symptoms of pollen allergy, and how pollution and climate change can worsen allergy symptoms by increasing the amount of pollen produced by plants such as ragweed and by making the pollen more allergenic. I reviewed the research on supplements that may help, including a tour of the fascinating strains of probiotics that have been shown to relieve symptoms of allergic rhinitis.

We met Grace, the world-traveling buyer for a luxury retailer. She was constantly in contact with clothing and the formaldehyde it often contains, which exacerbated her nasal allergies. By reducing her exposure to mold, adjusting her diet, and healing her digestion, we were able to get her on the road to recovery.

For your own journey to recovery, I highly recommend you go over the material in this chapter with your doctor, to collaborate with her or him on your care.

CHAPTER 12

EVERY BREATH YOU TAKE: ASTHMA

Sarah, a high-school senior, was gasping for air and could hardly get a breath. The vital airways that bring life-giving oxygen to the lungs were being cut off by a severe asthma attack. Her blonde hair stuck to her forehead and her face grew very pale. There was desperation in her green eyes; she had suffered asthma attacks before and was gripped by fear. She needed medical care and needed it fast.

Her parents drove her in the dark to the hospital at breakneck speed, the car swerving around corners and barreling down the straightaways, Sarah wheezing loudly in the backseat. It was six miles to the hospital downtown, but it felt like forever. Driving up to the big hospital, they scanned the building for the Emergency sign. They got Sarah out of the backseat and rushed her inside, their eyes momentarily blinded by the bright fluorescent lights. A crowd of people of all ages, some in their pajamas, waited for care.

A scene like this takes place two million times a year in U.S. emergency rooms.

The villains we met in Chapter 2, "How Did We Get So Sick?", and Chapter 5, "Mission Detoxable"—air pollution, tobacco smoke, and toxic chemicals—return here with a vengeance, ready to wreak havoc on our airways. These villains are powered by a vast industrial machine that never rests. Their menace spans the globe, making us sick with allergies, asthma, and innumerable other diseases. Who is lined up on the other side? The individual trying to protect her or his health. This is David versus Goliath.

The Asthma Epidemic

More than 300 million people worldwide suffer from asthma, reports a study from Tulane University and Oregon Health Sciences University. The National Center for Health Statistics, part of the Centers for Disease Control and Prevention, reports that 25 million people have asthma in the United States. Asthma in the U.S. population has been increasing steadily and is now at its highest level ever: one person out of ten will experience asthma at some time in his or her life. The *New England Journal of Medicine* article "The Asthma Epidemic" highlighted the scope of the problem. There are more than two million visits to emergency rooms for asthma each year in the U.S. and about 4,500 asthma deaths.[1] These lives could be saved.

Asthma is a complex and heterogeneous disease. The main symptoms of acute asthma—wheezing, shortness of breath, chest tightness, and cough—are caused by two principal events: 1) the cells that line the bronchial tubes produce excess mucus and promote inflammation, and 2) the muscles that line the walls of the bronchial tubes constrict. Both these events together produce a critical but reversible narrowing of the airways.

Between 50 and 80 percent of asthma cases are the result of allergies.[2] Asthma is the most complicated allergic disorder of all, because there are so many types of asthmatic reactions. Both Type 1 and Type 4 allergy may cause asthma. The two types may operate together or separately, and the nature of the reaction is influenced by a multitude of factors including, but not limited to, the level of pollution in the air you're breathing, whether or not you're overweight or subject to esophageal reflux, and whether you have sinusitis or nasal polyps. Both late-phase and delayed allergic reactions can scar the delicate architecture of your lungs through a process called airway remodeling.

Environmental stimuli like dust, mites, animal dander, mold, and pollens are the most common allergic triggers in asthma. In addition, food allergies occur in 10 to 50 percent of asthmatics.[3] Food allergies can play a critical role in aggravating asthmatic reactions, and the presence of asthma increases the risk that a food-allergic person may suffer a fatal reaction from food allergen exposure. People with asthma must not follow the Re-entry Food Challenge described in Chapter 7: asthmatics *must* avoid foods to which they may be allergic.

Conventional asthma treatment is based on the use of steroids to control inflammation and bronchodilators to prevent narrowing of the bronchial tubes. About 10 percent of people with asthma develop severe chronic disease that does not respond to steroids or bronchodilators.

What Is Asthma Control?

Control of asthma has been defined as not having any restriction in activities, not waking at night with asthma, not needing bronchodilator therapy to relieve symptoms more than three times per week, not missing school or work because of asthma, and not having severe acute asthmatic reactions. Data from several studies has shown that only between one in three and one in four people with asthma enjoy that level of control.[4] Clearly, much more needs to be done.

In this chapter I'll discuss the nutritional factors that scientific research and human clinical trials have found to be most helpful for reversing or controlling asthma. The takeaways from these studies are:

- Avoid foods that provoke asthmatic reactions.
- Eat detoxifying, antioxidant-rich vegetables and fruits.
- Eat beneficial fats from nuts, seeds, and seafood.
- Use probiotics to enhance immune balance.

- Consume foods and dietary supplements that increase the activity of glutathione, your body's most important antioxidant.

While these factors have been found to be effective in numerous studies, there is growing recognition that the immune amplification mechanisms in asthmatics are not the same for everyone, so an individualized approach to treatment is essential.[5] The complex and multifaceted nature of asthma underscores the need to work with your doctor on any treatment plan.

Asthma in the White House: Theodore Roosevelt

Before he was a student at Harvard, a boxer, a legendary hunter, a cowboy in North Dakota, the author of more than a dozen books, a Rough Rider in Cuba, or the governor of New York State, before he was Secretary of the Navy, before he served as Vice President and then President of the United States, and before he won the Nobel Peace Prize, Theodore Roosevelt was a little boy with asthma.

Born in 1858 on East 20th Street in Manhattan, he was plagued by illness as a child. "I was a sickly, delicate boy, suffered much from asthma, and frequently had to be taken away on trips to find a place where I could breathe," he wrote in his autobiography.

When the attacks came, they were terrifying, making him feel as if he were going to die. He gasped for breath and had the sensation that he was being strangled. He overheard his parents saying that he wasn't expected to live very long. He found himself afraid to leave the house, gripped by a terrible fear and in need of a way to cope with that fear.

His father told him that to overcome the terrible affliction of asthma, he would need to "make his body." Teddy's mission became strengthening himself in body and mind. On the outdoor balcony of the family home he undertook a rigorous training program, spending hour after hour on gymnastics. Boxing lessons followed, and then hunting, hiking, horseback riding, swimming, the long jump, running, rowing, and wrestling. He developed a lifelong love of the outdoors and believed in the restorative power of time spent in nature.

He read books constantly, eventually devouring an estimated 20,000 titles. He was without a doubt a man on a mission to build himself up. Teddy Roosevelt strove to get as much done as quickly as possible, with his illness teaching him that life itself was precious. His mottoes became "Get Action!" and "Do Things."

As governor of New York State, he bucked the entrenched political establishment and sought to use his power to solve problems for people. He backed progressive legislation that limited working hours for women and children, taxed corporations, and protected land in the Catskill and Adirondack Mountains.

When hostilities broke out with Spain, he insisted on participating personally, by joining the U.S. Army, and famously led his Rough Riders up San Juan Hill in Cuba. His exploits catapulted him to national fame, and he became a hero to millions of Americans who felt he embodied the vigorous ideals of the young country. Living at a breakneck pace, he became the youngest president of the United States at 42 years of age.

During a time of rapid industrial development, when entire forests were being cut down for lumber and huge areas were being destroyed by coal mining and drilling for oil, Roosevelt recognized that natural resources were finite, that even on a continent as big as North America nature needed protection and needed it right away. Although he was a voracious hunter, his experience taught him that nature had its limits, that even the teeming wildlife of the American plains could eventually be pushed to extinction. Ultimately, this led him to champion the establishment of the National Park System, so that vital wilderness could be forever protected against development.

Roosevelt's example is that you can improve your condition if you take an active role in your care and your health. As the most famous case of asthma in American history, he taught that weakness of the body can be overcome. Everything else you wish to accomplish will be enabled or greatly enhanced by taking excellent care of your health.[6]

Oxidative Stress, Allergy, and Asthma

One thing that the lungs of all asthmatics have in common is a condition called oxidative stress, which increases with the severity of asthma.[7]

Your body uses oxygen to burn fuel for energy and to destroy dangerous bacteria. The process, called oxidation, is like a well-controlled fire, similar in concept to a combustion engine. Your body also has an antioxidant defense system, which controls the fire and keeps it from damaging your own cells.

Oxidative stress results from an imbalance between these two essential activities, oxidation and antioxidation. Because all the oxygen in your tissues enters your body through the respiratory system, your lungs are especially prone to oxidative stress, and nothing aggravates that tendency more than inflammation.

Oxidative stress has been proven to directly stimulate bronchial muscle constriction, induce airway hyper-irritability, and increase mucus secretion.[8] It also plays a key role in the well-known link between air pollution and allergic asthma. Air pollution is an important factor in both the development and the worsening of asthma; it can trigger oxidative stress in anyone, but current research reveals that people with asthma have an exaggerated inflammatory response to air pollution–induced oxidative stress.[9]

It is critically important that people with asthma minimize their exposure to air pollutants, cigarette smoke in particular. Cigarette smoke contains more than 4,700 chemical compounds and very high concentrations of oxidants (ten trillion molecules per puff). Some of these become trapped in the cells that line the respiratory tract and continue to cause damage for a long time after smoke exposure ends.[10]

Nutrition vs. Asthma: Antioxidants

Over the past decade, scientists have been carefully researching the role of antioxidants in preventing or controlling asthma. This research is exciting and holds out great possibilities. I use its findings extensively in *The Allergy Solution*.

Once you've eliminated food allergens from your diet, your next step in overcoming asthma is ensuring a high intake of antioxidants from natural foods. Here's the science:

- People with asthma have reduced levels of dietary antioxidants such as vitamins A, C, and E in their blood.[11] These levels can improve with supplementation. In addition, people with more severe asthma have greater deficits in dietary antioxidant levels than do those with milder asthma.[12] It's not yet clear whether this occurs because the oxidative stress of asthma destroys these antioxidants or because asthmatics have less nutritionally sound diets to begin with. Either way, a higher intake of dietary antioxidants from food may be helpful for prevention and control of asthma.

- People who consume diets rich in antioxidants from fruits and vegetables have a reduced incidence of asthma compared with people consuming a typical Western diet, low in vegetables and fruit. A Finnish study with more than 10,000 participants showed a significant inverse relationship between dietary consumption of antioxidants called flavonoids, found in fruits and vegetables, and the development of asthma.[13]

Fruits and Vegetables Help Asthma, Research Finds

In an article published in *The American Journal of Clinical Nutrition*, Australian scientists demonstrated the potential of antioxidants from vegetables and fruits in preventing asthma attacks by placing adults with asthma on two diets: a high-antioxidant diet containing five servings of vegetables and two servings of fruit a day, and a low-antioxidant diet containing no more than two servings of vegetables and one serving of fruit a day.[14]

After two weeks, the people in the study consuming the high-antioxidant diet showed better lung function on breathing tests than did the people on the low-antioxidant diet. After 14 weeks, those on the low-antioxidant diet not only showed poorer lung function, they also showed higher blood levels of C-reactive protein (CRP), an important marker of systemic inflammation.

The Australian scientists then demonstrated that adding tomato juice (about two glasses a day) to the low-antioxidant diet produced a decrease in lung inflammation.[15] Tomatoes are an excellent dietary source of carotenoids and vitamin C. Those asthmatics who had tomato juice added to their low-antioxidant diet showed a decrease in the levels of white blood cells in mucus compared with those on the low-antioxidant diet who did not get supplemental tomato juice. Tomato juice alone, however, did not improve airflow. The whole-foods high-antioxidant diet was more effective than tomato juice for that purpose.

The Two Faces of Vitamin E

Vitamin E is probably the best-known dietary antioxidant. It's actually not one substance but eight, each of which may have different effects on your body. Research indicates that vitamin E from food or supplements may either prevent or aggravate asthma, depending upon the form of vitamin E being consumed.

There are eight forms of vitamin E in nature, of which two predominate in human tissues: alpha-tocopherol and gamma-tocopherol. These have similar antioxidant effects in test tubes, but your cells preferentially take up alpha-tocopherol and break down gamma-tocopherol, so that the concentration of alpha-tocopherol is typically ten times higher than the concentration of gamma-tocopherol in your tissues.[16]

Alpha- and gamma-tocopherol also differ in the way they combat inflammation. In laboratory experiments with animals and humans, gamma-tocopherol has been shown to have unique effects that can benefit acute nonallergic inflammation caused by exposure to bacteria, smoke, or ozone.[17]

However, researchers at Northwestern University in Chicago demonstrated that in allergic mice, gamma-tocopherol increases bronchial hyperreactivity and increases the recruitment of inflammatory eosinophils (Eos) into lung tissue, whereas alpha-tocopherol does the opposite.[18] They conclude that in chronic allergic asthma, as opposed to acute lung infection or injury, alpha-tocopherol is anti-inflammatory and blocks airway hyperactivity, whereas gamma-tocopherol is pro-inflammatory, increasing airway hyperactivity and interfering with the beneficial effects of alpha-tocopherol.[19]

The Northwestern researchers note that the past 40 years have witnessed an increase in gamma-tocopherol in the U.S. diet and in infant formulas, largely due to increased consumption of soybean oil, which is high in gamma-tocopherol.[20] Other vegetable oils, like olive oil, in contrast, contain minimal gamma-tocopherol. Since many vitamin E supplements use soybean oil as a carrier, vitamin E supplements (even if they are labeled as alpha-tocopherol) may act as hidden sources of gamma-tocopherol.

Several studies have found reduced levels of alpha-tocopherol in the blood of asthmatics.[21] The Northwestern researchers conducted a study of 4,500 individuals and found that higher levels of gamma-tocopherol in blood were associated with poorer lung function, whereas higher levels of alpha-tocopherol were associated with improved lung function.[22] They also worked out what they believe is the mechanism for the opposing effects of these two forms of vitamin E in asthmatics: The two forms have opposite effects on an enzyme called PKCa (protein kinase C alpha), which transports inflammatory cells into tissues during inflammation.[23] PKCa increases inflammation in asthma and increases the airway remodeling that accompanies the late-stage asthmatic response.[24] In the lungs of allergic mice, alpha inhibits and gamma enhances activity of PKCa.

Support for the Northwestern researchers' theory comes from a study done at Vanderbilt University in Nashville in which people with allergic asthma were given a high dose of natural alpha-tocopherol, 1,500 milligrams a day for four months.[25] The researchers chose the dietary form of alpha-tocopherol called d-alpha-tocopherol, derived from a natural source, rather than the synthetic form found in many supplements, which is called d,l-alpha-tocopherol. This distinction is important because only d-alpha tocopherol performs the normal functions of vitamin E. The effect of supplementation was to increase blood levels of alpha-tocopherol and decrease blood levels of gamma-tocopherol. Along with this change in vitamin E, levels of allergic mediators and oxidative stress markers in the lungs decreased. Airway reactivity to methacholine, a chemical that causes bronchial constriction, also decreased. This clinical study supports the contention of the Northwestern researchers that alpha-tocopherol may be good for asthmatics and gamma-tocopherol may actually be harmful.

Clinical trials with low-dose vitamin E (usually as alpha-tocopherol) have shown mixed results; the greatest benefits appear to occur in people who are exposed to air pollutants like ozone or sulphur dioxide. Vitamin E in that setting seems able to prevent the increase in airway inflammation produced by air pollution.[26]

This research has shaped the way I think about vitamin E in asthma and allergic disorders, although more research is needed, especially clinical trials. I don't believe that vitamin E should be used as a stand-alone supplement in people with asthma. For one thing, high-dose vitamin E supplementation when used alone can have a pro-oxidant effect rather than an antioxidant effect and may increase oxidative stress over time.[27] Also, vitamin E supplementation can reduce blood levels of coenzyme Q10, a nutrient that is essential for cell function. A European study demonstrated reduced coenzyme Q10 levels in the blood of people with asthma.[28] When supplements of coenzyme Q10 (120 milligrams/day) were given to people who needed inhaled steroids to control their asthma, there was a significant reduction in steroid dose needed.[29]

The bottom line: vitamin E supplements should be carefully chosen. The best form of vitamin E for asthmatics may be natural d-alpha-tocopherol in a soy-free base. It should not be used alone but only as part of a total dietary antioxidant program, like the Immune Balance Diet, described in Chapter 8. If high-dose vitamin E supplements are taken, coenzyme Q10 in a dose of 120 milligrams a day or more may also be needed.

Nutrition vs. Asthma: Controlling NOX

One of the major sources of oxidative stress in asthmatics is an enzyme called NOX, which stands for NADPH oxidase. NOX is found in mast cells and white blood cells. It is useful for fighting infection, but there are many human diseases, including asthma, in which NOX activity causes both inflammation and oxidative stress.

Pollen grains have been shown to contain their own version of NOX, so that high pollen counts may aggravate asthma even in people who are not allergic to the specific pollen. When pollen grains are deposited in airways along with diesel exhaust, the oxidative stress is amplified in a synergistic fashion: the combined inflammatory effect is greater than the sum of either pollen grains or diesel particles alone.[30]

A study from the University of Lecce, in Italy, found that flavonoids in vegetables, fruits, herbs, and spices can inhibit excessive

NOX activity. Omega-3 fatty acids in fish oils (EPA, or eicosapen-
taeonic acid, and DHA, or docosahexaenoic acid) have also shown
potential for inhibiting excessive NOX activity. This may explain
why numerous clinical trials have described a beneficial effect of
omega-3 supplementation in people with asthma.[31]

Fish oils seem to be especially effective in subduing the late-
phase allergic reaction in people with asthma. A long-term (20-
year) study of young Americans (ages 18 to 30) supported by
the National Heart, Lung, and Blood Institute of the National
Institutes of Health found that low dietary intake of omega-3s
from fish more than doubled the risk of developing asthma.[32]

Do You Need an Oil Change?

Dietary fat has a significant effect on the risk of asthma, and
changing the nature of the fat you consume through food choices
or supplementation can have a major impact on asthma control.

Fats are composed of components called fatty acids, which
are divided into two major categories: saturated and unsaturated.
These terms describe their chemical structure. Unsaturated fatty
acids contain double bonds between atoms. Monounsaturates have
one double bond. Polyunsaturates contain two or more double
bonds. Foods that are mostly made up of saturated fatty acids tend
to be solid at room temperature. Butter is a good example. Foods
that are mostly made up of unsaturated fatty acids are liquid at
room temperature, like vegetable oils. The more unsaturated the
fat, the colder its melting point, so the more likely it will stay
liquid, even when cold:

- Olive oil, which is primarily made up of oleic acid,
  a monounsaturated fatty acid, is liquid at room
  temperature but turns solid in the refrigerator.

- Corn oil, which is mostly made up of
  polyunsaturated fatty acids, stays liquid in the
  refrigerator but may solidify in the freezer.

- Fish oils, which are even more polyunsaturated than
  corn oil, stay liquid in the freezer.

Most unsaturated fatty acids have a chemical configuration called *cis*, which lines up atoms on the same side of a double bond, creating a bend in the molecule. Some processed and manufactured fats have a configuration called *trans*, which lines atoms up on opposite sides of a double bond, creating a molecule that is straight rather than curved. *Trans*-fatty acids are produced when polyunsaturated *cis* fatty acids are subjected to a process called hydrogenation, which is the food industry's attempt to prolong shelf life. Natural hydrogenation also occurs in the rumens of cattle, so that beef and milk contain trans-fatty acids at low levels.

I warned parents about the dangers of trans-fatty acids in my first book, *Superimmunity for Kids*, published in 1988. Since then, abundant research has confirmed the deleterious effects of dietary trans fats on health. A global study of half a million children, the International Study of Asthma and Allergies in Childhood (ISAAC), identified greater trans-fatty acid consumption as the most important dietary factor associated with developing asthma.[33] A more modest European study found that consumption of margarine, a major source of trans-fatty acids, produced an increased risk of developing asthma among adults.[34]

The Essential Fatty Acids: Omega-6 and Omega-3

Your body has the ability to make saturated and monounsaturated fatty acids, but it cannot make the major polyunsaturated fatty acids. These are called essential fatty acids (EFAs), and they are divided into two families, called omega-6 and omega-3, based upon their chemical structures.

I've been writing and lecturing about the impact of EFAs on health and illness for most of my medical career. In 1986 I wrote a scholarly article that was published in *The Journal of the American College of Nutrition*. It explained that people with allergies have an increased need for EFAs because of a block in the way their cells utilize them.[35] One of the fundamental principles is that you must get your EFAs from food, and both plants and animals can supply you with omega-6s or omega-3s. The difference between plant and animal sources is that EFAs found in animal foods are usually more unsaturated than those found in plants.

Omega-3s have attracted so much interest because they have effects on your body that tend to be anti-inflammatory. But the effects of omega-6s, which are the predominant category of EFA, are not so straightforward; they may either favor or inhibit inflammation. Certain omega-6 EFAs may benefit people with asthma, especially when balanced with the appropriate intake of omega-3s. In my experience, balance is the key, and more is not necessarily better.

Balancing Omegas to Help Asthma

Research I conducted in the 1980s in association with Dr. David Horrobin, an EFA pioneer, and Dr. Ross Rocklin, a professor of allergy and immunology at Tufts University, confirmed defective omega-6 metabolism in people with allergies, suggesting that some allergic individuals may require special omega-6 supplements to achieve proper balance.[36] This concept has been applied with significant benefits in the clinical trials described later in this chapter.

As mentioned earlier, a study of young American adults found that the 20-year incidence of asthma was directly linked to a reduced consumption of omega-3 fats from fish; in other words, omega-3 consumption and onset of asthma were inversely related.[37] As I explained in a review article I authored on diet and inflammation for the journal *Nutrition in Clinical Practice*, higher dietary omega-3 levels have been associated with decreased evidence of inflammation in the general population. This has also been observed in people with asthma: higher omega-3 intake from food produces less inflammation. It also produces better asthma control, whereas a high dietary omega-6 to omega-3 ratio produces poorly controlled asthma.[38]

I discussed the best way to balance dietary fats by eliminating trans fats, increasing omega-3s, and reducing omega-6s in my book *The Fat Resistance Diet*, which was written to help people lose weight with an anti-inflammatory diet. The basic principles, described in "The Allergy Solution Oil Change" on page 216, are simple and easy to implement.

The Allergy Solution Oil Change

To move from the modern Western diet to a balanced, allergy-fighting diet, consider the following choices. If you are allergic to any of the selections listed here, avoid it and make another choice.

- Eat adequate amounts of omega-3 foods. The chief form of omega-3s in plants is alpha-linolenic acid. Fish contain two other types of omega-3s, EPA (eicosapentaenoic acid) and DHA (docosahexaenoic acid), and your body has the ability to convert some alpha-linolenic acid to EPA and DHA. All forms of omega-3s appear to have health benefits. Good sources of alpha-linolenic acid are:

  Seeds like chia, flax, hemp, and sabja (or sweet basil). I feature chia seeds in the Immune Balance Smoothie.

  English walnuts. Walnut oil makes a tasty gourmet salad dressing.

  Leafy green vegetables like spinach and kale. Although they're low in total fats, leafy greens can supply ample omega-3s if eaten regularly. The spinach leaves in the Immune Power Smoothie will provide about 300 milligrams per serving.

- Eat omega-3-rich fish twice a week, unless you're allergic to fish. Good sources of EPA and DHA include salmon, sardines, trout, mackerel, herring, and anchovies. Caution: Tuna is naturally high in mercury because it's a large predator fish. Do not eat tuna more than once a month.

- Avoid trans-fats by avoiding foods made with hydrogenated or partially hydrogenated vegetable oil, which is found in margarines and many baked goods. Don't trust a label that says "Zero Trans Fats" or "Trans Fat Free." Manufacturers can make that claim if there is less than 500 milligrams of trans fat per serving. By making the serving size small enough, many foods containing these toxic fats can claim to be free of them.

- Make extra-virgin olive oil your main food oil. Skip high-omega-6 oils like corn, safflower, sunflower, and soybean. I have special concerns about soybean oil, as researchers at Northwestern University have linked increased consumption of soybean oil to increased risk of asthma. (See "The Two Faces of Vitamin E" on page 210.)

EFA Supplements and Asthma: The Promise of Clinical Trials

Diet is the best way to initiate an anti-asthmatic oil change, but its effects can be amplified by judicious use of omega-3 supplements. Researchers around the world have looked at how omega-3 consumption relates to symptoms, airflow, and inflammation in people with asthma. Most of these studies were done using supplements but without dietary changes. I believe that for optimal healing, supplements can be used in addition to diet, rather than as a substitute.

The studies done to date have looked at different parameters. What matters most to people are their symptoms. What matters most to doctors are changes in lung function, which is generally measured as airflow. Researchers may measure symptoms and airflow, but they also measure other endpoints. These include evidence of inflammation in respiratory secretions, as well as reactivity of the bronchial tubes to various challenges administered in a laboratory, like methacholine, a chemical that constricts bronchial tubes, or to inhaled allergens.

Laboratory measurements usually improve well before there's a change in symptoms or in airflow measured outside the laboratory. Clinically meaningful endpoints may take time.

Omega-3s: Studies from around the World

Almost all the studies described here used a double-blind, randomized, placebo-controlled protocol. As I've stated before, that is considered the gold standard for clinical research.

- In one of the earliest studies, French researchers administered fish oil to a group of asthmatics and followed them for one year. After nine months, there was a significant improvement in measured airflow among those receiving fish oil when compared with those receiving placebos.[39]

- A Japanese study found that fish oil supplements helped asthmatics. After ten months of supplements, asthma symptom scores and airway hypersensitivity had significantly decreased.[40]

- Italian scientists tested people with seasonal asthma due to airborne allergens. They administered 3 grams a day of omega-3s to asthmatics for 30 days and saw a significant decrease in bronchial hyperreactivity compared with placebo. They retested their patients 30 days after the omega-3 supplementation was stopped and found that airway hyperreactivity had returned to pre-treatment levels, suggesting that omega-3 supplementation may need to be continued.[41]

- Scientists in England and in Germany tested the effects of fish oil supplements on the asthmatic response to inhaled allergens.

German researchers administered a relatively low dose of omega-3s (690 milligrams a day for five weeks) to people with asthma that was caused by allergy to dust mites. They observed a decrease in measures of bronchial inflammation when the patients were challenged with an aerosol containing dust mite allergen.[42]

English researchers administered six grams a day of omega-3s for ten weeks and demonstrated a significant improvement in the late-phase asthmatic response when their subjects were exposed to inhaled allergens.[43]

- U.S. researchers in the Human Performance Laboratory at Indiana University tested the effect of omega-3s on exercise-induced asthma. They administered 5.2 grams a day of omega-3s from fish oil for three weeks to asthmatics whose asthma consistently worsened with physical exertion. They found that fish oil aided in the prevention of exercise-induced asthma, reduced the measures of bronchial inflammation studied, and decreased the need for bronchodilator medication with exercise for the subjects in the study. They found similar effects among elite athletes who suffered from exercise-induced asthma.[44]

- Danish researchers conducted the kind of long-term experiment that can most readily be accomplished in a setting such as Scandinavia, where careful lifetime health records are maintained on everyone. Pregnant women were given 2.7 grams per day of omega-3s from fish oil, or were given an olive oil placebo, from week 30 of pregnancy until delivery.[45] The researchers followed the offspring of those pregnancies for sixteen years and found that in the teenagers whose mothers had taken fish oil late in pregnancy, the development of allergic asthma was 87 percent lower than in the control group.

- Swedish researchers at the Karolinska Institut, home of the Nobel Prize, demonstrated that fish oil supplements not only reduced the omega-6 to omega-3 ratio in blood but also decreased the production of potent mediators of inflammation in people with asthma.[46]

What these studies suggest is that omega-3 supplementation can help diminish asthmatic responses in diverse groups of people across the world. Changes in airway hyperreactivity can occur within a few weeks, but clinically significant improvement in asthmatic symptoms may take several months.

Alternative Sources of Omega-3s

Fish oils are not the only source of omega-3s that may help people with asthma. The research team at Indiana University's Human Performance Laboratory and another research group at Pavlov Medical University in St. Petersburg, Russia, tested omega-3s extracted from the New Zealand green-lipped mussel.

With the mussel omega-3s, the American team demonstrated a decrease in symptoms of asthma and in the use of asthma medication, along with decreased production of chemical mediators of inflammation and greater resistance to exercise-induced asthma.[47]

The Russian team found a significant decrease in daytime wheezing and in measures of oxidative stress and an increase in morning airflow in the mussel extract group, compared with the placebo group; the dose of omega-3s was only 100 milligrams a day.[48] Research conducted at the Okayama University Medical School in Japan compared the effects of perilla seed oil, a vegetarian source of omega-3s, with the effects of corn oil, which lacks omega-3s but is rich in omega-6s.[49] After two weeks, the perilla oil group showed reduced levels of asthma-provoking leukotrienes compared to the corn oil group. After four weeks, lung function was significantly better in the perilla oil group than in the corn oil group.

When Omega-3s Are Not Enough

Researchers at the University of Wyoming found a subgroup of asthmatics who actually got worse with high dose omega-3s. Unlike the good omega-3 responders, the poor responders showed no decrease in inflammatory leukotriene levels after receiving fish oils.[50]

One explanation for this paradoxical response to omega-3s can be found in the research I mentioned earlier that I conducted with Professors Horrobin and Rocklin in the 1980s. Some people with allergies may actually need special sources of omega-6 fats because of a block in the way their bodies utilize omega-6s. For these people, increasing omega-3 intake without addressing their omega-6 problem may make the omega-6 block even worse.

The solution might be to combine omega-3s with a unique anti-inflammatory omega-6 fatty acid called gamma-linolenic acid (GLA), which is found in evening primrose oil, black currant seed oil, and borage seed oil. Breastfed infants receive GLA in their mothers' milk. GLA can help overcome the block in omega-6 metabolism that my colleagues and I demonstrated in allergic individuals during the 1980s.

Medical research highlights:

- A mixture of GLA (750 mg/day) plus EPA (a purified omega-3, at only 500 mg/day) given for four weeks as a liquid emulsion to allergic asthmatics, produced a significant reduction in leukotriene production by white blood cells and also decreased asthma symptoms and the use of bronchodilator inhalers when compared with placebos. As a result, asthma-related quality of life was significantly improved.[51]

- At National Jewish Medical Center in Denver, one of the world's leading institutions for the study and treatment of respiratory diseases, a mixture of fish oil and borage seed oil, which is a source of GLA, was added to a liquid formula containing milk protein, whey, vitamins, and minerals and given to asthmatic children for 12 weeks.[52] The group receiving the oils had a greater decrease in oxidative stress and a greater increase in measured airflow than the group receiving whey and milk protein only.

- Egyptian physicians found that asthmatics responded better when vitamin C (200 mg/day) and zinc (15 mg/day) were given along with fish oil than when fish oil was given alone.[53]

I like to use omega-3s and sometimes GLA as part of a nutritional program such as the Immune Balance Diet, and I often add zinc, and select antioxidants as well.

The Ecology of Asthma

Your body is like a rain forest. It teems with life. A hundred trillion microbes carpet every surface, outside and in. There are many more microbes in your body than human cells, and their presence is essential for your health. They stimulate your immune system, help regulate your hormones, and protect you from unwanted inflammation. Your relationship with them is every bit as complicated as the ecology of the Amazon Basin—and it's in as much danger, from:

- The modern diet, packed with sugar and fat and depleted of fiber and flavonoids

- Continuous exposure to antibiotics, which permeate our food supply

- The use of antimicrobial soaps and shampoos

- The effects of chronic inflammation

All these factors disturb the relationship that has evolved between us and our old microbial friends. Our microbes are under siege, and we are paying the price. The allergy epidemic is part of that price. Asthma is one outcome.

Research on the impact of your body's ecology on asthma is just getting started, but there are two interesting research findings that I'd like to share with you now, because I've found them very important in my clinical practice.

- The microbes that colonize the airways of asthmatics are different from the microbes that colonize the airways of people without asthma. This is true not only for bacteria, but also for yeasts.[54] These differences may be the result of having asthma and not the initial cause of asthma itself. The types of microbes growing in asthmatic airways are more likely to provoke inflammation than the microbes growing in the airways of people without asthma. I've been studying the body's microbial ecology for more than 30 years, and I've seen that same pattern over and over again. Inflammation in any part of the body creates a local environment that favors the growth of microbes that promote further inflammation. This state is called dysbiosis. From the microbes' perspective, it makes perfect sense. They thrive on inflammation, so they provoke more of it. It doesn't really matter if microbes caused the problem to begin with. They become the problem.

- Intestinal microbes may have a profound effect on the development of allergy. Just as the loss of biodiversity weakens a rain forest, diminished diversity of gut microbes predisposes people to the development of allergy, probably by weakening protective immune responses.[55] This raises the possibility that the right probiotics may help people with allergies and with asthma.

Can Probiotics Help with Asthma?

Having a pet changes the ecology of your home and your body. Families with pets are more likely to share the same microbes, probably because everyone is cuddling the same pet. They're likely to have a greater diversity of microbes. And having a pet will change the microbes found in house dust.

Researchers at the University of California–San Francisco exposed mice to house dust obtained from a home with a pet dog and to house dust from a home without any pets. They then attempted to provoke allergic asthma in the mice by sensitizing them to cockroaches and egg white. Mice fed dust from the home with a dog were able to resist the development of allergy. When their gut microbes were examined, they had a much greater diversity of bacteria than mice fed dust from the home with no pets. One particular species of bacteria, *Lactobacillus johnsonii*, was strikingly present in the allergy-resistant mice. When the scientists fed *Lactobacillus johnsonii* to a fresh group of mice, feeding that single probiotic protected the mice against the development of allergic asthma.[56]

Study results in humans depend on the probiotic used and the design of the clinical trial. Here are two interesting research studies:

- Lactobacillus gasseri strain A5, given for eight weeks to children in Taiwan, significantly improved all the outcomes studied: lung function, symptoms, and measures of inflammation in blood.[57]

- *Lactobacillus reuteri* strain DSM 17938 was given for two weeks to Italian children with dust mite allergy who had well-controlled asthma. The probiotic was shown to reduce airway inflammation without influencing lung function.[58] This trial was too short. As we saw in the studies with omega-3s, two weeks is enough time to reduce inflammation but not enough time to improve lung function.

Research studies suggest that probiotic supplementation with selected strains of *Lactobacillus* or *Bifidobacteria* may be a helpful adjunct in reducing inflammation and symptoms of people with allergic asthma. The greatest benefits for any kind of supplementation are likely to occur when it's used as part of the full Allergy Solution program.

It was the full program that allowed my patient Alexa to keep her dream job.

Breathing Easy Again

Alexa was a 40-year-old reporter for a major news magazine who landed a job as bureau chief for India. This required that she spend a great deal of time in New Delhi, which is one of the most polluted cities in the world. Within weeks of starting her new job, an old childhood ailment that had been gone for decades reappeared: allergic asthma. Alexa's symptoms—wheezing, coughing, and difficulty breathing—were worse outdoors and fluctuated in severity with the level of air pollution.

She consulted a local physician and was treated with monteleukast pills and an inhaler that consisted of a steroid combined with a long-acting bronchodilator. This controlled her symptoms until a trip to Calcutta, during which she developed a lung infection, was hospitalized, and required oral steroids for control of her asthma. Back in New Delhi, she found that she could not discontinue the steroid pills. Each time she reduced the dose, her asthma would flare.

I first met Alexa during her vacation, when she visited New York to spend time with family. Her asthma improved somewhat in New York City, but she still noticed that automotive exhaust would make her nose burn, she'd wheeze in the subways, and she'd cough much of the night. Shortness of breath still kept her from exercising. She told me she felt like she couldn't escape the pollution and the symptoms it produced. Her case highlights the global nature of the air pollution problem.

When I examined Alexa, I could hear the wheezing in her lungs and see evidence of allergy in her nose, which had a pale and swollen lining, characteristic of people with nasal allergy. Her tongue had a heavy white coating. Culture of the coating grew out the yeast *Candida albicans*. High *Candida* growth in her mouth was undoubtedly a result of her use of steroids and had probably been aggravated by the antibiotics she'd been given in Calcutta the year before.

A skin test revealed that she was allergic to *Candida*, a finding that occurs in about a third of people with severe asthma.[59] Inhalation of *Candida* fragments from yeast growing in the mouth can provoke asthmatic symptoms in asthmatics with yeast allergy.[60] I've found this to be an important aggravating factor for many asthmatics over the course of my medical career.

In Alexa's case, I didn't think that *Candida* allergy was the primary trigger for her asthma. It was a secondary factor that resulted from the effects of medication, but it had to be addressed, because it was part of the vicious cycle of inflammation and dysbiosis that made it impossible for her to discontinue steroids.

I had four weeks to help Alexa restore her health so that she could return to work. We needed to enhance her ability to detoxify, build up her antioxidant defenses, and correct the dysbiosis that had resulted from her treatment with steroids and antibiotics.

I prescribed an antifungal medication to clear up the yeast overgrowth in her mouth. A single dose increased her wheezing, a sign of how severely allergic she was to the yeast growing in her body. As the organisms began to die, they released allergens that aggravated her asthma. That reaction let me know that *Candida* allergy was a critical trigger for Alexa.

I decided that antifungal medication would have to wait. We'd have to gently reduce her burden of yeast with herbs. I chose berberine, a very thoroughly studied compound that is a component of several widely used herbs. Not only can berberine kill yeast, it has antioxidant and anti-inflammatory effects and can suppress allergic responses in the blood cells of patients with food allergy.[61] Berberine was effective for Alexa, and after two weeks she was able to use the antifungal drug I'd originally prescribed.

As the month went on, she began tapering down her dose of steroids and discontinued monteleukast. I began to focus on building up her levels of the antioxidant glutathione, using methods I will explain in the next chapter. Alexa was not allergic to milk products and found that plain yogurt improved her breathing.

By the end of her vacation, Alexa was no longer taking steroids. She had no symptoms of asthma and her lung function was normal. She was following the Immune Balance Diet, and I explained to her how to continue this diet in India. Anti-inflammatory vegetables and spices are abundant there. Sabja seeds could replace chia seeds in the Smoothie. Yogurt is an Indian staple, so she might not even need a probiotic supplement.

She left for India and I held my breath. A month later she called to give me the good news: no cough, no wheezing, no shortness of breath. On the bad air days, she'd stay indoors, just to be safe. She left New Delhi shortly after, and her condition remained improved.

Alexa's view of her illness went like this:

- Air pollution inflamed her lungs and depleted her of antioxidants.

- Steroids and antibiotics created a dysbiosis that pushed her over the edge.

- *Candida* allergy coupled with *Candida* overgrowth created a downward spiral.

- The Allergy Solution Program helped her restore her health.

$190 Million for Research into Inner-City Asthma

Asthma prevalence is disproportionately high in the big cities. In the United States, you are more likely to have asthma if you:

Live in an inner city

Are part of a minority group

Are economically disadvantaged

Suffer from high levels of stress

Now a small ray of hope is headed to places that are being hit hard by the asthma epidemic. Funding to the tune of $190 million is coming from the National Institute of Allergy and Infectious Diseases to support the Inner-City Asthma Consortium.[62] This consortium is a multicenter effort to understand the causes of the asthma epidemic in urban centers and to develop treatments for prevention and control. The research is being led by scientists at the University of Wisconsin. Clinical centers participating include Johns Hopkins University, Columbia University, University of California–San Francisco, the University of Texas, and many others. They will explore:

- Risk factors for asthma in inner cities

- Treatment approaches to mouse and cockroach allergies

- Safety and efficacy of new treatments

Conclusion

Sarah's asthma attack and trip to the emergency room opened this chapter. Two million such visits to the hospital for asthma occur each year in the United States. Studies confirm that only a fraction of asthma cases are considered well controlled.

I presented highlights of the research on nutrition in managing asthma, then explored the role of oxidative stress; this led to a discussion of the potential of antioxidants from food to help reduce oxidative stress. I described a fascinating Australian study that showed how antioxidants from vegetables and fruits may help asthma. Next I shared the science on omega-3s and asthma, which suggests that many people could use an oil change.

I also looked at the relationship between the microbiome and asthma. Finally, the problem of air pollution and asthma was highlighted by the case of Alexa, a reporter whose asthma returned when she was confronted by air pollution.

Asthma requires the care of a health care professional, so I encourage you to bring this book with you when you see your doctor.

CHAPTER 13

THE SUPER-ALLERGY-FIGHTING ANTIOXIDANT

Rebecca works as a respiratory therapist at a hospital in New York City and ironically developed asthma about a year after starting work. At first glance this seems strange, because the job of a respiratory therapist is to help people with acute or chronic lung diseases breathe better. In fact, the science shows that Rebecca's case is not unusual. Respiratory therapists are three to five times more likely to develop asthma *after* they begin to work in respiratory care as before, an article in the prestigious journal *Annals of Internal Medicine* explains.[1]

In another study, an international team led by a University of Texas physician sought to uncover the reasons for the elevated level of asthma risk in health-care workers. Knowing environmental exposures to be a prime suspect, they looked into hospitals and found cleaning and disinfecting chemicals, building cleaning solutions, and various adhesives. They determined that "occupational exposures are important contributors to asthma in health care providers." In addition, they cite earlier research linking administration of aerosolized medications to higher asthma risk for health-care workers.[2]

I explained to Rebecca that all sorts of chemical aerosols, even household cleaning sprays, increase the risk of developing or aggravating asthma, as we saw in Chapter 5.

Rebecca was being treated daily with a combination of drugs—a steroid and a bronchodilator—that kept her asthma under control. As a respiratory therapist she knew the potential side effects of the medications and did not want to rely on them for the rest of her life. In order to help her overcome dependence on medication, I had to understand all the factors contributing to her chronic asthma.

Rebecca had lifelong allergies to dust and dust mites, those microscopic, spiderlike insects that feed on the debris from human skin. Exposure to these gave her a stuffed nose, which she still experienced most mornings. She also had chronically dry skin, which is common among people with allergies. She kept her apartment very clean and dust-free, used household cleansers labeled "all natural" and "nontoxic," and ran a humidifier all winter hoping that her skin would stay moist. I saw a problem there, and also a solution.

Indoor humidity encourages the growth of dust mites, as we saw in Chapter 5. So my first recommendation to Rebecca was that she measure the relative humidity in her apartment with an inexpensive device sold in most hardware stores. Technically it's called a hygrometer, but asking for a humidity meter is more likely to get you to the right place in the store. Mites thrive when the relative humidity is greater than 50 percent.

I recommended that Rebecca keep her home's humidity between 30 and 40 percent and that we find other ways to keep her skin moist—nutritional ways. For example, supplementation with fish oils and evening primrose oil, described in Chapter 12, not only can help asthmatic symptoms but may also help to keep skin moist, working from the inside. I also recommended mite control measures, as discussed in Chapter 5.

Although Rebecca had less control over her environment at work, there were important protective measures she could take: cleaning her equipment only in a well-ventilated space, avoiding spray cleaners as much as possible, and being careful to minimize the spread of nebulized medication into the air when administering aerosol treatments.

Next, I needed to understand Rebecca's diet and lifestyle. She lived with her boyfriend, enjoyed her work, went running three or four times a week, and ate a relatively healthy diet, low in sugar and better than the average North American diet, but with considerable room for improvement.

Because Rebecca was a runner, I thought she might be hyperventilating. About a third of all people hyperventilate—that is, they overbreathe from time to time—and hyperventilation due to exercise or psychological stress can trigger asthma attacks.[3] I told Rebecca about a simple, effective method of breath control that has been shown to help asthmatics reduce their reliance on medication.[4] It was developed by a Russian physician, Konstantin Buteyko, and is described in a book to which I wrote the foreword, *Breathing Free*, by Teresa Hale, founder of London's Hale Clinic. Instructional videos are available through Buteyko Centers in several countries.

As a professional respiratory therapist, Rebecca grasped Buteyko's method quickly and wondered why she'd never learned about it in her training.

Before thinking about next steps, I wanted to suggest some dietary changes. Once we determined that there wasn't a problem food for Rebecca I turned my attention to enriching her diet for enhanced respiratory health.

I asked her to increase consumption of cruciferous vegetables like broccoli, cauliflower, brussels sprouts, and kale, eating 170 to 225 grams of food from that family every day. I asked her to eat saltwater fish three times a week and to use nuts, like almonds and walnuts, as her main snack food. I asked her to avoid products containing soybean oil, telling her about the research at Northwestern University that I described in the last chapter.

The final step involved the powerful antioxidant glutathione. To enhance glutathione, Rebecca began using undenatured whey protein every day and 600 milligrams of the amino acid NAC three times a day. When her chronically stuffed nose began to clear, I decided it was okay to wean her slowly and cautiously off her asthma inhalers, first eliminating the bronchodilator, then the inhaled steroid, according to a closely monitored schedule. She's been off the inhalers for three years now.

Which component of Rebecca's treatment had the greatest impact: environmental changes, breathing control, diet, or glutathione enhancement? My view is that they were all important and worked together in synergy. And glutathione's contribution was crucial.

Your Body's Best Friend

Glutathione is your body's best antioxidant friend. You've already made its acquaintance in some of the earlier chapters of this book. Unseen and unsung, this friend has been working tirelessly behind the scenes to help you detoxify, balance your immune system, and much more. It's a key weapon in your arsenal for fighting allergic reactions, and now research from around the world is unlocking the potential for glutathione to help improve the condition of asthma as well.

Glutathione is the rock star of antioxidants. It is also a team player, supporting the functioning of vitamin C, vitamin E, and selenium in the body. Glutathione plays an especially important role in helping to maintain the health of your lungs, nose, and sinuses. In fact, it is the major antioxidant in the respiratory tract.

The research suggests that glutathione could be as important for people with nasal allergies and sinus problems as for asthmatics. Levels of glutathione in the nasal lining of people with chronic sinusitis are only half the levels found in people without sinusitis, observed a study from University Hospital Vrije Universiteit in Amsterdam. The greater the degree of inflammation, the lower the level of glutathione.[5]

Scientific studies usually examine only one variable at a time. In real life there are multiple variables that impact a condition like asthma all the time. I use multiple approaches to enhance glutathione levels because the combination can yield better results than any single approach.

Enhancing Glutathione with Food or Supplements

Foods and supplements that increase the body's stores of glutathione have been shown in research studies to help provide various potential benefits, which I highlight below. Decisions about whether and how to use them must be individualized. Just as health status and nutritional requirements vary from person to person, the most appropriate methods of enhancing glutathione will vary as well. Always consult your doctor before changing your nutrition routine or taking nutritional supplements.

Whey Protein

Whey supplies the amino acid cysteine, one of the building blocks your body uses to make glutathione. Availability of cysteine is a well-documented limiting factor for glutathione production. Consumption of whey protein at a dose of 30 to 45 grams a day (about two to three level tablespoons) by healthy young adults significantly raised the glutathione levels of their white blood cells in a study done at McGill University in Montreal.[6]

In adults with exercise-induced asthma, 30 grams of undenatured whey protein a day for four weeks improved postexercise airflow in a randomized, double-blind, placebo-controlled study.[7]

These research studies suggest that whey protein is potentially a beneficial source of antioxidants for people with asthma and can improve bronchial airflow. However, I do not recommend the use of whey protein by people with cow's milk allergy, because whey is derived from cow's milk. Milk allergy may occur in 10 percent of asthmatics.

NAC, a Building Block of Glutathione

N-acetylcysteine (NAC) is a rapidly absorbed form of the amino acid cysteine and is available as a dietary supplement. Its main antioxidant benefit derives from its conversion to glutathione.[8] Because NAC administration rapidly increases the synthesis of glutathione, it is used in hospitals to raise glutathione levels of people with liver failure from an overdose of the painkiller acetaminophen, which is best known by the brand name Tylenol. Acetaminophen has been shown to increase the risk of asthma, probably by depleting glutathione (see "Painkillers May Aggravate Asthma" on the next page).

Research on NAC vs. Air Pollution

Research is being done around the world on the potential of NAC to help alleviate asthma, especially when air pollution is involved. One of the major respiratory irritants in provoking asthma is diesel fumes from trucks, buses, and automobiles: asthmatics respond to these fumes with increased asthma symptoms, airway hyperirritability, and inflammation. Recent research has demonstrated the ability of NAC in pill form to help reverse the aggravation of asthma produced by exposure to diesel fumes. This effect is probably caused by increasing glutathione levels in the respiratory tract.

Scientists at the University of British Columbia studied the protective effect of NAC for asthmatics who were exposed to diesel exhaust. They also measured the restriction in airflow produced by exposure to the chemical methacholine, which causes bronchial narrowing.[9] They found that taking 600 milligrams of NAC three times a day for six days reduced baseline bronchial reactivity to methacholine by 20 percent and prevented the increase in hyperreactivity provoked by diesel fumes for the participants in the study. These protective effects of NAC were associated with a decrease in measures of oxidative stress.[10] Of course you should always avoid diesel fumes and other sources of air pollution.

NAC, taken for three months, has also been shown to be helpful in promoting healing of laryngopharyngeal reflux, a disturbance in upper gastrointestinal function that is closely linked to asthma (see Chapter 9).[11]

Laboratory studies from the University of Valencia in Spain suggest that NAC inhibits activation of eosinophils and could be a useful treatment of allergic inflammation.[12] And NAC may prevent some aspects of the scarring and airway remodeling that occur in chronic asthma, according to laboratory research done in Japan.[13] All these effects are likely to be due to the ability of NAC to serve as a precursor of glutathione.

The timing of supplementing with NAC is important. It has a short life span in the blood. A single dose disappears rapidly, and more effective levels are achieved if NAC is given at a moderate dose three times a day rather than at a high dose once a day. At 600 milligrams of NAC three times a day for five days, glutathione levels in red blood cells increase by 50 percent.[14]

Warning: NAC may interfere with the action of some drugs used to treat cancer. If you are undergoing treatment for cancer, discuss all use of dietary supplements with your doctor.

Painkillers May Aggravate Asthma

Painkillers of different types may aggravate asthma. Aspirin and drugs like ibuprofen (Advil and Motrin) and naproxen (Aleve and Naprosyn) have long been known to precipitate asthma attacks in susceptible people, especially those with nasal polyps. Acetaminophen (Tylenol) has a subtler long-range influence on asthma. Your liver converts it to a highly toxic chemical that requires glutathione for its removal. Taking acetaminophen increases your need for glutathione, and if that need is not met, glutathione deficiency readily results, with disastrous consequences. By depleting glutathione, daily use of acetaminophen reduces total antioxidant capacity in your blood in as little as two weeks.[15]

Exposure to acetaminophen during the first year of life is associated with an increased risk of developing childhood asthma, according to research from the University of Coimbra in Portugal. Use of acetaminophen by children with a family history of asthma is also associated with an increased risk of developing asthma, as is regular use of the drug by adults. A recent scientific review stated: "There is substantial epidemiological evidence in adults and children that acetaminophen use is associated with asthma symptoms."[16]

Helping Glutathione Do Its Job

Your friend glutathione needs co-factors—vitamins and minerals that help it work properly. You can think of them as a friend of a friend. They help glutathione to perform its antioxidant functions in your body.

Selenium from Food Sources

Selenium is an essential mineral, with a recommended daily allowance (RDA) for healthy adults of 55 micrograms per day. The foods richest in selenium are Brazil nuts (two a day can supply the RDA), saltwater fish, and whole grains grown in selenium-rich soil.

Selenium is not itself an antioxidant, but it plays a critical role in allowing glutathione to do its job. When glutathione works as an antioxidant, it essentially sacrifices itself. It helps to restore the oxidant/antioxidant balance in cells by allowing itself to become oxidized. In doing so, it goes from its active antioxidant form, called GSH, to its oxidized and less active state, called GSSG. The enzyme that permits this is glutathione peroxidase (GPx). GPx depends on selenium for its activity.

Selenium and Asthma

Several studies have found reduced dietary intake or blood levels of selenium in asthmatics when compared with controls.[17] A few clinical trials have found beneficial effects of selenium supplementation at a level of 200 micrograms per day in adults with asthma. The benefits, according to the research, may include improvement in airflow, decreased need for inhaled steroids, and decreased inflammation as measured by the levels of chemical mediators called soluble adhesion molecules, which are part of the late-phase asthmatic reaction.[18]

After Brazil nuts, which may contain as much as 544 micrograms of selenium per 28 grams (almost ten times the recommended daily allowance in 20 nuts), the richest food sources of selenium are seafood and organ meats. Other sources include muscle meats, cereals and other grains, and dairy products.

The amount of selenium in plants depends on the amount of selenium in the soil and several other factors, such as soil pH, amount of organic matter in the soil, and whether the selenium is in a form that is amenable to plant uptake. As a result, selenium concentrations in plant-derived foods vary widely by geographic location. Because the selenium content of soil affects the amount of selenium in the plants that animals eat, the quantity of selenium in animal products can also vary widely.

Magnesium from Food Sources

Magnesium is an essential mineral that affects the activity of hundreds of enzymes in your body. Its major dietary sources are green vegetables, nuts, seeds, beans, and seafood. People can maintain good magnesium levels by eating foods rich in magnesium.

The top food sources of magnesium are:

- **Vegetables:** buckwheat, kidney beans, navy beans, soybeans, green beans, spinach, black-eyed peas, Swiss chard, broccoli, kale

- **Fruits:** bananas, watermelon, mangoes, dates, dried figs, blackberries

- **Nuts and seeds:** almonds, cashews, Brazil nuts, hazelnuts

Magnesium and Asthma

Higher dietary magnesium in the general population is associated with a decreased risk of inflammation and a decreased risk of wheezing and bronchial hyperreactivity. In people with chronic lung disease, reduced magnesium in the blood is linked to impairment of antioxidant defenses.[19]

When children with allergic asthma were given 12 weeks of magnesium supplementation (200 to 300 milligrams per day, depending upon age), the level of GSH in their red blood cells increased and their need for asthma inhalers decreased.[20]

Studies done in several countries have demonstrated similar benefits for magnesium supplementation in adolescents and adults. For teenagers with allergic asthma who needed steroid inhalers, 300 milligrams of magnesium per day for eight weeks reduced asthmatic symptoms and bronchial reactivity to methacholine, permitting decreased steroid doses, and also diminished allergen-induced skin test responses.[21] Improvement in symptoms and lung function has been seen in adults with mild to moderate asthma who received 340 milligrams of magnesium per day.[22] This level of magnesium intake is readily achieved through a healthy, plant-based diet. The Immune Balance Smoothie, consumed just once a day, meets half the magnesium needs of a healthy adult.

Stress can deplete your body's stores of magnesium by increasing its excretion through your kidneys. This appears to be the result of stress hormones like adrenaline, which blocks the uptake of magnesium into cells. High stress and low magnesium create a vicious cycle. People with low magnesium levels are more susceptible to the jarring effects of stress and produce more adrenaline when stressed, which aggravates the magnesium deficit in their cells. Improved stress management is a key part of the Allergy Solution, as described in Chapter 10.

Adrenaline: A Two-Edged Sword

Adrenaline is a powerful bronchodilator, and injections of adrenaline are given to treat acute asthma attacks. Adrenaline has some powerful side effects, however, which include rapid heartbeat, high blood pressure, and anxiety.

Bronchodilators are drugs with adrenaline-like effects taken as inhaled aerosols for treating asthma. They have the same side effects as injected adrenaline. The most common bronchodilator is albuterol.

A study done in the emergency department of Denver General Hospital found that frequent use of albuterol by nebulizer resulted in a significant decline in serum magnesium levels over 90 minutes.[23] When inhaled or oral bronchodilators are used as the only treatment for asthma, there is an increased risk of serious side effects.[24] A Canadian study found that people who relied on inhaled bronchodilators as the primary treatment of asthma had a higher rate of hospitalization and emergency room visits.[25] Magnesium depletion might be one mechanism for the side effects of bronchodilators.

To improve your magnesium status, increase your consumption of magnesium-rich foods: green vegetables like broccoli and leafy greens, beans, and nuts, picking those to which you have no allergy.

Vitamin C, Enzymes, and GSH

The effects of vitamin C in asthma appear to be quite variable and may depend upon its close relationship with glutathione, the level of air pollution, and the enzymes that utilize glutathione for detoxification and antioxidation, rather than any direct antioxidant effect of vitamin C in the lung.

Supplementation with vitamin C raises glutathione levels but has no effect on levels of vitamin C itself in respiratory secretions.[26] Vitamin C's antioxidant effect may be due to its ability to enhance GSH. A little-known effect of vitamin C supplementation is to increase the activity of GPx and also to increase activity of the enzyme that recycles GSSG back to GSH, an enzyme called glutathione reductase (GR).[27] This effect increases the ability of glutathione to function as an antioxidant.

Research on the health benefits of vitamin C in asthma has shown inconsistent results. These inconsistencies may be related to genetics and environment. People are most likely to need supplemental vitamin C if they have genetic deficiencies of detoxifying enzymes called glutathione-S-transferase enzymes (GSTs) and are also exposed to higher levels of air pollution.

GSTs use glutathione to enhance detoxification. They attach glutathione to a toxic substance so that it can be eliminated from the body. People with genetic defects of GSTs develop reduced levels of vitamin C in blood, probably because their level of oxidative stress is greater.[28] In some populations they are more susceptible to developing asthma.[29] Asthmatic children with defective GST genes are more susceptible to the irritant effects of ozone than are asthmatic children with normal GST genes. They are also more strongly harmed by reduced dietary vitamin C than are asthmatics with normal GST genes.[30]

The first step in improving vitamin C status is to increase intake of foods, like tomatoes and citrus fruit, that are rich in vitamin C. If you are exposed to higher levels of air pollution and have defects in the enzymes of detoxification, you may also benefit from vitamin C supplements.

Conclusion

This section focused on the globe-spanning research into glutathione, the superstar of antioxidants. Glutathione plays a key role in detoxification and is the major antioxidant in the respiratory tract. It works together with vitamin C and other antioxidants to protect against inflammatory damage to your body's cells and tissues.

I reviewed the research on enhancing glutathione levels and effects through nutrition. I introduced the nutrients that assist glutathione in its important functions, magnesium and selenium, and pointed out delicious food sources of them. We saw that inflammation is linked to lower glutathione levels and that common painkillers can deplete the body of glutathione.

I encourage you to bring the advances in nutrition and lifestyle presented here with you when you see your doctor. Always consult your doctor before changing your nutrition routine or taking nutritional supplements.

CHAPTER 14

WHAT HAPPENS IN YOUR GUT DOESN'T STAY IN YOUR GUT

Anne's first migraine occurred on her first day of middle school, which was more than 20 years ago. Her parents chalked it up to nerves. Anne coped with each headache by taking over-the-counter ibuprofen and lying down in a dark room until it passed. Fortunately, they were few and far between.

But when a blinding headache prevented Anne from completing the SATs, her doctor referred her to a neurologist, who prescribed Imitrex, a drug that specifically targets migraine headache. After that, Anne was always careful to keep a blister pack of this migraine medicine in her purse, because migraine medication often works best if taken at the onset of symptoms.

Anne's headaches were usually preceded by changes in vision. Objects would begin to look uneven and jagged, as if she were viewing them in a broken mirror. This forerunner of headache is called an aura. Once Anne noticed a migraine aura, she had about 15 minutes to pop an Imitrex before excruciating pain would begin penetrating one side of her head.

If the Imitrex didn't work quickly enough, she'd take the pain reliever naproxen a half hour later. The drugs usually relieved her headaches. The migraines were infrequent and easily controlled, for the time being.

Anne married right after college and gave birth to twins a year later. Once they were in school full-time, Anne began work as a paralegal at a new law firm in Montclair, New Jersey, where she lived. She shared her job with another local woman, which gave them both flexibility in balancing the responsibilities of work and motherhood.

Anne's children and the law practice grew at the same time, and Anne began working longer and longer hours. Then her migraine headaches began to interfere with her work. First their frequency increased. She found herself taking migraine medication every week. Then the medication stopped working well.

Anne saw a headache specialist, who changed the medications and gave her a list of foods to avoid: aged cheeses, chocolate, citrus fruits, hot dogs, aged meats, wine, beer, vinegar, onions, nuts, and food containing the flavor enhancer MSG (monosodium glutamate) or the artificial sweetener aspartame. The doctor's theory was that certain foods trigger migraines because they contain chemicals that cause blood vessels around the brain to constrict.[1]

Anne began to notice a connection between food and headaches, but headache control was not nearly as simple as just avoiding the foods on the list. Initially orange juice and chocolate seemed to be the main triggers. Then she discovered that cottage cheese was just as likely to trigger a headache as aged cheddar. When she avoided one group of foods, her headaches would improve for a few weeks and then get worse as new foods seemed to become triggers. She also realized that not eating anything for six hours might trigger a headache. This discovery just added to her confusion.

Unable to establish a clear set of migraine triggers, Anne gave up on dietary control. Her neurologist prescribed a series of drugs for headache prevention. Each one produced troublesome side effects, which ranged from fatigue to weight gain to anxiety, depending on the drug. She took a leave from her job. These headaches also placed enormous stress on Anne's marriage. She seemed to have so many inconsistent migraine triggers that her husband began to doubt whether the headaches were real.

When I met Anne, I realized that the first problem we had to confront was her confusion about food. Like most people who suffer from migraines, she had numerous triggers, but the advice she'd received about diet had not been thorough enough. It was based on the idea that certain chemicals found in foods could trigger migraines directly, acting like drugs to change blood flow to the brain. Although that theory is frequently stated, it is not supported by research.[2] As I'll explain below, the mechanism of food-induced migraine is usually allergy, a reaction in which the immune system amplifies the effect of a trigger.

I first explained to Anne that food-induced migraine is a very real disorder. The Women's Health Study, conducted at Harvard Medical School, followed 65,000 female health professionals for about ten years. Almost 15 percent of these women experienced migraine headaches. Among the women with migraines, almost half noted that specific foods triggered them. Having food as a trigger was strongly associated with greater migraine severity.[3]

Scientists have shown that food-induced migraine is actually an allergic disorder, not just a disorder of the brain's chemistry. Consider these research findings:

- All four types of allergic reaction described in Chapter 3 have been identified in people with migraine during and between attacks.[4]

- Migraines are strongly associated with other allergic illnesses, like asthma and rhinitis, which may go undetected if they're not searched for carefully.[5]

- Allergy desensitization treatment can decrease the frequency and severity of migraines.[6]

Although Anne was not aware of having nasal allergies, my examination revealed a telltale sign of allergic rhinitis: the lining of her nose looked swollen and pale. When I questioned her, she thought for a moment and then said, "Actually, my nose is stuffed up most of the time. I guess I'm just used to it."

I also observed that her abdomen was somewhat distended and tender. This reflected another set of common symptoms that had passed under Anne's radar: abdominal discomfort and gas. The Women's Health Study found that symptoms like abdominal bloating occur in about a quarter of women with migraines and, like food sensitivity, are associated with greater severity of headache.

I explained to Anne that to really understand the root causes of her migraines, we'd have to start by analyzing the function of her GI tract.

She didn't say anything, but the look on her face said, "I'm seeing you about headaches and you want to start with my gut?"

So I explained that whenever I evaluate a patient with multiple food sensitivities, the first question I ask is: What's happening in this person's gastrointestinal tract? The specific symptoms vary. The person might have headaches, eczema, hives, joint pain, mood swings, attention deficit disorder, hyperactivity, fatigue, abdominal pain, or dizziness.

If numerous foods are triggers, I will usually find a disturbance in the small intestine that's been called leaky gut. What happens in the gut doesn't stay in the gut. It travels throughout your body. Treatment that heals a leaky gut often heals food allergies.

The Surprising Truth about Your Gut

You think of your gut as the place where you digest food and absorb nutrients. That's only natural. Digestion and absorption are your GI tract's most critical activities. Your brain lets you know when they're needed by sending you a signal that says, "Feed me. I'm hungry."

But the jobs performed by your gut are actually much larger and more extensive than you ever imagined:

- Your gut is the largest organ of your immune system. Over two-thirds of your body's lymphocytes are found in the lining of the small intestine. From that base they travel throughout your body sending signals that influence immunity in all other organs. Your small intestine is where oral tolerance begins. As I described in Chapter 3, oral tolerance is the normal, healthy way for your body to respond to food, absorbing the nutrients and not reacting to the allergens. It's an active process, controlled by your T-reg cells.

- Your GI tract has its own nervous system, called the enteric nervous system (ENS). The ENS has been called the second brain. It contains as many nerve cells as your spinal cord and is in constant communication with your brain. In fact, crosstalk between your brain and your ENS accounts for some of the benefits of mind-body therapies in alleviating allergy. A fascinating experiment conducted in the Netherlands demonstrated that a mind-body training program could decrease the inflammatory response to gut-derived toxins.[7]

- Your gut is home to trillions of microbes, which include a thousand different species of bacteria, a few dozen types of yeast and an unknown number of viruses. Collectively, these are called the gut flora, or microbiome. Discovering how these microbes influence human health and illness has been a major quest of mine for over three decades. In the past few years, research into gut flora has blossomed into one of the most important areas of applied medical science. Creating a healthy floral population is the main goal of the technique I call reflorastation, which I describe later in this chapter.

- The gastrointestinal tract is an organ of detoxification. The intestinal lining is rich in detoxifying enzymes. Your gut and your liver work together to prevent noxious substances from reaching your tissues and to remove them from your body. Intestinal lining cells and the intestinal immune system create a protective barrier that defends your body against the damaging effects of toxins and allergens found in your gut.

These multiple functions of the digestive system interact with each other and with the food you eat to regulate your immune responses, your nutritional state, your metabolism, your pattern of sleep, and even your moods.

Leaky Gut Leads to Migraines

With leaky gut, there is excessive absorption of gut-derived toxins and food-derived allergens. The ability of the intestinal lining to create a protective barrier is compromised and oral tolerance fails, creating a vicious cycle. Exposure to food allergens now creates an allergic response that further inflames the lining of the small intestine and makes the leaky gut lining even leakier.

I've been writing and lecturing about leaky gut syndromes for 25 years. During that time, the recognition that leaky gut plays a significant role in allergy and inflammatory diseases has moved into the medical mainstream. At one time patients would tell me, "My doctor says there's no such thing as a leaky gut." Now the term appears in the most prestigious and conservative scientific journals.

European researchers have found links between migraine headache and leaky gut:

- Dutch scientists observed associations between migraines and gastrointestinal disorders. They state: "People who regularly experience GI symptoms have a higher prevalence of headaches . . . [U]nderlying mechanisms of migraine and GI diseases could be increased gut permeability and inflammation."[8] "Increased gut permeability" is the polite term for leaky gut.

- Josef Egger, the German neurologist whose outstanding research I described earlier in this book, provided a clear explanation for the links between food allergy, leaky gut, and migraine headache, which explains why headache may not develop until 48 hours after exposure to the food trigger.[9] He suggested that eating a food to which you're allergic causes inflammation in your intestines that makes the intestinal lining leaky. The leaky gut then allows excessive absorption of toxic substances produced by intestinal bacteria or derived from food. It is these toxins that are the ultimate cause of pain.

Sugar can also cause an increase in intestinal permeability, which may be additive with the effects of allergy. The synergy between sugar and allergens may explain why so many people with food allergies find that eating sugar makes their allergies worse.

A colleague of mine at Purdue University, Laura Stevens, has done important research bringing to light nutritional aspects of attention deficit/hyperactivity disorder in children. She's written about the toxic effects of food dyes on the brain, which are well substantiated by scientific evidence. Laura and I have both found that exposure to dietary sugar or food allergens can make children more susceptible to the toxic effects of food dyes. We believe that increased intestinal permeability due to sugar or allergen exposure allows increased penetration of these food additives into the body, producing changes in behavior.[10] Allergy and toxicity are therefore part of a vicious cycle in which allergy drives the forces that permit increased toxicity.

Testing for Leaky Gut

In order to fully assess Anne's GI function, I ordered two tests. The first was a test for intestinal permeability: Anne would need to drink a special solution and then collect her urine to see how much of that solution was being absorbed. The second test was a specialized stool test designed to analyze multiple components of her gut flora and the efficiency of her digestion.

The results were definitive. Anne had a marked increase in intestinal permeability (that is, a very leaky gut). She also had a complete absence of two groups of normal bacteria called *Lactobacillus* and *Bifidobacteria*. You may know the genus *Lactobacillus* through its best known species, *L. acidophilus*. I discussed the potential benefits of *Lactobacillus* and *Bifidobacteria* taken as probiotics for relieving symptoms of nasal allergies in Chapter 11 and asthma in Chapter 12.

Finally, Anne had reduced levels of pancreatic enzymes in her stool, with an elevation of undigested dietary fat, indicating impaired pancreatic function and malabsorption. Poor digestive function was likely to account for a fourth set of abnormalities, which were found in the blood tests I ordered: Anne showed very low blood levels of vitamin D and zinc.

All these abnormalities were undoubtedly related to one another. Probiotics like *Lactobacillus*, for example, can support the maintenance of normal intestinal permeability.[11] Pain relievers like ibuprofen and naproxen have been shown to greatly reduce the levels of *Lactobacilli* in the GI tract. This may be one mechanism by which they produce the well-known side effect of damage in the gut.[12] For the best treatment response, we'd need to correct all these abnormalities.

Armed with this information, I prepared a plan for reducing Anne's migraines by healing her gut. I call it the ARC program, which stands for:

- Avoidance
- Reflorastation
- Cultivation

I've used this program to treat many different kinds of allergic, inflammatory, and autoimmune disorders. It's not a treatment for any one disease. It's a treatment for one underlying cause of many different diseases.

The ARC of Healing

Stage One: Avoidance

The first step in healing a leaky gut is elimination of any exposure that damages the intestinal lining. The most common such exposures are drugs, infections, and foods.

- **Drugs** that increase intestinal permeability are mostly in the class called NSAIDS, which includes aspirin and pain relievers like ibuprofen and naproxen. A list of these is shown in the box on page 250. Anne had used several of these to control the pain of headache.

  Anne's path to healing: I advised her to stop pain relievers and rely on her migraine-specific medication while she completed other parts of the Allergy Solution program.

- **Infections** of the gut create a state of GI inflammation that increases intestinal permeability. For people with food allergy, the most important infections in my experience are caused by single-cell parasites, like *Giardia lamblia* and various amoebas, and by yeasts like *Candida albicans*.[13] In earlier chapters I gave examples of patients for whom these infections caused allergic illness. I search for infections like these in every patient I see with multiple food sensitivities. Some of the most dramatic reversals of allergy in my years of clinical practice have resulted from the identification and treatment of unsuspected GI infections.

- **Foods** may create a leaky gut in two distinct ways:

  - A typical Western diet, high in sugar and saturated fats, increases intestinal permeability and produces a state of systemic inflammation that's been called metabolic endotoxemia.[14] Daily alcohol consumption can also create a leaky gut with systemic inflammation.[15] The Immune Balance Diet is an antidote for both of these. I designed it to be a foundation for gut healing.

- Consuming foods to which you're allergic produces inflammation in the GI tract that makes it leaky. The Power Wash and Re-entry protocols are intended to help you identify and eliminate those foods while adopting a varied and nutritious diet.

  Anne's path to healing: Anne needed the systematic approach offered by Power Wash, Re-entry, and the Immune Balance Diet to identify the best foods for her to eat. She discovered that dairy, yeast, and corn were her principal trigger foods. By avoiding them and eating a nutritious, well-balanced, and varied diet according to the principles outlined in Chapter 8, she brought the frequency and severity of her headaches down to a manageable level.

Nonsteroidal Anti-inflammatory Drugs (NSAIDs)

Aspirin
Choline and magnesium salicylates
Choline salicylate
Celecoxib
Diclofenac
Diflunisal
Etodolac
Fenoprofen
Flurbiprofen
Ibuprofen

Indomethacin
Ketoprofen
Magnesium salicylate
Meclofenamate sodium
Mefenamic acid
Meloxicam
Nabumetone
Naproxen
Oxaprozin
Piroxicam
Salsalate
Sodium salicylate
Sulindac
Tolmetin sodium

Stage Two: Reflorastation

Gut bacteria can have a profound effect on intestinal permeability. Beneficial microbes stimulate your cells to produce a healthy intestinal barrier. Their absence is one cause of a leaky gut.

Belgian scientists explored the role of gut flora and leaky gut in alcohol addiction and withdrawal.[16] Using a laboratory measure of intestinal permeability, they divided their study population of chronic alcoholics into those with high permeability and those with normal permeability. The high-permeability (leaky gut) group had higher scores of depression, anxiety, and alcohol craving than the normal-permeability group. The leaky gut group also showed greater levels of systemic inflammation and a distinct pattern of changes in their gut flora. Compared to alcoholics with normal permeability, those with high permeability were deficient in *Bifidobacteria*, which are known for their anti-inflammatory effects. These scientists propose that for some alcoholics (about half of the total), drinking alcohol alters gut flora to deplete protective bacteria, increasing intestinal permeability and producing systemic inflammation, which aggravates the psychological disturbances found with alcohol addiction.

Can Probiotics Help Leaky Gut?

Several teams of scientists have studied the impact of probiotic supplements on intestinal permeability in people under different conditions of stress:

- Italian physicians administered *Lactobacillus rhamnosus* strain GG to subjects with abdominal pain for eight weeks. Compared with the placebo, the probiotic improved intestinal permeability and produced a significant reduction in pain.[17]

- When scientists in Finland gave the same probiotic strain to subjects with eczema caused by food allergy, they demonstrated a decrease in intestinal inflammation and improvement in severity of eczema.[18]

- A German team administered two strains of *Lactobacilli*, *L. rhamnosus* 19070-2 and *L. reuteri* DSM 12246, to subjects with severe allergic eczema. The probiotic combination improved intestinal permeability and reduced GI symptoms.[19]

Several different types of probiotics can help to heal a leaky gut. My clinical experience has shown me that there is no ideal probiotic strain for this purpose. The effects differ from person to person. For some people, fermented foods like yogurt, sauerkraut, or kimchi may be the best sources of probiotic bacteria.

For others, specific probiotic supplements can make the difference. Although you can't feel the leakiness of your gut, you can feel digestive symptoms like gas, bloating, and the quality of bowel movements. What you want from your gut is an absence of symptoms. When it works well, it does its job quietly, without talking back to you, and you barely know that it exists. The right probiotics for you can help you achieve that state. Any probiotic that aggravates gas, bloating, gurgling, constipation, or diarrhea is probably wrong for your gut.

I recommended two probiotics for Anne. One was a mixture of *Lactobacilli* that included *L. plantarum.* As its name implies, *L.*

plantarum comes from plants and is found in naturally fermented foods like sauerkraut; several strains have been shown to tighten the intestinal barrier, reversing leaky gut in human clinical trials.[20] The other was *Bifidobacterium infantis*, which has been shown to heal leaky gut in laboratory animals.[21] *B. infantis* also stimulates activity of T-reg cells.[22] You may remember from Chapter 3 that T-regs are lymphocytes that work to counteract and prevent allergic reactions. They are a critical component of the protective immune response that leads to oral tolerance.

The most rapid effect of these probiotics was to reduce Anne's gut discomfort.

Stage Three: Cultivation

Think of your gut as a garden. Weeding, seeding, and planting are not enough. You need to cultivate the soil. A nutritious diet, rich in plant fiber, is an essential step in healing a leaky gut. Other components of the Immune Balance Diet, specifically designed for the Allergy Solution program, provide additional enhancement of normal intestinal permeability, as demonstrated in laboratory studies. These components include:

- The anti-inflammatory spice turmeric, which flavors the Immune Balance Soup[23]

- The tea flavonoid, found in oolong and green tea[24]

- Sulforaphane, the broccoli compound found in the Immune Balance Smoothie when broccoli sprout powder is added; sulforaphane is also liberated from cooked broccoli by the addition of fresh daikon radish to the Immune Balance Soup[25]

Sometimes supplements of vitamins or minerals are needed, especially when there's a preexisting deficiency. Two supplements were important for Anne's treatment: vitamin D and zinc.

Vitamin D, Allergy, and Leaky Gut

Lack of vitamin D impairs intestinal barrier function, contributing to leaky gut.[26] Because food sources of vitamin D are few and its main source is sunlight, low blood levels of vitamin D are very common outside the tropics. It's unclear whether vitamin D deficiency is a cause of allergies, but some studies indicate that vitamin D supplementation can alleviate symptoms associated with allergy:

- A study done at the University of Nebraska looked at the effects of vitamin D supplementation for people suffering from chronic urticaria (hives). Vitamin D at a dose of 4,000 international units (IU) a day reduced the number and severity of hives and the degree of itching, so that sleep quality improved.[27]

- Patients with migraine headache and low vitamin D levels were shown to experience a dramatic reduction in migraine frequency when vitamin D supplementation was added to their migraine medication.[28] The doses administered ranged from 400 to 4,000 IU per day, depending upon the severity of the deficiency.

- Vitamin D supplementation for asthmatics allowed a reduction of up to 75 percent in the doses of inhaled steroids needed to control asthma. As blood levels of vitamin D went up, the rate of asthma attacks went down.[29] This study was conducted at 20 U.S. medical centers, coordinated by the National Institutes of Health, and published in *JAMA*, the Journal of the American Medical Association. It was widely reported in the media to show no benefits of vitamin D supplementation for asthmatics, but a careful reading of the results indicates that the press reports misrepresented the actual findings. If you have asthma and your blood levels of vitamin D are low, raising those blood levels can help you achieve better asthma control with less medication.

- Children with asthma due to dust mite allergy were given vitamin D supplementation (650 IU per day) in addition to allergy desensitization shots. The addition of vitamin D doubled the rate at which children were able to discontinue their use of inhaled steroids. Higher vitamin D levels seem to generate greater activity of T-reg cells.[30]

Zinc vs. Leaky Gut

Low blood levels of zinc frequently accompany a leaky gut. Zinc is an essential mineral with critical effects on immune function. Lack of zinc causes a breakdown of all barrier cells in your body, from the gut to the skin. Supplementation with zinc helps to correct excessive intestinal permeability and reduce gut inflammation in children with diarrhea.[31]

Scientists at Imperial College London demonstrated the potency of zinc in preventing the increased intestinal permeability caused by a powerful NSAID, indomethacin. Of all NSAID pain relievers, indomethacin does the most GI damage. The British researchers gave indomethacin to healthy human volunteers and demonstrated a tripling of intestinal permeability in just five days. When they co-administered a special form of zinc called zinc carnosine, there was no increase in intestinal permeability with indomethacin.[32]

Zinc has also shown potential for asthma. When asthmatics with low zinc levels were given 50 milligrams of zinc a day for eight weeks, they showed a significant improvement in lung function and a decrease in symptoms like cough, wheezing, and shortness of breath.[33]

What Are Prebiotics?

Probiotics are beneficial microbes taken as food or supplements. I've discussed their use in the treatment of nasal allergies and asthma. Prebiotics are something else: complex carbohydrates that your GI tract does not digest or absorb, so they travel intact through your small and large intestines and selectively encourage the growth of beneficial bacterial flora. Mother's milk is rich in prebiotics that encourage the growth of *Bifidobacteria*. The prebiotics in mother's milk are responsible for many of the health benefits of breastfeeding.

Fiber and resistant starch are components of solid foods with prebiotic effects. Resistant starch, as its name implies, resists digestion. It's found in foods such as bananas, plantains, beans, peas, and sweet potatoes. Many commercial prebiotics contain inulin, which is derived from chicory.

Italian researchers from the Laboratory of Experimental Biochemistry at the National Institute for Digestive Diseases in Bari fed inulin-enriched pasta to healthy volunteers who had no GI problems. It enhanced intestinal permeability and actually made "normal" laboratory results become even more normal.[34] HIV infection, the cause of AIDS, produces a marked increase in intestinal permeability. Prebiotics can help to reverse the leaky gut of people with HIV and improve their immune function.[35]

Because Anne had low blood levels of vitamin D and zinc, I had her supplement with vitamin D3 and zinc carnosine. I also recommended that she add a prebiotic powder to the Immune Balance Smoothie. There are many types of prebiotics available. For intestinal healing and allergy reversal, one choice is to use one based on a complex sugar called galacto-oligosaccharides, which is the main prebiotic in human breast milk.

By the time she began supplementation, Anne had already removed the food triggers for migraines from her diet and had significantly decreased the frequency and severity of her headaches. Adding probiotics, prebiotics, zinc, and vitamin D helped her to restore normal intestinal permeability over the next three months.

Within six months there was a dramatic reduction in her food allergies. As her gut healed, she became able to eat numerous trigger foods without developing any symptoms.

Anne's treatment was not a treatment for migraine headaches. It was a treatment to heal a leaky gut and alleviate food allergy. Restoring normal intestinal permeability freed her of her headaches.

The Allergy Solution Program for a Healthy Gut Microbiome

Leaky gut and the depletion of beneficial intestinal microbes through exposure to antibiotics and pesticides in food, and from a lack of dietary fiber and diversity, is an emerging factor in the rise of allergies. The solution is a whole-food, plant-based way of eating that I present in this book, which is designed to greatly improve detoxification, boost antioxidant status, and restore a healthy gut microbiome, with the help of probiotics and prebiotics.

The race to uncover the mysteries of the human microbiome and the profound implications for our health is one of the hottest areas of medical inquiry today. What has been discovered thus far offers a tantalizing glimpse into how we evolved together with these microbes and share our bodies and the earth with them. Our health destiny may very well depend on how well we can nurture our relationship with this community.

How can *you* maintain a healthy diversity of bacteria in your gut?

- Eat a varied, high-fiber diet that is rich in fruits and vegetables. The flavonoids found in fruits and vegetables act like conductors to encourage the growth of diverse bacteria. Fermented foods, like sauerkraut, kimchi, and yogurt, and raw foods also tend to increase diversity of gut bacteria. Resistant starch, found in bananas, plantains, beans, peas, and sweet potatoes, encourages the growth of a diversified microbiome.

- Avoid unnecessary exposure to antibiotics. Eighty percent of the antibiotics used in this country are fed to farm animals, not given to people. Select meat, eggs, and dairy products from animals that have not been treated with antibiotics.

- Eat organic as much as you can, and avoid genetically modified foods. Organic farming increases the diversity of bacteria in soil, which then affects the diversity of the bacteria you ingest with your food. Pesticides and herbicides kill more than pests. They can also kill good bacteria and encourage the growth of harmful bacteria. Unless you're scrubbing for surgery, avoid antibacterial soaps and shampoos. They just encourage the growth of resistant organisms and impact negatively on healthy bacteria.

- You may also benefit from probiotics. Before you start taking them, or any supplement, consult a doctor or nutritionist who's experienced in their use.

Conclusion

Your gut does far more than simply process food in and out of your body. In this segment we learned how the long and winding digestive tract can play a surprising role in allergies. Medications, infections, and food can lead to a disturbance in the small intestine called leaky gut and contribute to allergies. Something as simple and common as sugar can lead to a leaky gut.

We met Anne, the paralegal, whose case illuminated a fundamental truth that sometimes gets overlooked about allergies and our health: that the body is intrinsically interconnected. Her migraine headaches, an extremely painful and often debilitating condition, were actually a manifestation of what was going on within her digestive system: a leaky gut. I led her through my ARC of Healing: avoidance, reflorastation, and cultivation to address her leaky gut and alleviate her headaches.

We drilled down to glimpse the tremendous scope of the work the digestive tract performs. Your gut is the largest organ of your immune system. It is home to trillions of microbes and is a key facilitator in detoxification. As such, the gut regulates your immune responses, your metabolism, your sleep, and your moods. We examined the research on fostering a healthy gut with nutrition, probiotics, vitamin D, and zinc. This is quite a lot of data to digest, so please bring this book with you to discuss with your doctor.

BE PART OF
THE SOLUTION

My son Jonathan and I wrote *The Allergy Solution* to change how the world thinks about allergy, health, and our relationship to the environment. We have revealed the science that says allergies are not just annoying symptoms that can be covered over by medications, and the environment is not just a convenient place to put our car exhaust, toss our garbage, and spray our pesticides. The environment is all around us *and* within us, inside our digestive tract, respiratory system, and whole body.

We've shown you that three levels of environment impact our allergies and our health: the outdoor environment; the indoor environment, where we spend 90 percent of our time; and the internal environment, within our digestive system. And we have exposed the truth that just as the earth's environment is out of balance, our bodies have become out of balance.

The allergy epidemic is our bodies' response to living in a world where diesel-powered school buses belch out asthma-inducing soot; where secondhand smoke, formaldehyde, and cleaning products form a toxic indoor cloud that creates allergies and undermines health; and where eating fast food raises allergy risk.

Outdoor pollution contributes to the rising tide of allergic diseases. Ozone, nitric oxide, and diesel exhaust particles damage the respiratory lining, increase oxidative stress, and act in synergy with allergen exposure to create or aggravate allergic reactions.

Indoor pollutants that provoke the development of allergy include phthalates, formaldehyde, volatile organic hydrocarbons, triclosan, dust mites, and mold.

In the internal environment, depletion of beneficial intestinal microbes by exposure to antibiotics and pesticides in food and by lack of dietary fiber and diversity is an emerging factor in the rise of allergies.

There are *two* allergy epidemics that we have brought to light in these pages. In addition to the allergic diseases such as asthma, hay fever, eczema, and food allergies that now afflict one billion people worldwide, we also reveal the shocking rise of hidden allergies that lead to unexplained weight gain, anxiety, fatigue, ADHD, depression, digestive problems, brain fog, and many more complaints. Astonishing new research shows how all of these are linked to immune imbalance, which is at the center of allergy.

We are honored that we've been able to bring you the cutting-edge science that can help you understand the root causes of allergies and address them at their sources—or, as the book's subtitle says, to understand why you are sick and how to get well. We are encouraged by the role that vitamins and other nutrients in foods can play to help support and balance immunity, and by the ability of mind-body practices such as meditation to beat stress and reduce inflammation, which are central to healthy immunity.

Your Health, and the Environment, under Threat

But there is still much work to be done, because the environment we all depend on is threatened as never before. We have seen a preview of the future, and it is happening right now. The year 2015 was the hottest on record; in recent years thousands died in record-setting heat waves in Europe; multiyear droughts bake California and the Southwest; forest fires burn in the United States, Europe, Russia, and Australia; glaciers in mountain ranges across the globe are shrinking and disappearing; the ice in Greenland is melting; sea levels are rising; hurricanes and typhoons are becoming bigger and more dangerous.

Rising temperatures and smoke from forest fires make air pollution worse, exacerbating asthma and directly harming our health, while greenhouse gases are increasing pollen outputs. With carbon dioxide levels high and rising, global warming is set to continue, and the threat to our health continues to grow.

Just as we came to the end of writing *The Allergy Solution*, in June 2015, a central message of the book became a big story. The critical connection between global warming and health splashed across the front pages of major media.

"Climate Catastrophe Predicted by U.S. as Obama Urges UN Action," screamed Bloomberg News.[1]

"White House, EPA Say Climate Change a Dire Threat to Economy, Human Health," warned *USA Today*.[2]

That same month, the White House hosted a Summit on Climate Change and Health. "We know climate change is not a distant threat," a White House statement said. "We are already seeing impacts in communities across the country. In the past three decades, the percentage of Americans with asthma has more than doubled, and climate change is putting these individuals and many other vulnerable populations at greater risk of landing in the hospital."[3]

At the summit, U.S. Surgeon General Vivek Murthy underscored the urgency by saying that "climate change poses a serious, immediate, and global threat to human health." Rising temperatures are leading to earlier springs and longer pollen seasons, as well as more smog and ozone and worse air for cities, which means more hospital admissions and clinic visits for asthma, allergies, and respiratory diseases, he explained.[4]

The EPA, in its recent report *Climate Change in the United States: Benefits of Global Action*, said if greenhouse gas emissions are curtailed it could help avoid 13,000 premature deaths in 2050, and 57,000 premature deaths in 2100.[5]

Also in June, *The Lancet*, one of the world's most prestigious medical journals, published a major study, *Health and Climate Change: Policy Responses to Protect Public Health*, stating: "The effects of climate change are being felt today, and future projections represent an unacceptably high and potentially catastrophic risk to human health." It urged governments around the world to respond to this risk by reducing carbon emissions through a transition to renewable energy, a reduction in driving, and a rapid phase-out in the use of coal.[6]

Mother Nature Is Calling

In a fictional near future depicted in the film *Interstellar*, crop blight threatens the survival of civilization, as giant dust storms engulf the United States. The American farm, once a symbol of abundance and prosperity, is now a wasteland, and people have to wear masks to protect themselves from the thick dust.

In the hope of finding a new planet for people to live on, a NASA professor played by Michael Caine recruits an astronaut played by Matthew McConaughey to pilot a daring mission of discovery. Caine says, "Your daughter's generation will be the last to survive on Earth. Get out there and save the world." It is desperate, dramatic, and heroic, the stuff of great Hollywood movies.

But what if we turned all that passion for getting to the next planet into taking better care of this one? Could we all work together to turn around air pollution, giving those with asthma— and those without—a better chance to breathe free? Reductions in air pollution could also curb the rising levels of pollen, helping those with hay fever feel more comfortable.

Producing and using fewer toxic chemicals would reduce the burden on the environment. Maybe taking a train or bus or simply walking to work doesn't sound as dramatic as launching into outer space. But isn't each action we take to "save the planet" just as noble and heroic as those taken by astronauts in the movies?

Your allergies are connected to the food you eat, the air you breathe, and the environment you live in. Stand up for your health and protect nature as if your life depends on it. Join us and be part of the solution.

Learn more about natural health by joining our community at www.drgalland.com. Follow Dr. Galland on Facebook (facebook .com/leogallandmd) and Twitter (@leogallandmd), and follow Jonathan Galland at facebook.com/jonathangallandjd and on Twitter @ JonathanGalland.

NOTES

Introduction

1. Eriksson NE. Food sensitivity reported by patients with asthma and hay fever. A relationship between food sensitivity and birch pollen allergy and between food sensitivity and acetylsalicylic acid intolerance. *Allergy.* 1978 Aug;33(4):189–96.

Chapter 1

1. Millichap JG, Yee MM. The diet factor in pediatric and adolescent migraine. *Pediatr Neurol.* 2003 Jan;28(1):9–15; Vally H, Misso NL, Madan V. Clinical effects of sulphite additives. *Clin Exp Allergy.* 2009 Nov;39(11):1643–51; Petitpain N, Goffinet L, Cosserat F, Trechot P, Cuny JF. Recurrent fever, chills, and arthralgia with local anesthetics containing epinephrine-metabisulfite. *J Clin Anesth.* 2008 Mar;20(2):154.

2. Sass JO, Gunduz A, Araujo Rodrigues Funayama C, Korkmaz B, Dantas Pinto KG, Tuysuz B, Yanasse Dos Santos L, Taskiran E, de Fátima Turcato M, Lam CW, Reiss J, Walter M, Yalcinkaya C, Camelo Junior JS. Functional deficiencies of sulfite oxidase: Differential diagnoses in neonates presenting with intractable seizures and cystic encephalomalacia. *Brain Dev.* 2010 Aug;32(7):544–9; Abumrad NN, Schneider AJ, Steel D, Rogers LS. Amino acid intolerance during prolonged total parenteral nutrition reversed by molybdate therapy. *American Journal of Clinical Nutrition* 1981;34:255–2559; Ragg R, Natalio F, Tahir MN, Janssen H, Kashyap A, Strand D, Strand S, Tremel W. Molybdenum trioxide nanoparticles with intrinsic sulfite oxidase activity. *ACS Nano.* 2014 May 27;8(5):5182–9.

3. Añíbarro B, Caballero T, García-Ara C, Díaz-Pena JM, Ojeda JA. Asthma with sulfite intolerance in children: a blocking study with cyanocobalamin. *J Allergy Clin Immunol.* 1992 Jul;90(1):103–9; Stormont JM, Flaherty M, Condemi J. Hepatic metabisulfite sensitivity in a patient with sclerosing cholangitis. *Ann Allergy Asthma Immunol.* 2003 Sep;91(3):314–7.

4. Crook WG, Harrison WW, Crawford SE, Emerson BS. Systemic manifestations due to allergy. Report of fifty patients and a review of the literature on the subject (sometimes referred to as allergic toxemia and the allergic tension-fatigue syndrome). *Pediatrics.* 1961 May;27:790-9; Young EJ. The allergic tension-fatigue syndrome. Calif Med. 1970 Jun;112(6):46; Weinberg EG, Tuchinda M. Allergic tension-fatigue syndrome. *Ann Allergy.* 1973 Apr;31(4):209-11; Valverde E, Vich JM, Garcia-Calderon JV, Garcia-Calderon PA. In vitro response of lymphocytes in patients with allergic tension-fatigue syndrome. *Ann Allergy.* 1980 Sep;45(3):185-8; Kondo N, Fukutomi O, Agata H, Yokoyama Y. Proliferative responses of lymphocytes to food antigens are useful for detection of allergens in nonimmediate types of food allergy. *J Investig Allergol Clin Immunol.* 1997 Mar-Apr;7(2):122-6.

5. Papoutsakis C, Priftis KN, Drakouli M, Prifti S, Konstantaki E, Chondronikola M, Antonogeorgos G, Matziou V. Childhood overweight/obesity and asthma: is there a link? A systematic review of recent epidemiologic evidence. *J Acad Nutr Diet.* 2013 Jan;113(1):77-105; Wang J, Shi GP. Mast cell stabilization: novel medication for obesity and diabetes. *Diabetes Metab Res Rev.* 2011 Nov;27(8):919-24 (Mice fed a Western diet were able to reduce obesity through treatment with anti-allergic drugs that stabilize mast cells [cromolyn and ketotifen]); Ciprandi G, Caimmi D, Raschetti R, Miraglia Del Giudice M, Salpietro C, Caimmi S, Castellazzi AM. Adipokines and their role in allergies. *Int J Immunopathol Pharmacol.* 2011 Oct;24(4 Suppl):136; Litonjua AA, Gold DR. Asthma and obesity: common early-life influences in the inception of disease. *J Allergy Clin Immunol.* 2008 May;121(5):1075-84.

6. Hasler G, Gergen PJ, Ajdacic V, Gamma A, Eich D, Rössler W, Angst J. Asthma and body weight change: a 20-year prospective community study of young adults. *Int J Obes* (Lond). 2006 Jul;30(7):1111-8. (Multivariate longitudinal analyses revealed that asthma was associated with increased later weight gain and later obesity among women after controlling for potentially confounding variables, whereas weight gain and obesity were not associated with later asthma.)

7. Ratliff JC, Barber JA, Palmese LB, Reutenauer EL, Tek C. Association of prescription H1 antihistamine use with obesity: results from the National Health and Nutrition Examination Survey. *Obesity* (Silver Spring). 2010 Dec;18(12):2398-400. (Users of antihistamines have a greater prevalence of obesity than non-users.)

8. Cleveland CH Jr, Fisher RH, Brestel EP, Esinhart JD, Metzger WJ. Chronic rhinitis: an underrecognized association with fibromyalgia. *Allergy Proc.* 1992 Sep-Oct;13(5):263-7.

9. Bellanti JA, Sabra A, Castro HJ, Chavez JR, Malka-Rais J, de Inocencio JM. Are attention deficit hyperactivity disorder and chronic fatigue syndrome allergy related? what is fibromyalgia? *Allergy Asthma Proc.* 2005 Jan-Feb;26(1):19-28; Stejskal V, Ockert K, Bjørklund G. Metal-induced inflammation triggers fibromyalgia in metal-allergic patients. *Neuro Endocrinol Lett.* 2013;34(6):559-65.

10. Tollefsen E, Langhammer A, Bjermer L, Romundstad P, Holmen TL. Allergy: a systemic disease? The HUNT and Young-HUNT study, Norway. *Pediatr Allergy Immunol.* 2008 Dec;19(8):730-6.

11. Ruoppi P. Mold problem in the work environment—an otorhinolaryngologist's view. *Duodecim.* 2009;125(9):983-9.

12. Golding DN. Is there an allergic synovitis? *J R Soc Med.* 1990 May; 83(5): 312-4; Panush RS, Stroud RM, Webster EM. Food-induced (allergic) arthritis. Inflammatory arthritis exacerbated by milk. *Arthritis Rheum.* 1986 Feb;29(2):220-6; Panush RS. Food induced ("allergic") arthritis: clinical and serologic studies. *J Rheumatol.* 1990 Mar;17(3):291-4; Pulec JL. Allergic arthritis. *Ear Nose Throat J.* 1993 Feb;72(2):115.

13. Mansfield LE. Food allergy and headache. Whom to evaluate and how to treat. *Postgrad Med.* 1988 May 15;83(7):46-51, 55; Alam R. Is food allergy giving me a headache? *Immunol Allergy Clin North Am.* 2012 Feb;32(1):xiii-xiv; Martin VT, Taylor F, Gebhardt B, Tomaszewski M, Ellison JS, Martin GV, Levin L, Al-Shaikh E, Nicolas J, Bernstein JA. Allergy and immunotherapy: are they related to migraine headache? *Headache.* 2011 Jan;51(1):8-20; Stefanini GF, Marsigli L, Foschi FG, Emiliani F, Biselli M, Caputo F, Leefield GH, Castelli E, Gasbarrini G. Nonmigrainous headache from food allergy. *Allergy.* 1996 Sep;51(9):657-8.

14. Husby S, Høost A. Recurrent abdominal pain, food allergy and endoscopy. *Acta Paediatr.* 2001 Jan;90(1):3-4; Kokkonen J1, Ruuska T, Karttunen TJ, Niinimäki A. Mucosal pathology of the foregut associated with food allergy and recurrent abdominal pains in children. *Acta Paediatr.* 2001 Jan;90(1):16-21.

15. van Odijk J, Peterson CG, Ahlstedt S, Bengtsson U, Borres MP, Hulthén L, Magnusson J, Hansson T. Measurements of eosinophil activation before and after food challenges in adults with food hypersensitivity. *Int Arch Allergy Immunol.* 2006;140(4):334-41.

16. Arora AA, Weiler CR, Katzka DA. Eosinophilic esophagitis: allergic contribution, testing, and management. *Curr Gastroenterol Rep.* 2012 Jun;14(3):206-15; Wechsler JB, Schwartz S, Amsden K, Kagalwalla AF. Elimination diets in the management of eosinophilic esophagitis. *J Asthma Allergy.* 2014 May 24;7:85-94.

17. Kahn A, Mozin MJ, Casimir G, Montauk L, Blum D. Insomnia and cow's milk allergy in infants. *Pediatrics.* 1985 Dec;76(6):880-4; Kahn A, Rebuffat E, Blum D, Casimir G, Duchateau J, Mozin MJ, Jost R. Difficulty in initiating and maintaining sleep associated with cow's milk allergy in infants. *Sleep.* 1987 Apr;10(2):116-21; Kahn A, Mozin MJ, Rebuffat E, Sottiaux M, Muller MF. Milk intolerance in children with persistent sleeplessness: a prospective double-blind crossover evaluation. *Pediatrics.* 1989 Oct;84(4):595-603.

18. Sundbom F, Lindberg E, Bjerg A, Forsberg B, Franklin K, Gunnbjörnsdottir M, Middelveld R, Torén K, Janson C. Asthma symptoms and nasal congestion as independent risk factors for insomnia in a general population: results from the GA(2)LEN survey. *Allergy.* 2013 Feb;68(2):213-9; Jensen ME, Gibson PG, Collins CE, Hilton JM, Latham-Smith F, Wood LG. Increased sleep latency and reduced sleep duration in children with asthma. *Sleep Breath.* 2013 Mar;17(1):281-7; Terreehorst I, Duivenvoorden HJ, Tempels-Pavlica Z, Oosting

AJ, de Monchy JG, Bruijnzeel-Koomen CA, Post MW, Gerth van Wijk R. The unfavorable effects of concomitant asthma and sleeplessness due to the atopic eczema/dermatitis syndrome (AEDS) on quality of life in subjects allergic to house-dust mites. *Allergy.* 2002 Oct;57(10):919-25.

19. Chen MH, Su TP, Chen YS, Hsu JW, Huang KL, Chang WH, Chen TJ, Bai YM. Higher risk of developing major depression and bipolar disorder in later life among adolescents with asthma: a nationwide prospective study. *J Psychiatr Res.* 2014 Feb;49:25-30.

20. Goodwin RD, Galea S, Perzanowski M, Jacobi F. Impact of allergy treatment on the association between allergies and mood and anxiety in a population sample. *Clin Exp Allergy.* 2012 Dec;42(12):1765-71.

21. King DS. Can allergic exposure provoke psychological symptoms? A double-blind test. *Biol Psychiatry.* 1981 Jan;16(1):3-19.

22. Huang KP, Mullangi S, Guo Y, Qureshi AA. Autoimmune, atopic, and mental health comorbid conditions associated with alopecia areata in the United States. *JAMA Dermatol.* 2013 Jul;149(7):789-94; Barahmani N, Schabath MB, Duvic M; National Alopecia Areata Registry. History of atopy or autoimmunity increases risk of alopecia areata. *J Am Acad Dermatol.* 2009 Oct;61(4):581-91; Ucak H, Cicek D, Demir B, Erden I, Ozturk S. Prognostic factors that affect the response to topical treatment in patchy alopecia areata. *J Eur Acad Dermatol Venereol.* 2014 Jan;28(1):34-40.

23. Haye KR, Mandal D. Allergic vaginitis mimicking bacterial vaginosis. *Int J STD AIDS.* 1990 Nov;1(6):440-2; Dworetzky M. Allergic vaginitis. *Am J Obstet Gynecol.* 1989 Dec;161(6 Pt 1):1752-3; Ricer RE, Guthrie RM. Allergic vaginitis, a possibly new syndrome. A case report. *J Reprod Med.* 1988 Sep;33(9):781-3.

24. Loran OB, Pisarev SA, Klemenova NV, Sukhorukov VS. Allergic inflammation as one of the factors of pathogenesis of overactive urinary bladder. *Urologiia.* 2007 Mar-Apr;(2):37-41.

25. Skoner DP. Allergic rhinitis: definition, epidemiology, pathophysiology, detection, and diagnosis. *J Allergy Clin Immunol.* 2001 Jul;108(1 Suppl):S2-8.

26. **Arthritis:** Hvatum M, Kanerud L, Hällgren R, Brandtzaeg P. The gut-joint axis: cross reactive food antibodies in rheumatoid arthritis. *Gut.* 2006 Sep;55(9):1240-7; O'Farrelly C, Price R, McGillivray AJ, Fernandes L. IgA rheumatoid factor and IgG dietary protein antibodies are associated in rheumatoid arthritis. *Immunol Invest.* 1989 Jul;18(6):753-64; Karatay S, Erdem T, Kiziltunc A, Melikoglu MA, Yildirim K, Cakir E, Ugur M, Aktas A, Senel K. General or personal diet: the individualized model for diet challenges in patients with rheumatoid arthritis. *Rheumatol Int.* 2006 Apr;26(6):556-60; Karatay S, Erdem T, Yildirim K, Melikoglu MA, Ugur M, Cakir E, Akcay F, Senel K. The effect of individualized diet challenges consisting of allergenic foods on TNF-alpha and IL-1beta levels in patients with rheumatoid arthritis. *Rheumatology* (Oxford). 2004 Nov;43(11):1429-33. **Bronchitis:** Chawes BL. Upper and lower airway pathology in young children with allergic- and non-allergic rhinitis. *Dan Med Bull.* 2011 May;58(5):B4278. **Nephritis:** Shishkin AN. The role of immediate-type allergic reactions in the pathogenesis of the

nephrotic syndrome. *Ter Arkh.* 1996;68(6):19-21; Lagrue G, Laurent J, Rostoker G. Food allergy and idiopathic nephrotic syndrome. *Kidney Int Suppl.* 1989 Nov;27:S147-51; Lagrue G, Heslan JM, Belghiti D, Sainte-Laudy J, Laurent J. Basophil sensitization for food allergens in idiopathic nephrotic syndrome. *Nephron.* 1986;42(2):123-7; Kovács T, Mette H, Per B, Kun L, Schmelczer M, Barta J, Jean-Claude D, Nagy J. Relationship between intestinal permeability and antibodies against food antigens in IgA nephropathy. *Orv Hetil.* 1996 Jan 14;137(2):65-9. **Colitis:** Ruffner MA, Ruymann K, Barni S, Cianferoni A, Brown-Whitehorn T, Spergel JM. Food protein-induced enterocolitis syndrome: insights from review of a large referral population. *J Allergy Clin Immunol Pract.* 2013 Jul-Aug;1(4):343-9; D'Arienzo A, Manguso F, Astarita C, D'Armiento FP, Scarpa R, Gargano D, Scaglione G, Vicinanza G, Bennato R, Mazzacca G. Allergy and mucosal eosinophil infiltrate in ulcerative colitis. *Scand J Gastroenterol.* 2000 Jun;35(6):624-31.

27.   **Migraine:** Mitchell N, Hewitt CE, Jayakody S, Islam M, Adamson J, Watt I, Torgerson DJ. Randomised controlled trial of food elimination diet based on IgG antibodies for the prevention of migraine-like headaches. *Nutr J.* 2011 Aug 11;10:85. doi: 10.1186/1475-2891-10-85; Alpay K, Ertas M, Orhan EK, Ustay DK, Lieners C, Baykan B. Diet restriction in migraine, based on IgG against foods: a clinical double-blind, randomised, cross-over trial. *Cephalalgia.* 2010 Jul;30(7):829-37; Arroyave Hernández CM, Echavarría Pinto M, Hernández Montiel HL. Food allergy mediated by IgG antibodies associated with migraine in adults. *Rev Alerg Mex.* 2007 Sep-Oct;54(5):162-8. **Irritable bowel syndrome:** Carroccio A, Brusca I, Mansueto P, D'Alcamo A, Barrale M, Soresi M, Seidita A, La Chiusa SM, Iacono G, Sprini D. A comparison between two different in vitro basophil activation tests for gluten- and cow's milk protein sensitivity in irritable bowel syndrome (IBS)-like patients. *Clin Chem Lab Med.* 2013 Jun;51(6):1257-63; Stierstorfer MB, Sha CT, Sasson M. Food patch testing for irritable bowel syndrome. *J Am Acad Dermatol.* 2013 Mar;68(3):377-84; Guo H, Jiang T, Wang J, Chang Y, Guo H, Zhang W. The value of eliminating foods according to food-specific immunoglobulin G antibodies in irritable bowel syndrome with diarrhoea. *J Int Med Res.* 2012;40(1):204-10; Carroccio A, Brusca I, Mansueto P, Soresi M, D'Alcamo A, Ambrosiano G, Pepe I, Iacono G, Lospalluti ML, La Chiusa SM, Di Fede G. Fecal assays detect hypersensitivity to cow's milk protein and gluten in adults with irritable bowel syndrome. *Clin Gastroenterol Hepatol.* 2011 Nov;9(11):965-971.e3; Tobin MC, Moparty B, Farhadi A, DeMeo MT, Bansal PJ, Keshavarzian A. Atopic irritable bowel syndrome: a novel subgroup of irritable bowel syndrome with allergic manifestations. *Ann Allergy Asthma Immunol.* 2008 Jan;100(1):49-53. **Fibromyalgia:** Bellanti et al. 2005; Berstad A, Undseth R, Lind R, Valeur J. Functional bowel symptoms, fibromyalgia and fatigue: a food-induced triad? *Scand J Gastroenterol.* 2012 Sep;47(8-9):914-9. **Chronic fatigue syndrome:** Straus SE, Dale JK, Wright R, Metcalfe DD. Allergy and the chronic fatigue syndrome. *J Allergy Clin Immunol.* 1988 May;81(5 Pt 1):791-5; Bell KM, Cookfair D, Bell DS, Reese P, Cooper L. Risk factors associated with chronic fatigue syndrome in a cluster of pediatric cases. *Rev Infect Dis.* 1991 Jan-Feb;13 Suppl 1:S32-8. **Attention deficit disorder:** Hak E, de Vries TW, Hoekstra PJ, Jick SS. Association of childhood attention-deficit/hyperactivity disorder with atopic diseases and skin infections? A matched case-control study using the General Practice Research Database. *Ann Allergy Asthma Immunol.*

2013 Aug;111(2):102-106.e2; Tsai JD, Chang SN, Mou CH, Sung FC, Lue KH. Association between atopic diseases and attention-deficit/hyperactivity disorder in childhood: a population-based case-control study. *Ann Epidemiol.* 2013 Apr;23(4):185-8; Schmitt J, Apfelbacher C, Heinrich J, Weidinger S, Romanos M. Association of atopic eczema and attention-deficit/hyperactivity disorder - meta-analysis of epidemiologic studies. *Z Kinder Jugendpsychiatr Psychother.* 2013 Jan;41(1):35-42; Yaghmaie P, Koudelka CW, Simpson EL. Mental health comorbidity in patients with atopic dermatitis. *J Allergy Clin Immunol.* 2013 Feb;131(2):428-33; Chen MH, Su TP, Chen YS, Hsu JW, Huang KL, Chang WH, Bai YM. Attention deficit hyperactivity disorder, tic disorder, and allergy: is there a link? A nationwide population-based study. *J Child Psychol Psychiatry.* 2013 May;54(5):545-51. **Canker sores:** Wardhana, Datau EA. Recurrent aphthous stomatitis caused by food allergy. *Acta Med Indones.* 2010 Oct;42(4):236-40; Besu I, Jankovic L, Magdu IU, Konic-Ristic A, Raskovic S, Juranic Z. Humoral immunity to cow's milk proteins and gliadin within the etiology of recurrent aphthous ulcers? *Oral Dis.* 2009 Nov;15(8):560-4; Nolan A, Lamey PJ, Milligan KA, Forsyth A. Recurrent aphthous ulceration and food sensitivity. *J Oral Pathol Med.* 1991 Nov;20(10):473-5. **Burning mouth syndrome:** Lamey PJ, Lamb AB, Hughes A, Milligan KA, Forsyth A. Type 3 burning mouth syndrome: psychological and allergic aspects. *J Oral Pathol Med.* 1994 May;23(5):216-9; Pemberton M, Yeoman CM, Clark A, Craig GT, Franklin CD, Gawkrodger DJ. Allergy to octyl gallate causing stomatitis. *Br Dent J.* 1993 Aug 7;175(3):106-8; Whitley BD, Holmes AR, Shepherd MG, Ferguson MM. Peanut sensitivity as a cause of burning mouth. *Oral Surg Oral Med Oral Pathol.* 1991 Dec;72(6):671-4; Skoglund A, Egelrud T. Hypersensitivity reactions to dental materials in patients with lichenoid oral mucosal lesions and in patients with burning mouth syndrome. *Scand J Dent Res.* 1991 Aug;99(4):320-8. **Interstitial cystitis:** Pelikan Z, van Oers JA, Levens WJ, Fouchier SM. The role of allergy in interstitial cystitis. *Ned Tijdschr Geneeskd.* 1999 Jun 19;143(25):1289-92; Yamada T, Taguchi H, Nisimura H, Mita H, Sida T. Allergic study of interstitial cystitis. (1) A case of interstitial cystitis caused by squid and shrimp hypersensitivity. *Arerugi.* 1984 May;33(5):264-8. **Vulvodynia:** Harlow BL, He W, Nguyen RH. Allergic reactions and risk of vulvodynia. *Ann Epidemiol.* 2009 Nov;19(11):771-7; Ramirez De Knott HM, McCormick TS, Do SO, Goodman W, Ghannoum MA, Cooper KD, Nedorost ST. Cutaneous hypersensitivity to Candida albicans in idiopathic vulvodynia. *Contact Dermatitis.* 2005 Oct;53(4):214-8; O'Hare PM, Sherertz EF. Vulvodynia: a dermatologist's perspective with emphasis on an irritant contact dermatitis component. *J Womens Health Gend Based Med.* 2000 Jun;9(5):565-9. **Anxiety:** Patten SB, Williams JV. Self-reported allergies and their relationship to several Axis I disorders in a community sample. *Int J Psychiatry Med.* 2007;37(1):11-22; Euba R, Chalder T, Wallace P, Wright DJ, Wessely S. Self-reported allergy-related symptoms and psychological morbidity in primary care. *Int J Psychiatry Med.* 1997;27(1):47-56. (NOTE: Although people with anxiety disorders are more likely to report a history of allergy, people with allergies are not more likely to report anxiety or psychological distress. There are many ways to interpret this difference. One is that allergies contribute to psychological symptoms in some people (a sub-group of those who have psychological symptoms), but that people with allergies are not more prone to psychological symptoms in general. **Depression:** Parker G, Watkins T. Treatment-resistant depression: when antidepressant drug intolerance may indicate food intolerance. *Aust N Z J Psychiatry.* 2002 Apr;36(2):263-5.

28. **Asthma:** Confino-Cohen R, Brufman I, Goldberg A, Feldman BS. Vitamin D, Asthma Prevalence and Asthma exacerbations: A large adult population-based study. Allergy. 2014 Aug 19; Arshi S, Fallahpour M, Nabavi M, Bemanian MH, Javad-Mousavi SA, Nojomi M, Esmaeilzadeh H, Molatefi R, Rekabi M, Jalali F, Akbarpour N. The effects of vitamin D supplementation on airway functions in mild to moderate persistent asthma. *Ann Allergy Asthma Immunol.* 2014 Aug 1; Bonanno A, Gangemi S, La Grutta S, Malizia V, Riccobono L, Colombo P, Cibella F, Profita M. 25-Hydroxyvitamin D, IL-31, and IL-33 in children with allergic disease of the airways. *Mediators Inflamm.* 2014;2014:520241; Bener A, Ehlayel MS, Tulic MK, Hamid Q. Vitamin D deficiency as a strong predictor of asthma in children. *Int Arch Allergy Immunol.* 2012;157(2):168-75. **Food allergies and eczema:** Baek JH, Shin YH, Chung IH, Kim HJ, Yoo EG, Yoon JW, Jee HM, Chang YE, Han MY. The Link between Serum Vitamin D Level, Sensitization to Food Allergens, and the Severity of Atopic Dermatitis in Infancy. *J Pediatr.* 2014 Aug 6; Lee SA1, Hong S, Kim HJ, Lee SH, Yum HY. Correlation between serum Vitamin D level and the severity of atopic dermatitis associated with food sensitization. *Allergy Asthma Immunol Res.* 2013 Jul;5(4):207-10. doi: 10.4168/aair.2013.5.4.207. Epub 2013 Mar 13; Samochocki Z1, Bogaczewicz J, Jeziorkowska R, Sysa-Jędrzejowska A, Glińska O, Karczmarewicz E, McCauliffe DP, Woźniacka A. *Vitamin D effects in atopic dermatitis.* J Am Acad Dermatol. 2013 Aug;69(2):238-44. doi: 10.1016/j.jaad.2013.03.014. Epub 2013 May 2. **Nasal allergies:** Jung JW, Kim JY, Cho SH, Choi BW, Min KU, Kang HR. Allergic rhinitis and serum 25-hydroxyvitamin D level in Korean adults. *Ann Allergy Asthma Immunol.* 2013 Nov;111(5):352-7. **Allergy in general:** Sharief S, Jariwala S, Kumar J, Muntner P, Melamed ML. Vitamin D levels and food and environmental allergies in the United States: results from the National Health and Nutrition Examination Survey 2005-2006. *J Allergy Clin Immunol.* 2011 May;127(5):1195-202. doi: 10.1016/j.jaci.2011.01.017. Epub 2011 Feb 16.

29. Carneiro MF, Rhoden CR, Amantéa SL, Barbosa F Jr. Low concentrations of selenium and zinc in nails are associated with childhood asthma. *Biol Trace Elem Res.* 2011 Dec;144(1-3):244-52; Razi CH, Akelma AZ, Akin O, Kocak M, Ozdemir O, Celik A, Kislal FM. Hair zinc and selenium levels in children with recurrent wheezing. *Pediatr Pulmonol.* 2012 Dec;47(12):1185-91; Tahan F, Karakukcu C. Zinc status in infantile wheezing. *Pediatr Pulmonol.* 2006 Jul;41(7):630-4; David TJ, Wells FE, Sharpe TC, Gibbs AC. Low serum zinc in children with atopic eczema. *Br J Dermatol.* 1984 Nov;111(5):597-601; Jayaram L, Chunilal S, Pickering S, Ruffin RE, Zalewski PD. Sputum zinc concentration and clinical outcome in older asthmatics. *Respirology.* 2011 Apr;16(3):459-66.

30. Fabian E, Pölöskey P, Kósa L, Elmadfa I, Réthy LA. Nutritional supplements and plasma antioxidants in childhood asthma. *Wien Klin Wochenschr.* 2013 Jun;125(11-12):309-15; Razi et al 2012; Carneiro et al 2011.

31. Rosenlund H, Magnusson J, Kull I, Håkansson N, Wolk A, Pershagen G, Wickman M, Bergström A. Antioxidant intake and allergic disease in children. *Clin Exp Allergy.* 2012 Oct;42(10):1491-500; van Oeffelen AA, Bekkers MB, Smit HA, Kerkhof M, Koppelman GH, Haveman-Nies A, van der A DL, Jansen EH, Wijga AH. Serum micronutrient concentrations and childhood asthma: the PIAMA birth cohort study. *Pediatr Allergy Immunol.* 2011 Dec;22(8):784-93; Gontijo-Amaral C, Ribeiro MA, Gontijo LS, Condino-Neto A, Ribeiro JD. Oral magnesium supplementation in asthmatic children: a double-blind randomized placebo-controlled trial. *Eur J Clin Nutr.* 2007 Jan;61(1):54-60. Epub 2006 Jun 21; Sedighi M, Pourpak Z, Bavarian B, Safaralizadeh R, Zare A, Moin M. Low magnesium concentration in erythrocytes of children with acute asthma. *Iran J Allergy Asthma Immunol.* 2006 Dec;5(4):183-6; Alamoudi OS. Hypomagnesaemia in chronic, stable asthmatics: prevalence, correlation with severity and hospitalization. *Eur Respir J.* 2000 Sep;16(3):427-31; Hashimoto Y, Nishimura Y, Maeda H, Yokoyama M. Assessment of magnesium status in patients with bronchial asthma. J Asthma. 2000 Sep;37(6):489-96; Emmanouil E, Manios Y, Grammatikaki E, Kondaki K, Oikonomou E, Papadopoulos N, Vassilopoulou E. Association of nutrient intake and wheeze or asthma in a Greek pre-school population. *Pediatr Allergy Immunol.* 2010 Feb;21(1 Pt 1):90-5.

32. Wood LG, Gibson PG. Reduced circulating antioxidant defences are associated with airway hyper-responsiveness, poor control and severe disease pattern in asthma. *Br J Nutr.* 2010 Mar;103(5):735-41.

33. Nakamura K, Wada K, Sahashi Y, Tamai Y, Tsuji M, Watanabe K, Ohtsuchi S, Ando K, Nagata C. Associations of intake of antioxidant vitamins and fatty acids with asthma in pre-school children. *Public Health Nutr.* 2013 Nov;16(11):2040-5; Patel BD, Welch AA, Bingham SA, Luben RN, Day NE, Khaw KT, Lomas DA, Wareham NJ. Dietary antioxidants and asthma in adults. *Thorax.* 2006 May;61(5):388-93; Shidfar F, Baghai N, Keshavarz A, Ameri A, Shidfar S. Comparison of plasma and leukocyte vitamin C status between asthmatic and healthy subjects. *East Mediterr Health J.* 2005 Jan-Mar;11(1-2):87-95.

34. Makrides M, Gunaratne AW, Collins CT. Dietary n-3 LC-PUFA during the perinatal period as a strategy to minimize childhood allergic disease. *Nestle Nutr Inst Workshop Ser.* 2013;77:155-62; Montes R, Chisaguano AM, Castellote AI, Morales E, Sunyer J, López-Sabater MC. Fatty-acid composition of maternal and umbilical cord plasma and early childhood atopic eczema in a Spanish cohort. *Eur J Clin Nutr.* 2013 Jun;67(6):658-63; Miyake Y, Tanaka K, Okubo H, Sasaki S, Arakawa M. Maternal fat intake during pregnancy and wheeze and eczema in Japanese infants: the Kyushu Okinawa Maternal and Child Health Study. *Ann Epidemiol.* 2013 Nov;23(11):674-80; Li J, Xun P, Zamora D, Sood A, Liu K, Daviglus M, Iribarren C, Jacobs D Jr, Shikany JM, He K. Intakes of long-chain omega-3 (n-3) PUFAs and fish in relation to incidence of asthma among American young adults: the CARDIA study. *Am J Clin Nutr.* 2013 Jan;97(1):173-8.

35. Razi CH, Akin O, Harmanci K, Akin B, Renda R. Serum heavy metal and antioxidant element levels of children with recurrent wheezing. *Allergol Immunopathol* (Madr). 2011 Mar-Apr;39(2):85-9; Tamer L, Calikoğlu M, Ates NA, Yildirim H, Ercan B, Saritas E, Unlü A, Atik U. Glutathione-S-transferase gene polymorphisms (GSTT1, GSTM1, GSTP1) as increased risk

factors for asthma. *Respirology.* 2004 Nov;9(4):493-8; Karam RA1, Pasha HF, El-Shal AS, Rahman HM, Gad DM. Impact of glutathione-S-transferase gene polymorphisms on enzyme activity, lung function and bronchial asthma susceptibility in Egyptian children. *Gene.* 2012 Apr 15;497(2):314-9; Hanene C, Jihene L, Jamel A, Kamel H, Agnès H. Association of GST genes polymorphisms with asthma in Tunisian children. *Mediators Inflamm.* 2007;2007:19564.

36. Schaefer P Urticaria: evaluation and treatment. Am Fam Physician. 2011 May 1;83(9):1078-84.; Kulthanan K, Jiamton S, Thumpimukvatana N, Pinkaew S. Chronic idiopathic urticaria: prevalence and clinical course. *J Dermatol.* 2007;34(5):294–301.

37. Elamin E, Masclee A, Dekker J, Jonkers D. Ethanol disrupts intestinal epithelial tight junction integrity through intracellular calcium-mediated Rho/ROCK activation. *Am J Physiol Gastrointest Liver Physiol.* 2014 Apr 15;306(8):G677-85; Paganelli R, Fagiolo U, Cancian M, Scala E. Intestinal permeability in patients with chronic urticaria-angioedema with and without arthralgia. *Ann Allergy.* 1991 Feb;66(2):181-4.

38. Serrano H. Hypersensitivity to "Candida albicans" and other fungi in patients with chronic urticaria. *Allergol Immunopathol* (Madr). 1975 Sep-Oct;3(5):289-98; James J, Warin RP. An assessment of the role of Candida albicans and food yeasts in chronic urticaria. *Br J Dermatol.* 1971 Mar;84(3):227-37; Staubach P, Vonend A, Burow G, Metz M, Magerl M, Maurer M. Patients with chronic urticaria exhibit increased rates of sensitisation to Candida albicans, but not to common moulds. *Mycoses.* 2009 Jul;52(4):334-8.

39. Liu X, Han Y, Peng K, Liu Y, Li J, Liu H. Effect of traditional Chinese medicinal herbs on Candida spp. from patients with HIV/AIDS. *Adv Dent Res.* 2011 Apr;23(1):56-60; Iwazaki RS, Endo EH, Ueda-Nakamura T, Nakamura CV, Garcia LB, Filho BP. In vitro antifungal activity of the berberine and its synergism with fluconazole. *Antonie Van Leeuwenhoek.* 2010 Feb;97(2):201-5.

40. Davison HM. Cerebral allergy. *South Med J.* 1949 Aug;42(8):712-6.

41. Egger J, Stolla A, McEwen LM. Controlled trial of hyposensitisation in children with food-induced hyperkinetic syndrome. *Lancet.* 1992 May 9;339(8802):1150-3.

Chapter 2

1. Research needs in allergy: an EAACI position paper, in collaboration with EFA. *Clin Transl Allergy.* 2012; 2: 21. Published online Nov 2, 2012. doi: 10.1186/2045-7022-2-21.

2. World Allergy Association, "WAO White Book on Allergy 2011-2012: Executive Summary." http://www.worldallergy.org/UserFiles/file/WAO-White-Book-on-Allergy_web.pdf.

3. Eder W, Ege MJ, von Mutius E. University Children's Hospital, Munich, Germany. The asthma epidemic. *N Engl J Med*. 2006 Nov 23;355(21):2226-35.

4. Ellwood P et al. Do fast foods cause asthma, rhinoconjunctivitis and eczema? Global findings from the International Study of Asthma and Allergies in Childhood (ISAAC) phase three. *Thorax*. 2013 Apr;68(4):351-60. doi: 10.1136/thoraxjnl-2012-202285. Epub 2013 Jan 14.

5. Sjögren YM, Jenmalm MC, Böttcher MF, Björkstén B, Sverremark-Ekström E. *Clin Exp Allergy*. 2009 Apr;39(4):518-26. Altered early infant gut microbiota in children developing allergy up to 5 years of age.

6. Yang SN et al. The effects of environmental toxins on allergic inflammation. *Allergy Asthma Immunol Res*. 2014 Nov;6(6):478-84. doi: 10.4168/aair.2014.6.6.478. Epub 2014 Oct 15.

7. World Health Organization, "Climate change: An opportunity for public health." http://www.who.int/mediacentre/commentaries/climate-change/en/.

8. New York University Department of Economics, "Vehicle Ownership and Income Growth, Worldwide: 1960-2030," Joyce Dargay, Dermot Gately and Martin Sommer, January 2007. http://www.econ.nyu.edu/dept/courses/gately/DGS_Vehicle%20Ownership_2007.pdf.

9. Daniel Tencer, "Number of Cars Worldwide Surpasses 1 Billion; Can the World Handle This Many Wheels?" The Huffington Post Canada, August 23, 2011, http://www.huffingtonpost.ca/2011/08/23/car-population_n_934291.html.

10. Albertine JM et al. Projected carbon dioxide to increase grass pollen and allergen exposure despite higher ozone levels. *PLoS One*. 2014 Nov 5;9(11):e111712. doi: 10.1371/journal.pone.0111712. eCollection 2014.

11. D'Amato G. Effects of climatic changes and urban air pollution on the rising trends of respiatory allergy and asthma. *Multidiscip Respir Med*. 2011 Feb 28;6(1):28-37. doi: 10.1186/2049-6958-6-1-28.

12. Ibid.

13. Huang SK, Zhang Q, Qiu Z, Chung KF. Mechanistic impact of outdoor air pollution on asthma and allergic diseases. *J Thorac Dis*. 2015 Jan;7(1):23-33. doi: 10.3978/j.issn.2072-1439.2014.12.13.

14. Ibid.

15. Ibid.

16. Ibid.

17. Diaz-Sanchez D, Tsien A, Fleming J, Saxon A. Combined diesel exhaust particulate and ragweed allergen challenge markedly enhances human in vivo nasal ragweed-specific IgE and skews cytokine production to a T helper cell 2-type pattern. *J Immunol*. 1997 Mar 1;158(5):2406-13.

18. D'Amato 2001.

19. Bell ML, McDermott A, Zeger SL, Samet JM, Dominici F. Ozone and short-term mortality in 95 US urban communities, 1987-2000. *JAMA*. 2004 Nov 17;292(19):2372-8.

20. D'Amato 2001.

21. Beggs PJ, Bambrick HJ. Is the global rise of asthma an early impact of anthropogenic climate change? *Environ Health Perspect*. 2005 Aug;113(8):915-9.

22. Ayres JG, and colleagues, and the Environment and Health Committee of the European Respiratory Society, Institute of Occupational & Environmental Medicine, University of Birmingham, Birmingham, UK. Climate change and respiratory disease: European Respiratory Society position statement. *Eur Respir J*. 2009 Aug;34(2):295-302. doi: 10.1183/09031936.00003409. Epub 2009 Feb 27.

23. Rom WN, Pinkerton KE, Martin WJ, Forastiere F. Global warming: a challenge to all American Thoracic Society members. *Am J Respir Crit Care Med*. 2008 May 15;177(10):1053-4. doi: 10.1164/rccm.200801-052ED.

24. Patz JA et al. Climate change: challenges and opportunities for global health. *JAMA*. 2014 Oct 15;312(15):1565-80. doi: 10.1001/jama.2014.13186.

25. U.S. Environmental Protection Agency, "Climate Change Impacts on Human Health." http://www.epa.gov/climatechange/impacts/health.html.

26. Robine JM et al. Death toll exceeded 70,000 in Europe during the summer of 2003. *C R Biol*. 2008 Feb;331(2):171-8. doi: 10.1016/j.crvi.2007.12.001. Epub 2007 Dec 31.

27. Physicians for Social Responsibility, "More Extreme Heat Waves: Global Warming's Wake Up Call." http://www.psr.org/resources/more-extreme-heat-waves.html.

28. Ayres et al, 2009.

29. U.S. Environmental Protection Agency, "Climate Change Impacts on Human Health."

30. Ibid.

31. Ayres et al, 2009.

32. Rom et al, 2008.

33. Yang SN et al. The effects of environmental toxins on allergic inflammation. *Allergy Asthma Immunol Res*. 2014 Nov;6(6):478-84. doi: 10.4168/aair.2014.6.6.478. Epub 2014 Oct 15.

34. Ibid.

35. U.S. Fish and Wildlife Service, "Environmental Quality."

36. Yang et al, 2014.

37. Ibid.

38. The National Institute of Environmental Health Sciences, "Endocrine Disruptors." https://www.niehs.nih.gov/health/materials/endocrine_disruptors_508.pdf.

39. World Health Organization, "Children's environmental health." http://www.who.int/ceh/risks/cehemerging2/en/.

40. Ibid.

41. Australian Government Department of Health, "Diethylhexyl phthalate (DEHP) Fact Sheet." http://www.nicnas.gov.au/communications/publications/information-sheets/existing-chemical-info-sheets/diethylhexyl-phthalate-dehp-factsheet.

42. The National Institute of Environmental Health Sciences, "Endocrine Disruptors."

43. Yang et al, 2014.

44. World Health Organization. Concise International Chemical Assessment Document 17, "Butyl Benzyl Phthalate." http://www.who.int/ipcs/publications/cicad/en/cicad17.pdf.

45. Yang et al, 2014.

46. Ibid.

47. Ibid.

48. Minnesota Department of Health, "Formaldehyde in Your Home." http://www.health.state.mn.us/divs/eh/indoorair/voc/formaldehyde.htm.

49. U.S. Consumer Product Safety Commission, "An Update on Formaldehyde." http://www.cpsc.gov/PageFiles/121919/AN_UPDATE_ON_FORMALDEHYDE-update03102015.pdf.

50. Minnesota Department of Health, "Formaldehyde in Your Home."

51. U.S. Consumer Product Safety Commission, "An Update on Formaldehyde."

52. Australian Government Department of Health, "Formaldehyde Fact Sheet." http://www.nicnas.gov.au/communications/publications/information-sheets/existing-chemical-info-sheets/formaldehyde-factsheet.

53. Garrett MH et al. Increased risk of allergy in children due to formaldehyde exposure in homes. *Allergy.* 1999 Apr;54(4):330-7.

54. Rumchev KB et al. Domestic exposure to formaldehyde significantly increases the risk of asthma in young children. *Eur Respir J.* 2002 Aug;20(2):403-8.

55. Ibid.

56. Krzyzanowski M, Quackenboss JJ, Lebowitz MD. Chronic respiratory effects of indoor formaldehyde exposure. *Environ Res.* 1990 Aug;52(2):117-25.

Chapter 3

1. Thyssen JP. Nickel and cobalt allergy before and after nickel regulation—evaluation of a public health intervention. *Contact Dermatitis.* 2011 Sep;65Suppl 1:1-68.

2. Braga M, Quecchia C, Perotta C, Timpini A, Maccarinelli K, Di Tommaso L, Di Gioacchino M. Systemic nickel allergy syndrome: nosologic framework and usefulness of diet regimen for diagnosis. *Int J Immunopathol Pharmacol.* 2013 Jul-Sep;26(3):707-16.

3. Karlsson MR, Rugtveit J, Brandtzaeg P. Allergen-responsive CD4+CD25+ regulatory T cells in children who have outgrown cow's milk allergy. *J Exp Med.* 2004 Jun 21;199(12):1679-88.

4. Gourevitch D, Kossenkov AV, Zhang Y, Clark L, Chang C, Showe LC, Heber-Katz E. Inflammation and Its Correlates in Regenerative Wound Healing: An Alternate Perspective. *AdvWound Care* (New Rochelle). 2014 Sep 1;3(9):592-603; St John AL, Abraham SN. Innate immunity and its regulation by mast cells. *J Immunol.* 2013 May 1;190(9):4458-63; Metz M, Piliponsky AM, Chen CC, Lammel V, Abrink M, Pejler G, Tsai M, Galli SJ. Mast cells can enhance resistance to snake and honeybee venoms. Science. 2006 Jul 28;313(5786):526-30.

5. Wong GW, Zhuo L, Kimata K, Lam BK, Satoh N, Stevens RL. Ancient origin of mast cells. *Biochem Biophys Res Commun.* 2014 Aug 22;451(2):314-8.

6. Kita H. Eosinophils: multifunctional and distinctive properties. *Int Arch Allergy Immunol.* 2013;161Suppl 2:3-9.

7. Gell PGH, Coombs RRA. *Clinical Aspects of Immunology.* London: Blackwell, 1963.

8. Treviño RJ. Immunology of foods. *Otolaryngol Head Neck Surg.* 1986 Sep;95(2):171-6.

9. Berrens L, van Dijk AG, Weemaes CM. Complement consumption in eggwhite and fish sensitivity. *Clin Allergy.* 1981 Mar;11(2):101-9; Treviño RJ. Immunologic mechanisms in the production of food sensitivities. *Laryngoscope.* 1981 Nov;91(11):1913-36; Saalman R, Carlsson B, Fällström SP, Hanson LA, Ahlstedt S. Antibody-dependent cell-mediated cytotoxicity to beta-lactoglobulin-coated cells with sera from children with intolerance of cow's milk protein. *ClinExpImmunol.* 1991 Sep;85(3):446-52; Carini C, Fratazzi C, Aiuti F. Immune complexes in food-induced arthralgia. *Ann Allergy.* 1987 Dec;59(6):422-8; McCrory WW, Becker CG, Cunningham-Rundles C, Klein RF, Mouradian J, Reisman L. Immune complexglomerulopathy in a child with food hypersensitivity. *Kidney Int.* 1986 Oct;30(4):592-8; Paganelli R, Atherton DJ, Levinsky RJ. Differences between normal and

milk allergic subjects in their immune responses after milk ingestion. *Arch Dis Child*. 1983 Mar;58(3):201-6; Martelletti P, Sutherland J, Anastasi E, Di Mario U, Giacovazzo M. Evidence for an immune-mediated mechanism in food-induced migraine from a study on activated T-cells, IgG4 subclass, anti-IgG antibodies and circulating immune complexes. *Headache*. 1989 Nov;29(10):664-70.

10. Fineman SM. Optimal treatment of anaphylaxis: antihistamines versus epinephrine. *Postgrad Med*. 2014 Jul;126(4):73-81; Campbell RL, Luke A, Weaver AL, St Sauver JL, Bergstralh EJ, Li JT, Manivannan V, Decker WW. Prescriptions for self-injectable epinephrine and follow-up referral in emergency department patients presenting with anaphylaxis. *Ann Allergy Asthma Immunol*. 2008 Dec;101(6):631-6.

11. Sclar DA, Lieberman PL. Anaphylaxis: underdiagnosed, underreported, and undertreated. *Am J Med*. 2014 Jan;127(1 Suppl):S1-5.

12. Bublin M, Breiteneder H. Cross-reactivity of peanutallergens. *Curr Allergy Asthma Rep*. 2014 Apr;14(4):426; Zhuang Y, Dreskin SC. Redefining the major peanut allergens. *Immunol Res*. 2013 Mar;55(1-3):125-34.

13. Sicherer SH, Muñoz-Furlong A, Burks AW, Sampson HA. Prevalence of peanut and tree nut allergy in the US determined by a random digit dial telephone survey. *J Allergy Clin Immunol*. 1999 Apr;103(4):559-62.

14. Sicherer SH, Muñoz-Furlong A, Sampson HA. Prevalence of peanut and tree nut allergy in the United States determined by means of a random digit dial telephone survey: a 5-year follow-up study. *J Allergy Clin Immunol*. 2003 Dec;112(6):1203-7.

15. Sicherer SH, Sampson HA. Peanut allergy: Emerging concepts and approaches for an apparent epidemic. *J Allergy Clin Immunol*. 2007;120(3):491–503.

16. Grundy J, Matthews S, Bateman B, Dean T, Arshad SH. Rising prevalence of allergy to peanut in children: Data from 2 sequential cohorts. *J Allergy Clin Immunol*. 2002;110(5):784–9.

17. Lack G, Fox D, Northstone K, Golding J; Avon Longitudinal Study of Parents and Children Study Team. Factors associated with the development of peanut allergy in childhood. *N Engl J Med*. 2003 Mar 13;348(11):977-85.

18. Dixon V, Habeeb S, Lakshman R. Did you know this medicine has peanut butter in it, doctor? *Arch Dis Child*. Jul 2007;92(7): 654.

19. Fox AT, Sasieni P, du Toit G, Syed H, Lack G. Household peanut consumption as a risk factor for the development of peanut allergy. *J Allergy Clin Immunol*. 2009 Feb;123(2):417-23.

20. Strid J, Hourihane J, Kimber I, Callard R, Strobel S. Epicutaneous exposure to peanut protein prevents oral tolerance and enhances allergic sensitization. *Clin Exp Allergy*. 2005 Jun;35(6):757-66. (Here were their exact findings: Epicutaneous exposure to peanut protein induced potent Th2-type immunity with high levels of IL-4 and serum IgE. Primary skin exposure prevented the

subsequent induction of oral tolerance to peanut in an antigen-specific manner. Upon oral challenge, mice became further sensitized and developed strong peanut-specific IL-4 and IgE responses. Furthermore, animals with existing tolerance to peanut were partly sensitized following epicutaneous exposure.)

21. Pabst O, Mowat AM. Oral tolerance to food protein. *Mucosal Immunology* (2012) 5, 232–9.

22. Commins SP, Satinover SM, Hosen J, Mozena J, Borish L, Lewis BD, et al. Delayed anaphylaxis, angioedema, or urticaria after consumption of red meat in patients with IgE antibodies specific for galactose-α-1,3-galactose. *J Allergy Clin Immunol.* 2009;123:426–3.

23. Van Nunen SA, O'Connor KS, Clarke LR, Boyle RX, Fernando SL. An association between tick bite reactions and red meat allergy in humans. *Med J Aust.* 2009 May 4;190(9):510-1; Hamsten C, Starkhammar M, Tran TA, Johansson M, Bengtsson U, Ahlén G, Sällberg M, Grönlund H, van Hage M. Identification of galactose-α-1,3-galactose in the gastrointestinal tract of the tick Ixodes ricinus; possible relationship with red meat allergy. *Allergy.* 2013 Apr;68(4):549-52; Hamsten C, Tran TA, Starkhammar M, Brauner A, Commins SP, Platts-Mills TA, van Hage M. Red meat allergy in Sweden: association with tick sensitization and B-negative blood groups. *J Allergy Clin Immunol.* 2013 Dec;132(6):1431-4; Gonzalez-Quintela A, Dam Laursen AS, Vidal C, Skaaby T, Gude F, Linneberg A. IgE antibodies to alpha-gal in the general adult population: relationship with tick bites, atopy, and cat ownership. *Clin Exp Allergy.* 2014 Aug;44(8):1061-8; Wen L, Zhou J, Yin J, Sun JL, Sun Y, Wu K, Katial R. Delayed anaphylaxis to red meat associated with specific IgE antibodies to galactose. *Allergy Asthma Immunol Res.* 2015 Jan;7(1):92-4.

24. Steinke JW, Platts-Mills TA, Commins SP. The alpha-gal story: Lessons learned from connecting the dots. *J Allergy Clin Immunol.* 2015 Mar;135(3):589-96; Soh JY, Huang CH, Lee BW. Carbohydrates as food allergens. *Asia Pac Allergy.* 2015 Jan;5(1):17-24.

Chapter 4

1. Wan H, Winton HL, Soeller C, Tovey ER, Gruenert DC, Thompson PJ, Stewart GA, Taylor GW, Garrod DR, Cannell MB, Robinson C. *J Clin Invest.* 1999 Jul;104(1):123-33. Der p 1 facilitates transepithelial allergen delivery by disruption of tight junctions.

Chapter 5

1. Sheri Maxwell, B.S., Charles P. Gerba, Ph.D. "Shoe Study." Department of Soil, Water and Environmental Science, University of Arizona, Tucson, Arizona, March 31, 2008.

2. American College of Allergy, Asthma and Immunology. "Dust Allergy." http://www.acaai.org/allergist/allergies/types/dust-allergy-information/pages/default.

aspx; Asthma and Allergy Foundation of America. "Dust Mites."
http://www.aafa.org/display.cfm?id=9&sub=18&cont=228.

3. Wan et al, 1999.

4. Hewitt CR, Brown AP, Hart BJ, Pritchard DI. A major house dust mite allergen
    disrupts the immunoglobulin E network by selectively cleaving CD23: innate
    protection by antiproteases. *J Exp Med*. 1995 Nov 1;182(5):1537-44.

5. National Institute of Environmental Health Sciences. "Dust Mites." http://
    www.niehs.nih.gov/health/topics/agents/allergens/dustmites/index.cfm.

6. Wright LS, Phipatanakul W. Environmental remediation in the treatment
    of allergy and asthma: latest updates. *Curr Allergy Asthma Rep*. 2014
    Mar;14(3):419. doi: 10.1007/s11882-014-0419-7.

7. Martins-Green M et al. Cigarette smoke toxins deposited on surfaces:
    implications for human health. *PLoS ONE*. January 29, 2014.

8. Curtis W. Noonan Center for Environmental Health Sciences, The University
    of Montana. Asthma randomized trial of indoor wood smoke (ARTIS):
    Rationale and Methods. *Contemp Clin Trials*. Sep 2012; 33(5): 1080–1087.
    Published online Jun 23, 2012.

9. Bui DS et al. Ambient wood smoke, traffic pollution and adult asthma
    prevalence and severity. *Respirology*. 2013 Oct;18(7):1101-7. doi: 10.1111/
    resp.12108.

10. Steinemann AC, Gallagher LG, Davis AL, MacGregor IC. Chemical emissions
    from residential dryer vents during use of fragranced laundry products. *Air
    Qual Atmos Health*. 2013 Mar;6(1):151-6. doi: 10.1007/s11869-011-0156-1.

11. Ibid.

12. Zock JP et al. The use of household cleaning sprays and adult asthma:
    an international longitudinal study. *Am J Respir Crit Care Med*. 2007 Oct
    15;176(8):735-41. Epub 2007 Jun 21.

13. Le Moual N, Varraso R, Siroux V, Dumas O, Nadif R, Pin I, Zock JP, Kauffmann
    F; Epidemiological Study on the Genetics and Environment of Asthma.
    Domestic use of cleaning sprays and asthma activity in females. *Eur Respir J*.
    2012 Dec;40(6):1381-9. doi: 10.1183/09031936.00197611. Epub 2012 Apr 10.

14. Anne Marie Kelly. "Scented Ads: Not Just For Perfume Anymore." *Forbes*,
    January 17, 2012. http://www.forbes.com/sites/annemariekelly/2012/01/17/
    scented-ads-not-just-for-perfume-anymore.

15. Bruce Horovitz. "Dollars and Scents: Some Magazines Are Rethinking Those
    Perfume Ads." *Los Angeles Times,* November 17, 1992. http://articles.latimes.
    com/1992-11-17/business/fi-603_1_perfume-ads.

16. Cone JE, Shusterman D. Health effects of indoor odorants. *Environ Health
    Perspect*. Nov 1991; 95: 53–9.

17. Akdag M et al. Does usage of room air fresheners affect the nasal mucosa? *Am J Rhinol Allergy*. 2014 Sep 11.

18. DaSilva SC et al. Increased skin barrier disruption by sodium lauryl sulfate in mice expressing a constitutively active STAT6 in T cells. *Arch Dermatol Res*. 2012 Jan;304(1):65-71. doi: 10.1007/s00403-011-1168-2. Epub 2011 Sep 30.

19. Belkaid Y, Segre JA. Dialogue between skin microbiota and immunity. *Science*. 2014 Nov 21;346(6212):954-9.

20. Fyhrquist N, Ruokolainen L, Suomalainen A, Lehtimäki S, Veckman V, Vendelin J, Karisola P, Lehto M, Savinko T, Jarva H, Kosunen TU, Corander J, Auvinen P, Paulin L, von Hertzen L, Laatikainen T, Mäkelä M, Haahtela T, Greco D, Hanski I, Alenius H. Acinetobacter species in the skin microbiota protect against allergic sensitization and inflammation. *J Allergy Clin Immunol*. 2014 Dec;134(6):1301-1309.e11.

Chapter 6

1. Park HH, Lee S, Son HY, Park SB, Kim MS, Choi EJ, Singh TS, Ha JH, Lee MG, Kim JE, Hyun MC, Kwon TK, Kim YH, Kim SH. Flavonoids inhibit histamine release and expression of proinflammatory cytokines in mast cells. *Arch Pharm Res*. 2008 Oct;31(10):1303-11; Park HH, Lee S, Oh JM, Lee MS, Yoon KH, Park BH, Kim JW, Song H, Kim SH. Anti-inflammatory activity of fisetin in human mast cells (HMC-1). *Pharmacol Res*. 2007 Jan;55(1):31-7; Gong JH, Shin D, Han SY, Kim JL, Kang YH. Kaempferol suppresses eosionphil infiltration and airway inflammation in airway epithelial cells and in mice with allergic asthma. *J Nutr*. 2012 Jan;142(1):47-56 (Kaempferol is a natural flavonol-type flavonoid that has been isolated from citrus fruits, brussels sprouts, broccoli, apples, and other plant sources); Jung CH, Lee JY, Park JH, Cho BJ, Sim SS, Kim CJ. Flavonols attenuate the immediate and late-phase asthmatic responses to aerosolized-ovalbumin exposure in the conscious guinea pig. *Fitoterapia*. 2010 Oct;81(7):803-12. doi: 10.1016/j.fitote.2010.04.011. Epub 2010 May 10.

Chapter 7

1. Egger J, Carter CM, Soothill JF, Wilson J. Oligoantigenic diet treatment of children with epilepsy and migraine. *J Pediatr*. 1989 Jan;114(1):51-8.

Chapter 8

1. Kim W, Lee H. Advances in nutritional research on regulatory T-cells. Nutrients. Nov 2013; 5(11): 4305–4315; Issazadeh-Navikas S, Teimer R, Bockermann R. Influence of dietary components on regulatory T cells. *Mol Med*. 2012; 18(1): 95–110; Wong CP, Nguyen LP, Noh SK, Bray TM, Bruno RS, Ho E. Induction of regulatory T cells by green tea polyphenol EGCG. *Immunol Lett*. 2011 Sep 30;139(1-2):7-13.

2. Singh A, Holvoet S, Mercenier A. Dietary polyphenols in the prevention and treatment of allergic diseases. *Clin Exp Allergy.* 2011 Oct;41(10):1346-59.

3. Chiu TH, Huang HY, Chiu YF, Pan WH, Kao HY, Chiu JP, Lin MN, Lin CL. Taiwanese vegetarians and omnivores: dietary composition, prevalence of diabetes and IFG. *PLoS One.* 2014 Feb 11;9(2):e88547; Yen CE, Yen CH, Huang MC, Cheng CH, Huang YC. Dietary intake and nutritional status of vegetarian and omnivorous preschool children and their parents in Taiwan. *Nutr Res.* 2008 Jul;28(7):430-6; Krajcovicová-Kudláčková M, Simoncic R, Béderová A, Grancicová E, Magálová T. Influence of vegetarian and mixed nutrition on selected haematological and biochemical parameters in children. *Nahrung.* 1997 Oct;41(5):311-14.

4. Kuo KL, Weng MS, Chiang CT, Tsai YJ, Lin-Shiau SY, Lin JK. Comparative studies on the hypolipidemic and growth suppressive effects of oolong, black, pu-erh, and green tea leaves in rats. *J Agric Food Chem.* 2005 Jan 26;53(2):480-9.

5. Yun JM, Jialal I, Devaraj S. Effects of epigallocatechin gallate on regulatory T cell number and function in obese v. lean volunteers. *Br J Nutr.* 2010 Jun;103(12):1771-7.

6. Wang J, Ren Z, Xu Y, Xiao S, Meydani SN, Wu D. Epigallocatechin-3-gallate ameliorates experimental autoimmune encephalomyelitis by altering balance among CD4+ T-cell subsets. *Am J Pathol.* 2012 Jan;180(1):221-34.

7. Kuo CL, Chen TS, Liou SY, Hsieh CC. Immunomodulatory effects of EGCG fraction of green tea extract in innate and adaptive immunity via T regulatory cells in murine model. *Immunopharmacol Immunotoxicol.* 2014 Oct;36(5):364-70.

8. Pae M, Ren Z, Meydani M, Shang F, Smith D, Meydani SN, Wu D. Dietary supplementation with high dose of epigallocatechin-3-gallate promotes inflammatory response in mice. *J Nutr Biochem.* 2012 Jun;23(6):526-31.

9. Nerurkar A et al. When conventional providers recommend unconventional medicine: results of a national study. *Arch Intern Med.* May 9, 2011; 171(9): 862–864. doi: 10.1001/archinternmed.2011.160.

10. Ehren JL, Maher P. Concurrent regulation of the transcription factors Nrf2 and ATF4 mediates the enhancement of glutathione levels by the flavonoid fisetin. *Biochem Pharmacol.* 2013 Jun 15;85(12):1816-26.

11. Tada-Oikawa S, Murata M, Kato T. Preferential induction of apoptosis in regulatory T cells by tributyltin: possible involvement in the exacerbation of allergic diseases. *Nihon Eiseigaku Zasshi.* 2010 Sep;65(4):530-5.

12. Wu MY, Hung SK, Fu SL. Immunosuppressive effects of fisetin in ovalbumin-induced asthma through inhibition of NF-κB activity. *J Agric Food Chem.* 2011 Oct 12;59(19):10496-504; Goh FY1, Upton N, Guan S, Cheng C, Shanmugam MK, Sethi G, Leung BP, Wong WS. Fisetin, a bioactive flavonol, attenuates allergic airway inflammation through negative regulation of NF-κB. *Eur J Pharmacol.* 2012 Mar 15;679(1-3):109-16.

13. Maher P. Modulation of multiple pathways involved in the maintenance of neuronal function during aging by fisetin. *Genes Nutr.* 2009 Dec;4(4):297-307.

14. Reganold JP, Andrews PK, Reeve JR, Carpenter-Boggs L, Schadt CW, Alldredge JR, Ross CF, Davies NM, Zhou J. Fruit and soil quality of organic and conventional strawberry agroecosystems. *PLoS One.* 2010 Sep 1;5(9). pii: e12346. Erratum in *PLoS One.* 2010;5(10). doi: 10.1371/annotation/1eefd0a4-77af-4f48-98c3-2c5696ca9e7a.

15. Li RR, Pang LL, Du Q, Shi Y, Dai WJ, Yin KS. Apigenin inhibits allergen-induced airway inflammation and switches immune response in a murine model of asthma. *Immunopharmacol Immunotoxicol.* 2010 Sep;32(3):364-70.

Chapter 9

1. Tanaka A, Nomura Y, Matsuda A, Ohmori K, Matsuda H. Mast cells function as an alternative modulator of adipogenesis through 15-deoxy-delta-12, 14-prostaglandin J2. *Am J Physiol Cell Physiol.* 2011 Dec;301(6):C1360-7; Liu J, Divoux A, Sun J, Zhang J, Clement K, Glickman JN, Sukhova GK, Wolters PJ, Du J, Gorgun CZ, et al. Genetic deficiency and pharmacological stabilization of mast cells reduce diet-induced obesity and diabetes in mice. *Nat. Med.* 2009;15:940–5.

2. Sood A, Seagrave J, Herbert G, Harkins M, Alam Y, Chiavaroli A, Shohreh R, Montuschi P, Campen M, Harmon M, Qualls C, Berwick M, Schuyler M. High sputum total adiponectin is associated with low odds for asthma. *J Asthma.* 2014 Jun;51(5):459-66.

3. Yamamoto R, Ueki S, Moritoki Y, Kobayashi Y, Oyamada H, Konno Y, Tamaki M, Itoga M, Takeda M, Ito W, Chihara J. Adiponectin attenuates human eosinophil adhesion and chemotaxis: implications in allergic inflammation. *J Asthma.* 2013 Oct;50(8):828-35.

4. Grotta MB, Squebola-Cola DM, Toro AA, Ribeiro MA, Mazon SB, Ribeiro JD, Antunes E. Obesity increases eosinophil activity in asthmatic children and adolescents. *BMC Pulm Med.* 2013 Jun 18;13:39.

5. Rönmark E, Andersson C, Nyström L, Forsberg B, Järvholm B, Lundbäck B. Obesity increases the risk of incident asthma among adults. *Eur Respir J.* 2005 Feb;25(2):282-8 ("Increased body mass index was a significant risk factor for both males and females"); Zhang X, Morrison-Carpenter T, Holt JB, Callahan DB. Trends in adult current asthma prevalence and contributing risk factors in the United States by state: 2000-2009. *BMC Public Health.* 2013 Dec 10;13:1156; Sideleva O, Dixon AE. The many faces of asthma in obesity. *J Cell Biochem.* 2014 Mar;115(3):421-6 (NOTE: Obesity is a major risk factor for the development of asthma and causes severe, uncontrolled disease that responds poorly to therapy. The obese state alters early onset allergic asthma and leads to the development of a novel form of late-onset asthma secondary to obesity. The presentation of early onset allergic asthma is altered through effects on immune function. Factors such as mechanical loading, effects of adipokines on airways, altered diet, insulin resistance, and altered

metabolism of nitric oxide likely all contribute to increased airway reactivity in obesity, causing late onset asthma in obesity. Obesity also alters responses to environmental factors such as ozone and particulate matter. Focused studies to understand the importance of these factors in the pathogenesis of airway disease in obesity will be essential to develop therapies to intervene in this new epidemic of airway disease); Ma J, Xiao L. Association of general and central obesity and atopic and nonatopic asthma in US adults. *J Asthma*. 2013 May;50(4):395-402; Forno E, Acosta-Pérez E, Brehm JM, Han YY, Alvarez M, Colón-Semidey A, Canino G, Celedón JC. Obesity and adiposity indicators, asthma, and atopy in Puerto Rican children. *J Allergy Clin Immunol*. 2014 May;133(5):1308-14, 1314.e1-5 (Analysis of a large U.S. population database found that waist to height ratio was associated with the presence of allergic asthma in both women and men); Kilpeläinen M, Terho EO, Helenius H, Koskenvuo M. Body mass index and physical activity in relation to asthma and atopic diseases in young adults. *Respir Med*. 2006 Sep;100(9):1518-25 ("The risk of allergic rhinoconjunctivitis and atopic dermatitis increased quite linearly with BMI among women but not men. Low leisure time physical activity seems not to explain the greater risk of asthma among obese men and women. The quite linear association between BMI and both allergic rhinoconjunctivitis and wheezing among women suggests the independent effect of body fat on atopic diseases"); Silverberg JI, Silverberg NB, Lee-Wong M. Association between atopic dermatitis and obesity in adulthood. *Br J Dermatol*. 2012 Mar;166(3):498-504.

6. Chung SD, Chen PY, Lin HC, Hung SH. Comorbidity profile of chronic rhinosinusitis: a population-based study. *Laryngoscope*. 2014 Jul;124(7):1536-41.

7. Ratliff JC, Barber JA, Palmese LB, Reutenauer EL, Tek C. Association of prescription H1 antihistamine use with obesity: results from the National Health and Nutrition Examination Survey. *Obesity* (Silver Spring). 2010 Dec;18(12):2398-400.

8. Visness CM, London SJ, Daniels JL, Kaufman JS, Yeatts KB, Siega-Riz AM, Liu AH, Calatroni A, Zeldin DC. Association of obesity with IgE levels and allergy symptoms in children and adolescents: results from the National Health and Nutrition Examination Survey 2005-2006. *J Allergy Clin Immunol*. 2009 May;123(5):1163-9, 1169.e1-4.

9. Brumpton B, Langhammer A, Romundstad P, Chen Y, Mai XM. General and abdominal obesity and incident asthma in adults: the HUNT study. *Eur Respir J*. 2013 Feb;41(2):323-9; Von Behren J, Lipsett M, Horn-Ross PL, Delfino RJ, Gilliland F, McConnell R, Bernstein L, Clarke CA, Reynolds P. Obesity, waist size and prevalence of current asthma in the California Teachers Study cohort. *Thorax*. 2009 Oct;64(10):889-93; Shore SA. Obesity and asthma: location, location, location. *Eur Respir J*. 2013 Feb;41(2):253-4; Jensen ME, Gibson PG, Collins CE, Hilton JM, Wood LG. Diet-induced weight loss in obese children with asthma: a randomized controlled trial. *Clin Exp Allergy*. 2013 Jul;43(7):775-84; Scott HA, Gibson PG, Garg ML, Pretto JJ, Morgan PJ, Callister R, Wood LG. Dietary restriction and exercise improve airway inflammation and clinical outcomes in overweight and obese asthma: a randomized trial. *Clin Exp Allergy*. 2013 Jan;43(1):36-49.

10. Hanna BC, Wormald PJ. Gastroesophageal reflux and chronic rhinosinusitis. *Curr Opin Otolaryngol Head Neck Surg.* 2012 Feb;20(1):15-8.

11. DelGaudio JM. Direct nasopharyngeal reflux of gastric acid is a contributing factor in refractory chronic rhinosinusitis. *Laryngoscope.* 2005 Jun;115(6):946-57.

12. McCallister JW, Parsons JP, Mastronarde JG. The relationship between gastroesophageal reflux and asthma: an update. *Ther Adv Respir Dis.* 2011 Apr;5(2):143-50; Sontag SJ. The spectrum of pulmonary symptoms due to gastroesophageal reflux. *Thorac Surg Clin.* 2005 Aug;15(3):353-68; Komatsu Y, Hoppo T, Jobe BA. Proximal reflux as a cause of adult-onset asthma: the case for hypopharyngeal impedance testing to improve the sensitivity of diagnosis. *JAMA Surg.* 2013 Jan;148(1):50-8; Banaszkiewicz A1, Dembinski L, Zawadzka-Krajewska A, Dziekiewicz M, Albrecht P, Kulus M, Radzikowski A. Evaluation of laryngopharyngeal reflux in pediatric patients with asthma using a new technique of pharyngeal pH-monitoring. *Adv Exp Med Biol.* 2013;755:89-95; Kilic M, Ozturk F, Kirmemis O, Atmaca S, Guner SN, Caltepe G, Sancak R, Kalayci AG. Impact of laryngopharyngeal and gastroesophageal reflux on asthma control in children. *Int J Pediatr Otorhinolaryngol.* 2013 Mar;77(3):341-5.

13. Canani RB, Cirillo P, Roggero P, Romano C, Malamisura B, Terrin G, Passariello A, Manguso F, Morelli L, Guarino A; Working Group on Intestinal Infections of the Italian Society of Pediatric Gastroenterology, Hepatology and Nutrition (SIGENP). Therapy with gastric acidity inhibitors increases the risk of acute gastroenteritis and community-acquired pneumonia in children. *Pediatrics.* 2006 May;117(5):e817-20; Hauben M, Horn S, Reich L, Younus M. Association between gastric acid suppressants and Clostridium difficile colitis and community-acquired pneumonia: analysis using pharmacovigilance tools. *Int J Infect Dis.* 2007 Mar 2; Vestergaard P, Rejnmark L, Mosekilde L. Proton pump inhibitors, histamine H2 receptor antagonists, and other antacid medications and the risk of fracture. *Calcif Tissue Int.* 2006 Aug;79(2):76-83; Gulmez SE, Holm A, Frederiksen H, Jensen TG, Pedersen C, Hallas J. Use of proton pump inhibitors and the risk of community-acquired pneumonia: a population-based case-control study. *Arch Intern Med.* 2007 May 14;167(9):950-5; Jalving M, Koornstra JJ, Wesseling J, Boezen HM, DE Jong S, Kleibeuker JH. Increased risk of fundic gland polyps during long-term proton pump inhibitor therapy. *Aliment Pharmacol Ther.* 2006 Nov 1;24(9):1341-8; Laheij RJ, Sturkenboom MC, Hassing RJ, Dieleman J, Stricker BH, Jansen JB. Risk of community-acquired pneumonia and use of gastric acid-suppressive drugs. *JAMA.* 2004 Oct 27;292(16):1955-60; Dial S, Delaney JA, Barkun AN, Suissa S. Use of gastric acid-suppressive agents and the risk of community-acquired Clostridium difficile-associated disease. *JAMA.* 2005 Dec 21;294(23):2989-95; Dial S, Alrasadi K, Manoukian C, Huang A, Menzies D. Risk of Clostridium difficile diarrhea among hospital inpatients prescribed proton pump inhibitors: cohort and case-control studies. *CMAJ.* 2004 Jul 6;171(1):33-8; Laheij RJ, Van Ijzendoorn MC, Janssen MJ, Jansen JB. Gastric acid-suppressive therapy and community-acquired respiratory infections. *Aliment Pharmacol Ther.* 2003 Oct 15;18(8):847-51; Yang YX, Lewis JD, Epstein S, Metz DC. Long-term proton pump inhibitor therapy and risk of hip fracture. *JAMA.* 2006 Dec 27;296(24):2947-53.

14. Blake K, Teague WG. Gastroesophageal reflux disease and childhood asthma. *Curr Opin Pulm Med.* 2013 Jan;19(1):24-9; Writing Committee for the American Lung Association Asthma Clinical Research Centers, Holbrook JT, Wise RA, Gold BD, Blake K, Brown ED, Castro M, Dozor AJ, Lima JJ, Mastronarde JG, Sockrider MM, Teague WG. Lansoprazole for children with poorly controlled asthma: a randomized controlled trial. *JAMA.* 2012 Jan 25;307(4):373-81.

15. Yoshikawa I, Nagato M, Yamasaki M, Kume K, Otsuki M. Long-term treatment with proton pump inhibitor is associated with undesired weight gain. *World J Gastroenterol.* 2009 Oct 14;15(38):4794-8.

16. Untersmayr E, Bakos N, Schöll I, Kundi M, Roth-Walter F, Szalai K, Riemer AB, Ankersmit HJ, Scheiner O, Boltz-Nitulescu G, Jensen-Jarolim E. Anti-ulcer drugs promote IgE formation toward dietary antigens in adult patients. *FASEB J.* 2005 Apr;19(6):656-8.

17. DeMuth K, Stecenko A, Sullivan K, Fitzpatrick A. Relationship between treatment with antacid medication and the prevalence of food allergy in children. *Allergy Asthma Proc.* 2013 May-Jun;34(3):227-32.

18. Pali-Schöll I, Herzog R, Wallmann J, Szalai K, Brunner R, Lukschal A, Karagiannis P, Diesner SC, Jensen-Jarolim E. Antacids and dietary supplements with an influence on the gastric pH increase the risk for food sensitization. *Clin Exp Allergy.* 2010 Jul;40(7):1091-8.

19. Ramírez E, Cabañas R, Laserna LS, Fiandor A, Tong H, Prior N, Calderón O, Medrano N, Bobolea I, Frías J, Quirce S. Proton pump inhibitors are associated with hypersensitivity reactions to drugs in hospitalized patients: a nested case-control in a retrospective cohort study. *Clin Exp Allergy.* 2013 Mar;43(3):344-52.

20. Hak E, Mulder B, Schuiling-Veninga CC, de Vries TW, Jick SS. Use of acid-suppressive drugs in pregnancy and the risk of childhood asthma: bidirectional crossover study using the general practice research database. *Drug Saf.* 2013 Nov;36(11):1097-104.

21. Diesner SC, Pali-Schöll I, Jensen-Jarolim E, Untersmayr E. Mechanisms and risk factors for type 1 food allergies: the role of gastric digestion. *Wien Med Wochenschr.* 2012 Dec;162(23-24):513-8.

22. Pali-Schöll I, Jensen-Jarolim E. Anti-acid medication as a risk factor for food allergy. *Allergy.* 2011 Apr;66(4):469-77.

23. Rodriguez-Stanley S, Ahmed T, Zubaidi S, Riley S, Akbarali HI, Mellow MH, Miner PB. Calcium carbonate antacids alter esophageal motility in heartburn sufferers. *Dig Dis Sci.* 2004 Nov-Dec;49(11-12):1862-7; Rich H, Sohn UD, Behar J, Kim N, Biancani P. Experimental esophagitis affects intracellular calcium stores in the cat lower esophageal sphincter. *Am J Physiol.* 1997 Jun;272(6 Pt 1):G1523-9; Kovac JR, Preiksaitis HG, Sims SM. Functional and molecular analysis of L-type calcium channels in human esophagus and lower esophageal sphincter smooth muscle. *Am J Physiol Gastrointest Liver Physiol* 289: G998-G1006, 2005; Harnett KM, Cao W, Kim N, Sohn UD, Rich H, Behar

J, Biancani P. Signal transduction in esophageal and LES circular muscle contraction. *Yale J Biol Med*. 1999 Mar-Jun;72(2-3):153-68.

24. Lucendo AJ, Arias A. Treatment of adult eosinophilic esophagitis with diet. *Dig Dis*. 2014;32(1-2):120-5; Kagalwalla AF. Dietary treatment of eosinophilic esophagitis in children. *Dig Dis*. 2014;32(1-2):114-9.

25. Simon D, Straumann A, Dahinden C, Simon HU. Frequent sensitization to Candida albicans and profilins in adult eosinophilic esophagitis. *Allergy*. 2013 Jul;68(7):945-8.

26. Vidal C, Pérez-Carral C, Chomón B. Unsuspected sources of soybean exposure. *Ann Allergy Asthma Immunol*. 1997 Oct;79(4):350-2.

27. Shimada K, Kawarabayashi T, Tanaka A, Fukuda D, Nakamura Y, Yoshiyama M, Takeuchi K, Sawaki T, Hosoda K, Yoshikawa J. Oolong tea increases plasma adiponectin levels and low-density lipoprotein particle size in patients with coronary artery disease. *Diabetes Res Clin Pract*. 2004 Sep;65(3):227-34.

28. He RR, Chen L, Lin BH, Matsui Y, Yao XS, Kurihara H. Beneficial effects of oolong tea consumption on diet-induced overweight and obese subjects. *Chin J Integr Med*. 2009 Feb;15(1):34-41.

29. Jin T, Kim OY, Shin MJ, Choi EY, Lee SS, Han YS, Chung JH. Fisetin up-regulates the expression of adiponectin in 3T3-L1 adipocytes via the activation of silent mating type information regulation 2 homologue 1 (SIRT1)-deacetylase and peroxisome proliferator-activated receptors (PPARs). *J Agric Food Chem*. 2014 Oct 29;62(43):10468-74.

30. Jung CH, Kim H, Ahn J, Jeon TI, Lee DH, Ha TY. Fisetin regulates obesity by targeting mTORC1 signaling. *J Nutr Biochem*. 2013 Aug;24(8):1547-54.

31. Nisha VM, Anusree SS, Priyanka A, Raghu KG. Apigenin and quercetin ameliorate mitochondrial alterations by tunicamycin-induced ER stress in 3T3-L1 adipocytes. *Appl Biochem Biotechnol*. 2014 Oct;174(4):1365-75.

32. Jennings A, Welch AA, Spector T, Macgregor A, Cassidy A. Intakes of anthocyanins and flavones are associated with biomarkers of insulin resistance and inflammation in women. *J Nutr*. 2014 Feb;144(2):202-8.

33. Jennings et al, 2014; Yannakoulia M1, Yiannakouris N, Melistas L, Fappa E, Vidra N, Kontogianni MD, Mantzoros CS. Dietary factors associated with plasma high molecular weight and total adiponectin levels in apparently healthy women. *Eur J Endocrinol*. 2008 Oct;159(4):R5-10; Simão TN, Lozovoy MA, Simão AN, Oliveira SR, Venturini D, Morimoto HK, Miglioranza LH, Dichi I. Reduced-energy cranberry juice increases folic acid and adiponectin and reduces homocysteine and oxidative stress in patients with the metabolic syndrome. *Br J Nutr*. 2013 Nov;110(10):1885-94; Gulati S, Misra A, Pandey RM, Bhatt SP, Saluja S. Effects of pistachio nuts on body composition, metabolic, inflammatory and oxidative stress parameters in Asian Indians with metabolic syndrome: a 24-wk, randomized control trial. *Nutrition*. 2014 Feb;30(2):192-7; Ostrowska L, Fiedorczuk J, Adamska E. Effect of diet and other factors on serum adiponectin concentrations in patients with type 2 diabetes. *Rocz*

Panstw Zakl Hig. 2013;64(1):61-6; Yeung EH, Appel LJ, Miller ER 3rd, Kao WH. The effects of macronutrient intake on total and high-molecular weight adiponectin: results from the OMNI-Heart trial. *Obesity* (Silver Spring). 2010 Aug;18(8):1632-7; Lehtonen HM, Suomela JP, Tahvonen R, Vaarno J, Venojärvi M, Viikari J, Kallio H. Berry meals and risk factors associated with metabolic syndrome. *Eur J Clin Nutr.* 2010 Jun;64(6):614-21; Lozano A, Perez-Martinez P, Marin C, Tinahones FJ, Delgado-Lista J, Cruz-Teno C, Gomez-Luna P, Rodriguez-Cantalejo F, Perez-Jimenez F, Lopez-Miranda J. An acute intake of a walnut-enriched meal improves postprandial adiponectin response in healthy young adults. *Nutr Res.* 2013 Dec;33(12):1012-8.

34. Pereira R de S. Regression of gastroesophageal reflux disease symptoms using dietary supplementation with melatonin, vitamins and aminoacids: comparison with omeprazole. *J Pineal Res.* 2006 Oct;41(3):195-200; Werbach MR. Melatonin for the treatment of gastroesophageal reflux disease. *Altern Ther Health Med.* 2008 Jul-Aug;14(4):54-8; Kandil TS, Mousa AA, El-Gendy AA, Abbas AM. The potential therapeutic effect of melatonin in Gastro-Esophageal Reflux Disease. *BMC Gastroenterol.* 2010 Jan 18;10:7.

Chapter 10

1. Marshall GD Jr. Stress and allergic diseases—still underrecognized and undertreated. *Ann Allergy Asthma Immunol.* 2014 Apr;112(4):275.

2. Kiecolt-Glaser JK, Heffner KL, Glaser R, Malarkey WB, Porter K, Atkinson C, Laskowski B, Lemeshow S, Marshall GD. How stress and anxiety can alter immediate and late phase skin test responses in allergic rhinitis. *Psychoneuroendocrinology.* 2009 Jun;34(5):670-80.

3. Dave ND, Xiang L, Rehm KE, Marshall GD Jr. Stress and allergic diseases. *Immunol Allergy Clin North Am.* 2011 Feb;31(1):55-68.

4. Kilpeläinen M, Koskenvuo M, Helenius H, Terho EO. Stressful life events promote the manifestation of asthma and atopic diseases. *Clin Exp Allergy.* 2002 Feb;32(2):256-63.

5. Rosenkranz MA et al. A comparison of mindfulness-based stress reduction and an active control in modulation of neurogenic inflammation. *Brain Behav Immun.* 2013 Jan;27(1):174-84. doi: 10.1016/j.bbi.2012.10.013. Epub 2012 Oct 22.

6. Posner MI, Tang YY, Lynch G. Mechanisms of white matter change induced by meditation training. Front Psychol. 2014 Oct 27;5:1220; Moore A, Gruber T, Derose J, Malinowski P. Regular, brief mindfulness meditation practice improves electrophysiological markers of attentional control. *Front Hum Neurosci.* 2012 Feb 10;6:18.

7. Kozasa EH, Sato JR, Lacerda SS, Barreiros MA, Radvany J, Russell TA, Sanches LG, Mello LE, Amaro E Jr. Meditation training increases brain efficiency in an attention task. *Neuroimage.* 2012 Jan 2;59(1):745-9; van Leeuwen S, Singer W, Melloni L. Meditation increases the depth of information processing and

improves the allocation of attention in space. *Front Hum Neurosci.* 2012 May 15;6:133; Gard T, Taquet M, Dixit R, Hölzel BK, de Montjoye YA, Brach N, Salat DH, Dickerson BC, Gray JR, Lazar SW. Fluid intelligence and brain functional organization in aging yoga and meditation practitioners. *Front Aging Neurosci.* 2014 Apr 22;6:76.

8. Wolever RQ, Bobinet KJ, McCabe K, Mackenzie ER, Fekete E, Kusnick CA, Baime M. Effective and viable mind-body stress reduction in the workplace: a randomized controlled trial. *J Occup Health Psychol.* 2012 Apr;17(2):246-58.

9. Tonelli ME, Wachholtz AB. Meditation-based treatment yielding immediate relief for meditation-naïve migraineurs. *Pain Manag Nurs.* 2014 Mar;15(1):36-40; Keefer L, Blanchard EB. A one year follow-up of relaxation response meditation as a treatment for irritable bowel syndrome. *Behav Res Ther.* 2002 May;40(5):541-6.

10. Bae BG, Oh SH, Park CO, Noh S, Noh JY, Kim KR, Lee KH. Progressive muscle relaxation therapy for atopic dermatitis: objective assessment of efficacy. *Acta DermVenereol.* 2012 Jan;92(1):57-61.

11. Nickel C, Lahmann C, Muehlbacher M, Pedrosa Gil F, Kaplan P, Buschmann W, Tritt K, Kettler C, Bachler E, Egger C, Anvar J, Fartacek R, Loew T, Rother W, Nickel M. Pregnant women with bronchial asthma benefit from progressive muscle relaxation: a randomized, prospective, controlled trial. *Psychother Psychosom.* 2006;75(4):237-43; Nickel C, Kettler C, Muehlbacher M, Lahmann C, Tritt K, Fartacek R, Bachler E, Rother N, Egger C, Rother WK, Loew TH, Nickel MK. Effect of progressive muscle relaxation in adolescent female bronchial asthma patients: a randomized, double-blind, controlled study. *J Psychosom Res.* 2005 Dec;59(6):393-8.

12. Bidwell AJ, Yazel B, Davin D, Fairchild TJ, Kanaley JA. Yoga training improves quality of life in women with asthma. *J Altern Complement Med.* 2012 Aug;18(8):749-55; Pbert L, Madison JM, Druker S, Olendzki N, Magner R, Reed G, Allison J, Carmody J. Effect of mindfulness training on asthma quality of life and lung function: a randomised controlled trial. *Thorax.* 2012 Sep;67(9):769-76.

13. Henry M, de Rivera JL, Gonzalez-Martin IJ, Abreu J. Improvement of respiratory function in chronic asthmatic patients with autogenic therapy. *J Psychosom Res.* 1993 Apr;37(3):265-70.

14. Olness K, Hall H, Rozniecki JJ, Schmidt W, Theoharides TC. Mast cell activation in children with migraine before and after training in self-regulation. *Headache.* 1999 Feb;39(2):101-7.

15. Vempati R, Bijlani RL, Deepak KK. The efficacy of a comprehensive lifestyle modification programme based on yoga in the management of bronchial asthma: a randomized controlled trial. *BMC Pulm Med.* 2009 Jul 30;9:37.

16. Kuo FE. Parks and other green environments: Essential components of a healthy human habitat. *Australas.* Parks Leisure. 2010;14:1–48.

17. Epsom Salt Council. "About Epsom Salts." http://www.epsomsaltcouncil.org/ articles/universal_health_institute_about_epsom_salt.pdf.

18. Epsom Salt Council. "Report on Absorption of magnesium sulfate (Epsom salts) across the skin." http://www.epsomsaltcouncil.org/articles/report_on_ absorption_of_magnesium_sulfate.pdf.

19. Khalfa S et al. Effects of relaxing music on salivary cortisol level after psychological stress. *Ann N Y Acad Sci.* 2003 Nov;999:374-6.

20. **Fibromyalgia:** Baptista AS, Villela AL, Jones A, Natour J. Effectiveness of dance in patients with fibromyalgia: a randomized, single-blind, controlled study. *Clin Exp Rheumatol.* 2012 Nov-Dec;30(6 Suppl 74):18-23; Carbonell-Baeza A, Aparicio VA, Martins-Pereira CM, Gatto-Cardia CM, Ortega FB, Huertas FJ, Tercedor P, Ruiz JR, Delgado-Fernandez M. Efficacy of Biodanza for treating women with fibromyalgia. *J Altern Complement Med.* 2010 Nov;16(11):1191-200. **Depression:** Pinniger R, Brown RF, Thorsteinsson EB, McKinley P. Argentine tango dance compared to mindfulness meditation and a waiting-list control: a randomised trial for treating depression. *Complement Ther Med.* 2012 Dec;20(6):377-84; Akandere M, Demir B. The effect of dance over depression. *Coll Antropol.* 2011 Sep;35(3):651-6. **High blood pressure:** Aweto HA, Owoeye OB, Akinbo SR, Onabajo AA. Effects of dance movement therapy on selected cardiovascular parameters and estimated maximum oxygen consumption in hypertensive patients. *Nig Q J Hosp Med.* 2012 Apr-Jun;22(2):125-9. **Heart failure:** Belardinelli R, Lacalaprice F, Ventrella C, Volpe L, Faccenda E. Waltz dancing in patients with chronic heart failure: new form of exercise training. *Circ Heart Fail.* 2008 Jul;1(2):107-14. **Cancer-related fatigue and quality of life:** Sturm I, Baak J, Storek B, Traore A, Thuss-Patience P. Effect of dance on cancer-related fatigue and quality of life. *Support Care Cancer.* 2014 Aug;22(8):2241-9; Sandel SL, Judge JO, Landry N, Faria L, Ouellette R, Majczak M. Dance and movement program improves quality-of-life measures in breast cancer survivors. *Cancer Nurs.* 2005 Jul-Aug;28(4):301-9. **Parkinson's disease:** McKee KE, Hackney ME. The effects of adapted tango on spatial cognition and disease severity in Parkinson's disease. J Mot Behav. 2013;45(6):519-29; Volpe D, Signorini M, Marchetto A, Lynch T, Morris ME. A comparison of Irish set dancing and exercises for people with Parkinson's disease: a phase II feasibility study. *BMC Geriatr.* 2013 Jun 4;13:54; Duncan RP, Earhart GM. Randomized controlled trial of community-based dancing to modify disease progression in Parkinson disease. *Neurorehabil Neural Repair.* 2012 Feb;26(2):132-43. **Rheumatoid arthritis:** Moffet H, Noreau L, Parent E, Drolet M. Feasibility of an eight-week dance-based exercise program and its effects on locomotor ability of persons with functional class III rheumatoid arthritis. *Arthritis Care Res.* 2000 Apr;13(2):100-11; Van Deusen J, Harlowe D. The efficacy of the ROM Dance Program for adults with rheumatoid arthritis. *Am J Occup Ther.* 1987 Feb;41(2):90-5. **Asthma:** Wolf SI, Lampl KL. Pulmonary rehabilitation: the use of aerobic dance as a therapeutic exercise for asthmatic patients. *Ann Allergy.* 1988 Nov;61(5):357-60.

21. Verghese J, Lipton RB, Katz MJ, Hall CB, Derby CA, Kuslansky G, Ambrose AF, Sliwinski M, Buschke H. Leisure activities and the risk of dementia in the elderly. *N Engl J Med.* 2003 Jun 19;348(25):2508-16.

22. Christiane Northrup, *Goddesses Never Age* (Carlsbad, CA: Hay House, 2014), p. 261.

23. Jaremka LM et al. Loneliness promotes inflammation during acute stress. *Psychol Sci.* 2013 Jul 1;24(7):1089-97. doi: 10.1177/0956797612464059. Epub 2013 Apr 29.

24. Creswell JD, Irwin MR, Burklund LJ, Lieberman MD, Arevalo JM, Ma J, Breen EC, Cole SW. Mindfulness-Based Stress Reduction training reduces loneliness and pro-inflammatory gene expression in older adults: a small randomized controlled trial. *Brain Behav Immun.* 2012 Oct;26(7):1095-101.

25. Powell E. Does habitual stress cause sleep problems and daytime functioning impairments, or is stress the result of poor sleep? Research abstract presented on Wednesday, June 10, at SLEEP 2009, the 23rd Annual Meeting of the Associated Professional Sleep Societies.

26. Howatson G, Bell PG, Tallent J, Middleton B, McHugh MP, Ellis J. Effect of tart cherry juice (Prunuscerasus) on melatonin levels and enhanced sleep quality. *European Journal of Nutrition.* 2011 Oct 30.

Chapter 11

1. Nation J, Kaufman M, Allen M, Sheyn A, Coticchia J. Incidence of gastroesophageal reflux disease and positive maxillary antral cultures in children with symptoms of chronic rhinosinusitis. *Int J Pediatr Otorhinolaryngol.* 2014 Feb;78(2):218-22; de Bortoli N1, Nacci A, Savarino E, Martinucci I, Bellini M, Fattori B, Ceccarelli L, Costa F, Mumolo MG, Ricchiuti A, Savarino V, Berrettini S, Marchi S. How many cases of laryngopharyngeal reflux suspected by laryngoscopy are gastroesophageal reflux disease–related? *World J Gastroenterol.* 2012 Aug 28;18(32):4363-70. doi: 10.3748/wjg.v18. i32.4363.

2. Bernstein JA. Allergic and mixed rhinitis: Epidemiology and natural history. *Allergy Asthma Proc.* 2010 Sep-Oct;31(5):365-9.

3. Greiner AN, Hellings PW, Rotiroti G, Scadding GK. Allergic rhinitis. *Lancet.* 2011 Dec 17;378(9809):2112-22. doi: 10.1016/S0140-6736(11)60130-X. Epub 2011 Jul 23.

4. Bousquet J, Bullinger M, Fayol C, Marquis P, Valentin B, Burtin B. Assessment of quality of life in patients with perennial allergic rhinitis with the French version of the SF-36 Health Status Questionnaire. *J Allergy Clin Immunol.*1994;94(2 Pt 1):182–188.

5. Vuurman EF, Vuurman LL, Lutgens I, Kremer B. Allergic rhinitis is a risk factor for traffic safety. *Allergy.* 2014 Jul;69(7):906-12.

6. Wilken JA, Berkowitz R, Kane R. Decrements in vigilance and cognitive functioning associated with ragweed-induced allergic rhinitis. *Ann Allergy Asthma Immunol.* 2002 Oct;89(4):372-80.

7.	Ciprandi G, Passalacqua G. Allergy and the nose. *Clin Exp Immunol*. Sep 2008; 153(Suppl 1): 22–26; Ciprandi G, Tosca MA, Fasce L. Allergic children have more numerous and severe respiratory infections than non-allergic children. *Pediatr Allergy Immunol*.2006;17:389–91; Cirillo I, Marseglia GL, Klersy C, Ciprandi G. Allergic patients have more numerous and prolonged respiratory infections than non-allergic subjects. *Allergy*. 2007;62:1087–90.

8.	Jáuregui I, Mullol J, Dávila I, Ferrer M, Bartra J, del Cuvillo A, Montoro J, Sastre J, Valero A. Allergic rhinitis and school performance. *J Investig Allergol Clin Immunol*. 2009;19Suppl 1:32-9.

9.	Camelo-Nunes IC, Solé D. Allergic rhinitis: indicators of quality of life. *J Bras Pneumol*. 2010 Jan-Feb;36(1):124-33.

10.	Bianco A, Whiteman SC, Sethi SK, Allen JT, Knight RA, Spiteri MA. Expression of intercellular adhesion molecule-1 (ICAM-1) in nasal epithelial cells of atopic subjects: a mechanism for increased rhinovirus infection? *Clin Exp Immunol*. 2000 Aug;121(2):339-45.

11.	Novick SG, Godfrey JC, Pollack RL, Wilder HR. Zinc-induced suppression of inflammation in the respiratory tract, caused by infection with human rhinovirus and other irritants. *Med Hypotheses*. 1997 Oct;49(4):347-57.

12.	Hulisz D. Efficacy of zinc against common cold viruses: an overview. *J Am Pharm Assoc* (2003). 2004 Sep-Oct;44(5):594-603.

13.	Hamilos DL. Chronic rhinosinusitis: epidemiology and medical management. *J Allergy Clin Immunol*. 2011 Oct;128(4):693-70.

14.	Lotvall J, Ekerljung L, Lundback B. Multi-symptom asthma is closely related to nasal blockage, rhinorrhea and symptoms of chronic rhinosinusitis–evidence from the West Sweden Asthma Study. *Respir Res*. 2010;11:163; ten Brinke A, Sterk PJ, Masclee AA, et al. Risk factors of frequent exacerbations in difficult-to-treat asthma. EurRespir J. 2005;26:812–818; Bresciani M, Paradis L, Des Roches A, et al. Rhinosinusitis in severe asthma. *J Allergy Clin Immunol*. 2001;107:73–80; Braunstahl GJ. United airways concept: what does it teach us about systemic inflammation in airways disease? *Proc Am Thorac Soc*. 2009;6:652–654; Leynaert B, Neukirch C, Kony S, Guénégou A, Bousquet J, Aubier M, Neukirch F. Association between asthma and rhinitis according to atopic sensitization in a population-based study. *J Allergy Clin Immunol*. 2004 Jan;113(1):86-93; Ciprandi G, Cirillo I. The lower airway pathology of rhinitis. *J Allergy Clin Immunol*. 2006;118:1105–1109.

15.	Ziska LH, Gebhard DE, Frenz DA, Faulkner S, Singer BD, Straka JG. Cities as harbingers of climate change: common ragweed, urbanization, and public health. *J Allergy Clin Immunol*. 2003 Feb;111(2):290-5.

16.	Allergic fungal rhinosinusitis: a review. Glass D, Amedee RG. *Ochsner J*. 2011 Fall; 11(3): 271–275.

17.	Luong A, Davis LS, Marple BF. Peripheral blood mononuclear cells from allergic fungal rhinosinusitis adults express a Th2 cytokine response to fungal antigens. *Am J Rhinol Allergy*. 2009 May-Jun;23(3):281-7.

18. Mulligan JK, Bleier BS, O'Connell B, Mulligan RM, Wagner C, Schlosser RJ. Vitamin D3 correlates inversely with systemic dendritic cell numbers and bone erosion in chronic rhinosinusitis with nasal polyps and allergic fungal rhinosinusitis. *Clin Exp Immunol.* 2011 Jun;164(3):312-20.

19. Dennis DP. Chronic sinusitis: defective T-cells responding to superantigens, treated by reduction of fungi in the nose and air. *Arch Environ Health.* 2003 Jul;58(7):433-41.

20. Pang YT, Eskici O, Wilson JA. Nasalpolyposis: role of subclinical delayed food hypersensitivity. *Otolaryngol Head Neck Surg.* 2000 Feb;122(2):298-301.

21. Collins MM, Loughran S, Davidson P, Wilson JA. Nasalpolyposis: prevalence of positive food and inhalant skin tests. *Otolaryngol Head Neck Surg.* 2006 Nov;135(5):680-3.

22. Yang SB, Li TL, Chen X, An YF, Zhao CQ, Wen JB, Tian DF, Wen Z, Xie MQ, Yang PC. Staphylococcal enterotoxin B-derived haptens promote sensitization. *Cell Mol Immunol.* 2013 Jan;10(1):78-83.

23. Tilahun AY, Chowdhary VR, David CS, Rajagopalan G. Systemic inflammatory response elicited by superantigen destabilizes T regulatory cells, rendering them ineffective during toxic shock syndrome. *J Immunol.* 2014 Sep 15;193(6):2919-30; Ou LS, Goleva E, Hall C, Leung DY. T regulatory cells in atopic dermatitis and subversion of their activity by superantigens. *J Allergy Clin Immunol.* 2004 Apr;113(4):756-63.

24. Kirtsreesakul V, Atchariyasathian V. Nasalpolyposis: role of allergy on therapeutic response of eosinophil- and noneosinophil-dominated inflammation. *Am J Rhinol.* 2006 Jan-Feb;20(1):95-100.

25. Verhaar AP, Wildenberg ME, Duijvestein M, Vos AC, Peppelenbosch MP, Löwenberg M, Hommes DW, van den Brink GR. Superantigen-induced steroid resistance depends on activation of phospholipase Cβ2. *J Immunol.* 2013 Jun 15;190(12):6589-95.

26. Hisano M, Yamaguchi K, Inoue Y, Ikeda Y, Iijima M, Adachi M, Shimamura T. Inhibitory effect of catechin against the superantigen staphylococcal enterotoxin B (SEB). *Arch Dermatol Res.* 2003 Sep;295(5):183-9; Watson JL, Vicario M, Wang A, Moreto M, McKay DM. Immune cell activation and subsequent epithelial dysfunction by Staphylococcus enterotoxin B is attenuated by the green tea polyphenol (-)-epigallocatechin gallate. *Cell Immunol.* 2005 Sep;237(1):7-16; Rasooly R, Do PM, Friedman M. Inhibition of biological activity of staphylococcal enterotoxin A (SEA) by apple juice and apple polyphenols. *J Agric Food Chem.* 2010 May 12;58(9):5421-6; Benedik E, Skrt M, Podlipnik C, Ulrih NP. Binding of flavonoids to staphylococcal enterotoxin B. *Food Chem Toxicol.* 2014 Dec;74:1-8.

27. Syed AK, Ghosh S, Love NG, Boles BR. Triclosan promotes staphylococcus aureus nasal colonization. *M Bio.* 2014 Apr 8;5(2):e01015. doi: 10.1128/mBio.01015-13.

28. Drury B, Scott J, Rosi-Marshall EJ, Kelly JJ. Triclosan exposure increases triclosan resistance and influences taxonomic composition of benthic bacterial communities. *Environ Sci Technol*. 2013 Aug 6;47(15):8923-30; Luděk Bláha, Pavel Babica, and Blahoslav Maršálek. Toxins produced in cyanobacterial water blooms–toxicity and risks. Interdiscip Toxicol. 2009 Jun; 2(2): 36–41.

29. Simon-Nobbe B, Denk U, Pöll V, Rid R, Breitenbach M. The spectrum of fungal allergy. *Int Arch Allergy Immunol*. 2008;145(1):58-86.

30. Luccioli S, Malka-Rais J, Nsouli TM, Bellanti JA. Clinical reactivity to ingestion challenge with mixed mold extract may be enhanced in subjects sensitized to molds. *Allergy Asthma Proc*. 2009 Jul-Aug;30(4):433-42.

31. Zauli D, Tiberio D, Grassi A, Ballardini G. Ragweed pollen travels long distance. *Ann Allergy Asthma Immunol*. 2006 Jul;97(1):122-3.

32. Pascal M, Muñoz-Cano R, Reina Z, Palacín A, Vilella R, Picado C, Juan M, Sánchez-López J, Rueda M, Salcedo G, Valero A, Yagüe J, Bartra J. Lipid transfer protein syndrome: clinical pattern, cofactor effect and profile of molecular sensitization to plant-foods and pollens. *Clin Exp Allergy*. 2012 Oct;42(10):1529-39; Alvarado MI, Jimeno L, De La Torre F, Boissy P, Rivas B, Lázaro MJ, Barber D. Profilin as a severe food allergen in allergic patients overexposed to grass pollen. *Allergy*. 2014 Dec;69(12):1610-6.

33. Vieths S, Scheurer S, Ballmer-Weber B. Current understanding of cross-reactivity of food allergens and pollen. *Ann N Y Acad Sci*. 2002 May;964:47-68.

34. Bohle B. The impact of pollen-related food allergens on pollen allergy. *Allergy*. 2007 Jan;62(1):3-10.

35. Saarinen K, Jantunen J, Haahtela T. Birch pollen honey for birch pollen allergy—a randomized controlled pilot study. *Int Arch Allergy Immunol*. 2011;155(2):160-6.

36. Yagami T. Allergies to cross-reactive plant proteins. Latex-fruit syndrome is comparable with pollen-food allergy syndrome. *Int Arch Allergy Immunol*. 2002 Aug;128(4):271-9.

37. Kramer MF, Heath MD. Probiotics in the treatment of chronic rhinoconjunctivitis and chronic rhinosinusitis. *J Allergy* (Cairo). 2014;2014:983635; Klaenhammer TR, Kleerebezem M, Kopp MV, Rescigno M. The impact of probiotics and prebiotics on the immune system. *Nature Reviews Immunology*. 2012;12:728–734.

38. Perrin Y, Nutten S, Audran R, et al. Comparison of two oral probiotic preparations in a randomized crossover trial highlights a potentially beneficial effect of Lactobacillus paracasei NCC2461 in patients with allergic rhinitis. *Clinical and Translational Allergy*.2014;4(1, article 1).

39. Wassenberg J, Nutten S, Audran R, et al. Effect of Lactobacillus paracasei ST11 on a nasal provocation test with grass pollen in allergic rhinitis. *Clinical and Experimental Allergy.* 2011;41(4):565–573.

40. Perrin et al, 2014.

41. Wang MF, Lin HC, Wang YY, Hsu CH. Treatment of perennial allergic rhinitis with lactic acid bacteria. *Pediatric Allergy and Immunology.* 2004;15(2):152–158.

42. Costa DJ, Marteau P, Amouyal M, Poulsen LK, Hamelmann E, Cazaubiel M, Housez B, Leuillet S, Stavnsbjerg M, Molimard P, Courau S, Bousquet J. Efficacy and safety of the probiotic Lactobacillus paracasei LP-33 in allergic rhinitis: a double-blind, randomized, placebo-controlled trial (GA2LEN Study). *Eur J ClinNutr.* 2014 May;68(5):602-7.

43. Lin WY, Fu LS, Lin HK, Shen CY, Chen YJ. Evaluation of the effect of Lactobacillus paracasei (HF.A00232) in children (6–13 years old) with perennial allergic rhinitis: a 12-week, double-blind, randomized, placebo-controlled study. *Pediatrics & Neonatology.* 2013.

44. Lue KH, Sun HL, Lu KH, Ku MS, Sheu JN, Chan CH, Wang YH. A trial of adding Lactobacillus johnsonii EM1 to levocetirizine for treatment of perennial allergic rhinitis in children aged 7-12 years. *Int J Pediatr Otorhinolaryngol.* 2012 Jul;76(7):994-1001.

45. Lin TY, Chen CJ, Chen LK, Wen SH, Jan RH. Effect of probiotics on allergic rhinitis in Df, Dp or dust-sensitive children: a randomized double blind controlled trial. *Indian Pediatrics.* 2013;50(2):209–213.

46. Ishida Y, Nakamura F, Kanzato H, et al. Clinical effects of Lactobacillus acidophilus strain L-92 on perennial allergic rhinitis: a double-blind, placebo-controlled study. *Journal of Dairy Science.* 2005;88(2):527–533.

47. Singh A, Hacini-Rachinel F, Gosoniu ML, et al. Immune-modulatory effect of probiotic Bifidobacterium lactis NCC2818 in individuals suffering from seasonal allergic rhinitis to grass pollen: an exploratory, randomized, placebo-controlled clinical trial. *European Journal of Clinical Nutrition.* 2013;67(2):161–167.

48. Ouwehand AC, Nermes M, Collado MC, Rautonen N, Salminen S, Isolauri E. Specific probiotics alleviate allergic rhinitis during the birch pollen season. *World Journal of Gastroenterology.* 2009;15(26):3261–3268.

49. Xiao JZ, Kondo S, Yanagisawa N, et al. Effect of probiotic Bifidobacterium longum BBS36 in relieving clinical symptoms and modulating plasma cytokine levels of Japanese cedar pollinosis during the pollen season. A randomized double-blind, placebo-controlled trial. *Journal of Investigational Allergology and Clinical Immunology.* 2006;16(2):86–93; Xiao J-Z, Kondo S, Yanagisawa N, et al. Clinical efficacy of probiotic Bifidobacterium longum for the treatment of symptoms of Japanese cedar pollen allergy in subjects evaluated in an environmental exposure unit. *Allergology International.* 2007;56(1):67–75.

50. Hao Q, Lu Z, Dong BR, Huang CQ, Wu T. Probiotics for preventing acute upper respiratory tract infections. *Cochrane Database Syst Rev.* 2011 Sep 7;(9):CD006895; King S, Glanville J, Sanders ME, Fitzgerald A, Varley D. Effectiveness of probiotics on the duration of illness in healthy children and adults who develop common acute respiratory infectious conditions: a systematic review and meta-analysis. *Br J Nutr.* 2014 Jul 14;112(1):41-54.

51. Schlosser RJ, Soler ZM, Schmedes GW, Storck K, Mulligan JK. Impact of vitamin D deficiency upon clinical presentation in nasal polyposis. *Int Forum Allergy Rhinol.* 2014 Mar;4(3):196-9; Wang LF, Lee CH, Chien CY, Chen JY, Chiang FY, Tai CF. Serum 25-hydroxyvitamin D levels are lower in chronicrhinosinusitis with nasal polyposis and are correlated with disease severity in Taiwanese patients. *Am J Rhinol Allergy.* 2013 Nov-Dec;27(6):e162-5; Pinto JM, Schneider J, Perez R, DeTineo M, Baroody FM, Naclerio RM. Serum 25-hydroxyvitamin D levels are lower in urban African American subjects with chronicrhinosinusitis. *J Allergy Clin Immunol.* 2008 Aug;122(2):415-7.

52. Akbar NA, Zacharek MA. Vitamin D: immunomodulation of asthma, allergic rhinitis, and chronic rhinosinusitis. *Curr Opin Otolaryngol Head Neck Surg.* 2011 Jun;19(3):224-8.

53. Sheffner AL. The reduction in vitro in viscosity of mucoprotein solution by a new mucolytic agent, Nacetyl-L-cysteine. *Ann N Y AcadSci.* 1963;106:298310; Todisco T, Polidori R, Rossi F, et al. Effect of Nacetylcysteine in subjects with slow pulmonary mucociliary clearance. *Eur J Respir Dis Suppl.* 1985;139:136-141; Stafanger G, Bisgaard H, Pedersen M, et al. Effect of N-acetylcysteine on the human nasal ciliary activity in vitro. *Eur J Respir Dis.* 1987;70:157-162.

54. Seltzer AP. Adjunctive use of bromelains in sinusitis: a controlled study. *Eye Ear Nose Throat Mon.* 1967;46:1281-1288.

55. Taub SJ. The use of bromelains in sinusitis: a double-blind clinical evaluation. *Eye Ear Nose Throat Mon.* 1967;46:361-362.

56. Büttner L, Achilles N, Böhm M, Shah-Hosseini K, Mösges R. Efficacy and tolerability of bromelain in patients with chronic rhinosinusitis—a pilot study. *B-ENT.* 2013;9(3):217-25.

57. Rimoldi R, Ginesu F, Giura R. The use of bromelain in pneumological therapy. *Drugs Exp Clin Res.* 1978;4:55-66.

Chapter 12

1. Bice JB, Leechawengwongs E, Montanaro A. Biologic targeted therapy in allergic asthma. *Ann Allergy Asthma Immunol.* 2014 Feb;112(2):108-15; Akinbami LJ, Moorman JE, Liu X. Asthma prevalence, health care use, and mortality: United States, 2005-2009. *Natl Health Stat Report.* 2011 Jan 12;(32):1-14; Follenweider LM, Lambertino A. Epidemiology of asthma in the United States. *Nurs Clin North Am.* 2013 Mar;48(1):1-10.

2. Erle DJ, Sheppard D. The cell biology of asthma. *J Cell Biol*. 2014 Jun 9;205(5):621-31.

3. Bird JA, Burks AW. Food allergy and asthma. *Prim Care Respir J*. 2009 Dec;18(4):258-65.

4. Cowie RL, Conley DP, Underwood MF, Reader PG. A randomised controlled trial of the Buteyko technique as an adjunct to conventional management of asthma. *Respir Med*. 2008 May;102(5):726-32.

5. Stephen T Holgate. Stratified approaches to the treatment of asthma. *Br J Clin Pharmacol*. Aug 2013;76(2):277–291.

6. *Theodore Roosevelt, An Autobiography* (New York: Charles Scribner's Sons, 1913); http://www.pbs.org/wgbh/americanexperience/features/interview/ tr-mccullough; *The Roosevelts: An Intimate History*, A film by Ken Burns, 2014 (http://www.pbs.org/kenburns/films/the-roosevelts); Edmund Morris, *Theodore Rex* (New York: Random House, Reprint edition, 2010).

7. Murata K, Fujimoto K, Kitaguchi Y, Horiuchi T, Kubo K, Honda T. Hydrogen peroxide content and pH of expired breath condensate from patients with asthma and COPD. *COPD*. 2014 Feb;11(1):81-7; Holguin F. Oxidative stress in airway diseases. *Ann Am Thorac Soc*. 2013 Dec;10 Suppl:S150-7.

8. Zuo L, Otenbaker NP, Rose BA, Salisbury KS. Molecular mechanisms of reactive oxygen species-related pulmonary inflammation and asthma. *Mol Immunol*. 2013 Nov;56(1-2):57-63.

9. Auerbach A, Hernandez ML.The effect of environmental oxidative stress on airway inflammation. *Curr Opin Allergy Clin Immunol*. 2012 Apr;12(2):133-9.

10. Church DF, Pryor WA. Free-radical chemistry of cigarette smoke and its toxicological implications. *Environ Health Perspect*. 1985 Dec;64:111-26; Nakayama T, Church DF, Pryor WA. Quantitative analysis of the hydrogen peroxide formed in aqueous cigarette tar extracts. *Free Radic Biol Med*. 1989;7(1):9-15.

11. Guo CH, Liu PJ, Lin KP, Chen PC. Nutritional supplement therapy improves oxidative stress, immune response, pulmonary function, and quality of life in allergic asthma patients: an open-label pilot study. *Altern Med Rev*. 2012 Mar;17(1):42-56.

12. Wood LG, Gibson PG. Reduced circulating antioxidant defences are associated with airway hyper-responsiveness, poor control and severe disease pattern in asthma. *Br J Nutr*. 2010 Mar;103(5):735-41.

13. Knekt P, Kumpulainen J, Järvinen R, Rissanen H, Heliövaara M, Reunanen A, Hakulinen T, Aromaa A. Flavonoid intake and risk of chronic diseases. *Am J Clin Nutr*. 2002 Sep;76(3):560-8.

14. Wood LG, Garg ML, Smart JM, Scott HA, Barker D, Gibson PG. Manipulating antioxidant intake in asthma: a randomized controlled trial. *Am J Clin Nutr*. 2012 Sep;96(3):534-43.

15. Wood LG, Garg ML, Powell H, Gibson PG. Lycopene-rich treatments modify noneosinophilic airway inflammation in asthma: proof of concept. *Free Radic Res.* 2008 Jan;42(1):94-102.

16. Leonard SW, Paterson E, Atkinson JK, Ramakrishnan R, Cross CE, Traber MG. Studies in humans using deuterium-labeled alpha- and gamma-tocopherolsdemonstrate faster plasma gamma-tocopherol disappearance and greater gamma-metabolite production. *Free Radic Biol Med.* 2005;38:857–866.

17. Patel A, Liebner F, Netscher T, Mereiter K, Rosenau T. Vitamin E chemistry. Nitration of non-alpha-tocopherols: products and mechanistic considerations. *J Org Chem.* 2007;72:6504–6512; Fakhrzadeh L, Laskin JD, Laskin DL. Ozone-induced production of nitric oxide and TNF-alpha and tissue injury are dependent on NF-kappaB p50. *Am J Physiol Lung Cell Mol Physiol.* 2004;287:L279–L285; Hernandez ML, Wagner JG, Aline Kala R, Mills K, Wells HB, Alexis NE, Lay JC, Jiang Q, Zhang H, Zhou H, et al. Vitamin E, γ-tocopherol, reduces airway neutrophil recruitment after inhaled endotoxin challenge in rats and in healthy volunteers. *Free Radic Biol Med.* 2013;60:56–62; Wiser J, Alexis NE, Jiang Q, Wu W, Robinette C, Roubey R, Peden DB. In vivo gamma-tocopherol supplementation decreases systemic oxidative stress and cytokine responses of human monocytes in normal and asthmatic subjects. *Free Radic Biol Med.* 2008;45:40–49; Wagner JG, Harkema JR, Jiang Q, Illek B, Ames BN, Peden DB. Gamma-tocopherol attenuates ozone-induced exacerbation of allergic rhinosinusitis in rats. *Toxicol Pathol.* 2009;37:481–491; Wagner JG, Jiang Q, Harkema JR, Ames BN, Illek B, Roubey RA, Peden DB. Gamma-tocopherol prevents airway eosinophilia and mucous cell hyperplasia in experimentally induced allergic rhinitis and asthma. *Clin Exp Allergy.* 2008;38:501–511; Hamahata A, Enkhbaatar P, Kraft ER, Lange M, Leonard SW, Traber MG, Cox RA, Schmalstieg FC, Hawkins HK, Whorton EB, et al. Gamma-tocopherol nebulization by a lipid aerosolization device improves pulmonary function in sheep with burn and smoke inhalation injury. *Free Radic Biol Med.* 2008;45:425–433.

18. Berdnikovs S, Abdala-Valencia H, McCary C, Somand M, Cole R, Garcia A, Bryce P, Cook-Mills J. Isoforms of vitamin E have opposing immunoregulatory functions during inflammation by regulating leukocyte recruitment. *J Immunol.* 2009;182:4395–4405.

19. Cook-Mills JM, McCary CA. Isoforms of vitamin E differentially regulate inflammation. *Endocr Metab Immune Disord Drug Targets.* 2010;10:348–366; McCary CA, Abdala-Valencia H, Berdnikovs S, Cook-Mills JM. Supplemental and highly elevated tocopherol doses differentially regulate allergic inflammation: reversibility of alpha-tocopherol and gamma-tocopherol's effects. *J Immunol.* 2011;186:3674–3685; Cook-Mills JM, Marchese ME, Abdala-Valencia H. Vascular cell adhesion molecule-1 expression and signaling during disease: regulation by reactive oxygen species and antioxidants. *Antioxid Redox Signal.* 2011;15:1607–1638.

20. Cook-Mills JM, Abdala-Valencia H, Hartert T. Two faces of vitamin E in the lung. *Am J Respir Crit Care Med.* Aug 1, 2013; 188(3): 279–284.

21. Troisi RJ, Willett WC, Weiss ST, Trichopoulos D, Rosner B, Speizer FE. A prospective study of diet and adult-onset asthma. *Am J Respir Crit Care Med.* 1995;151:1401–1408; Dow L, Tracey M, Villar A, Coggon D, Margetts BM, Campbell MJ, Holgate ST. Does dietary intake of vitamins C and E influence lung function in older people? *Am J Respir Crit Care Med.* 1996;154:1401–1404; Kalayci O, Besler T, Kilinc K, Sekerel BE, Saraclar Y. Serum levels of antioxidant vitamins (alpha tocopherol, beta carotene, and ascorbic acid) in children with bronchial asthma. *Turk J Pediatr.* 2000;42:17–21; Kelly FJ, Mudway I, Blomberg A, Frew A, Sandstrom T. Altered lung antioxidant status in patients with mild asthma. *Lancet.* 1999;354:482–483; Schunemann HJ, Grant BJ, Freudenheim JL, Muti P, Browne RW, Drake JA, Klocke RA, Trevisan M. The relation of serum levels of antioxidant vitamins C and E, retinol and carotenoids with pulmonary function in the general population. *Am J Respir Crit Care Med.* 2001;163:1246–1255; Al-Abdulla NO, Al Naama LM, Hassan MK. Antioxidant status in acute asthmatic attack in children. *J Pak Med Assoc.* 2010;60:1023–1027.

22. Marchese ME, Kumar R, Colangelo LA, Avila PC, Jacobs DR Jr, Gross M, Sood A, Liu K, Cook-Mills JM. The vitamin E isoforms α-tocopherol and γ-tocopherol have opposite associations with spirometric parameters: the CARDIA study. *Respir Res* 2014 Mar 15;15:31.

23. Abdala-Valencia H, Berdnikovs S, Cook-Mills JM. Vitamin E isoforms differentially regulate intercellular adhesion molecule-1 activation of PKCα in human microvascular endothelial cells. *PLoS ONE.* 2012;7:e41054; McCary CA, Yoon Y, Panagabko C, Cho W, Atkinson J, Cook-Mills JM. Vitamin E isoforms directly bind PKCα and differentially regulate activation of PKCα. *Biochem J.* 2012;441:189–198.

24. Du CL, Xu YJ, Liu XS, Xie JG, Xie M, Zhang ZX, Zhang J, Qiao LF. Up-regulation of cyclin D1 expression in asthma serum-sensitized human airway smooth muscle promotes proliferation via proteinkinase C alpha. *Exp Lung Res.* 2010 May;36(4):201-10; Tang YJ, Xu YJ, Xiong SD, Zhao JP, Zhang ZX. The effect of inhaled glucocorticosteroid on proteinkinase C alpha expression and interleukin-5 production in induced sputum inflammatory cells of asthma patients. *Zhonghua Nei Ke Za Zhi.* 2004 Nov;43(11):849-52.

25. Hoskins A, Roberts JL 2nd, Milne G, Choi L, Dworski R. Natural-source d-α-tocopheryl acetate inhibits oxidant stress and modulates atopic asthma in humans in vivo. *Allergy.* 2012 May;67(5):676-82.

26. Romieu I, Sienra-Monge JJ, Ramírez-Aguilar M, Téllez-Rojo MM, Moreno-Macías H, Reyes-Ruiz NI, del Río-Navarro BE, Ruiz-Navarro MX, Hatch G, Slade R, Hernández-Avila M. Antioxidant supplementation and lung functions among children with asthma exposed to high levels of air pollutants. *Am J Respir Crit Care Med.* 2002 Sep 1;166(5):703-9; Trenga CA, Koenig JQ, Williams PV. Dietary antioxidants and ozone-induced bronchial hyperresponsiveness in adults with asthma. *Arch Environ Health.* 2001 May-Jun;56(3):242-9.

27. Pearson P, Lewis SA, Britton J, Young IS, Fogarty A. The pro-oxidant activity of high-dose vitamin E supplements in vivo. *Bio Drugs.* 2006;20(5):271-3.

28. Gazdík F1, Gvozdjáková A, Nádvorníková R, Repická L, Jahnová E, Kucharská J, Piják MR, Gazdíková K. Decreased levels of coenzyme Q(10) in patients with bronchial asthma. *Allergy*. 2002 Sep;57(9):811-4.

29. Gvozdjáková A, Kucharská J, Bartkovjaková M, Gazdíková K, Gazdík FE. Coenzyme Q10 supplementation reduces corticosteroids dosage in patients with bronchial asthma. *Biofactors*. 2005;25(1-4):235-40.

30. Taylor PE, Jacobson KW, House JM, Glovsky MM. Links between pollen, atopy and the asthma epidemic. *Int Arch Allergy Immunol*. 2007;144(2):162-70; Behrendt H, Becker WM. Localization, release and bioavailability of pollen allergens: the influence of environmental factors. *Curr Opin Immunol*. 2001 Dec;13(6):709-15.

31. Carluccio MA, Ancora MA, Massaro M, Carluccio M, Scoditti E, Distante A, Storelli C, De Caterina R. Homocysteine induces VCAM-1 gene expression through NF-kappaB and NAD(P)H oxidase activation: protective role of Mediterranean diet polyphenolic antioxidants. *Am J Physiol Heart Circ Physiol*. 2007 Oct;293(4):H2344-54; Schneider SM, Fung VS, Palmblad J, Babior BM. Activity of the leukocyte NADPH oxidase in whole neutrophils and cell-free neutrophil preparations stimulated with long-chain polyunsaturated fatty acids. *Inflammation*. 2001 Feb;25(1):17-23.

32. Arm JP, Horton CE, Spur BW, Mencia-Huerta JM, Lee TH. The effects of dietary supplementation with fish oil lipids on the airways response to inhaled allergen in bronchial asthma. *Am Rev Respir Dis*. 1989 Jun;139(6):1395-400 (The magnitude of the allergen-induced late asthmatic response was significantly attenuated from 2 to 7 h after allergen challenge following dietary supplementation with Max-EPA, supplying 5.5 grams EPA/day [p less than 0.005] but not with placebo); Arm JP, Horton CE, Mencia-Huerta JM, House F, Eiser NM, Clark TJ, Spur BW, Lee TH. Effect of dietary supplementation with fish oil lipids on mild asthma. *Thorax*. 1988 Feb;43(2):84-92 (The fish oil supplemented diet supplying 5.5 grams of omega-3's/day produced a 50% inhibition of total leukotriene B generation by ionophore stimulated neutrophils and neutrophil chemotaxis was substantially suppressed. Neutrophil function remained unchanged in the placebo group); Masuev KA. The effect of polyunsaturated fatty acids of the omega-3 class on the late phase of the allergic reaction in bronchial asthma patients. *TerArkh*. 1997;69(3):31-3 (Significant attenuation of late allergic response in patients who had taken fish oil for two weeks); Li J, Xun P, Zamora D, Sood A, Liu K, Daviglus M, Iribarren C, Jacobs D Jr, Shikany JM, He K. Intakes of long-chain omega-3 (n-3) PUFAs and fish in relation to incidence of asthma among American young adults: the CARDIA study. *Am J Clin Nutr*. 2013 Jan;97(1):173-8 (The objective was to prospectively investigate the association between long chain [LC] ω3 polyunsaturated fatty acids [PUFAs] and fish intake and incidence of asthma among American young adults. A 20-y follow-up longitudinal analysis was conducted in a biracial cohort of 4162 Americans, aged 18-30 y, with a history of asthma at baseline in 1985. Diet was assessed by a validated interviewer-administered quantitative food-frequency questionnaire at the examinations in 1985, 1992, and 2005. Incident self-reported asthma was defined as having a physician diagnosis of asthma and/or the use of asthma medications between 1985 and 2005.

During the 20-y follow-up, 446 incident cases of asthma were identified. LCω3PUFA intake was significantly inversely associated with incidence of asthma after adjustment for sociodemographic, major lifestyle, and dietary confounders. The multivariable-adjusted HR for the highest quintile of LCω3PUFA intake as compared with the lowest quintile was 0.46 [95% CI: 0.33, 0.64; P-trend < 0.01]. DHA showed a greater inverse association than did EPA. The association between LCω3PUFAs and incident asthma was not appreciably modified by sex, race, BMI, smoking status, or allergic status. This study showed that intakes of LCω3PUFAs are inversely longitudinally associated with the incidence of asthma in American young adults).

33. Asher MI, Stewart AW, Mallol J, Montefort S, Lai CK, Aït-Khaled N, Odhiambo J. Which population level environmental factors are associated with asthma, rhinoconjunctivitis and eczema? Review of the ecological analyses of ISAAC Phase One. *Respir Res.* 2010 Jan 21;11:8; Weiland SK, von Mutius E, Hüsing A, Asher MI. Intake of trans fatty acids and prevalence of childhood asthma and allergies in Europe. *Lancet.* 1999 Jun 12;353(9169):2040-1.

34. Nagel G, Linseisen J. Dietary intake of fatty acids, antioxidants and selected food groups and asthma in adults. *Eur J Clin Nutr.* 2005 Jan;59(1):8-15.

35. Galland L. Increased requirements for essential fatty acids in atopic individuals: a review with clinical descriptions. *J Am Coll Nutr.* 1986;5(2):213-28.

36. Rocklin RE, Thistle L, Galland L, Manku MS, Horrobin D. Altered arachidonic acid content in polymorphonuclear and mononuclear cells from patients with allergic rhinitis and/or asthma. *Lipids.* 1986 Jan;21(1):17-20.

37. Li et al, 2013.

38. Galland L. Diet and inflammation. NutrClinPract. 2010 Dec;25(6):634-40; Haidari F, Mohammadshahi M, Borsi SH, Haghighizadeh MH, Malgard S. Comparison of essential fatty acid intakes and serum levels of inflammatory factors between asthmatic and healthy adults: a case-control study. *Iran J Allergy Asthma Immunol.* 2014 Oct;13(5):335-42; Barros R1, Moreira A, Fonseca J, Delgado L, Castel-Branco MG, Haahtela T, Lopes C, Moreira P. Dietary intake of α-linolenic acid and low ratio of n-6:n-3 PUFA are associated with decreased exhaled NO and improved asthma control. Br J Nutr. 2011 Aug;106(3):441-50.

39. Dry J, Vincent D. Effect of a fish oil diet on asthma: results of a 1-year double-blind study. *Int Arch Allergy Appl Immunol.* 1991;95(2-3):156-7.

40. Nagakura T, Matsuda S, Shichijyo K, Sugimoto H, Hata K. Dietary supplementation with fish oil rich in omega-3 polyunsaturated fatty acids in children with bronchial asthma. *Eur Respir J.* 2000 Nov;16(5):861-5.

41. Villani F, Comazzi R, De Maria P, Galimberti M. Effect of dietary supplementation with polyunsaturated fatty acids on bronchial hyperreactivity in subjects with seasonal asthma. *Respiration.* 1998;65(4):265-9.

42. Schubert R, Kitz R, Beermann C, Rose MA, Lieb A, Sommerer PC, Moskovits J, Alberternst H, Böhles HJ, Schulze J, Zielen S. Effect of n-3 polyunsaturated fatty acids in asthma after low-dose allergen challenge. *Int Arch Allergy Immunol.* 2009;148(4):321-9.

43. Arm JP, Horton CE, Spur BW, Mencia-Huerta JM, Lee TH. The effects of dietary supplementation with fish oil lipids on the airways response to inhaled allergen in bronchial asthma. *Am Rev Respir Dis.* 1989 Jun;139(6):1395-400.

44. Mickleborough TD, Lindley MR, Ionescu AA, Fly AD. Protective effect of fish oil supplementation on exercise-induced bronchoconstriction in asthma. *Chest.* 2006 Jan;129(1):39-49; Mickleborough TD, Murray RL, Ionescu AA, Lindley MR. Fish oil supplementation reduces severity of exercise-induced bronchoconstriction in elite athletes. *Am J Respir Crit Care Med.* 2003 Nov 15;168(10):1181-9.

45. Olsen SF, Østerdal ML, Salvig JD, Mortensen LM, Rytter D, Secher NJ, Henriksen TB. Fish oil intake compared with olive oil intake in late pregnancy and asthma in the offspring: 16 y of registry-based follow-up from a randomized controlled trial. *Am J Clin Nutr.* 2008 Jul;88(1):167-75.

46. Lundström SL, Yang J, Brannan JD, Haeggström JZ, Hammock BD, Nair P, O'Byrne P, Dahlén SE, Wheelock CE. Lipid mediator serum profiles in asthmatics significantly shift following dietary supplementation with omega-3 fatty acids. *Mol Nutr Food Res.* 2013 Aug;57(8):1378-89.

47. Mickleborough TD, Vaughn CL, Shei RJ, Davis EM, Wilhite DP. Marine lipid fraction PCSO-524 (lyprinol/omega XL) of the New Zealand green lipped mussel attenuates hyperpnea-induced bronchoconstriction in asthma. *Respir Med.* 2013 Aug;107(8):1152-63.

48. Treatment of asthma with lipid extract of New Zealand green-lipped mussel: a randomised clinical trial. Emelyanov A, Fedoseev G, Krasnoschekova O, Abulimity A, Trendeleva T, Barnes PJ. *Eur Respir J.* 2002 Sep;20(3):596-600.

49. Okamoto M, Mitsunobu F, Ashida K, Mifune T, Hosaki Y, Tsugeno H, Harada S, Tanizaki Y. Effects of dietary supplementation with n-3 fatty acids compared with n-6 fatty acids on bronchial asthma. *Intern Med.* 2000 Feb;39(2):107-11.

50. Broughton KS, Johnson CS, Pace BK, Liebman M, Kleppinger KM. Reduced asthma symptoms with n-3 fatty acid ingestion are related to 5-series leukotriene production. *Am J Clin Nutr.* 1997 Apr;65(4):1011-7.

51. Surette ME, Koumenis IL, Edens MB, Tramposch KM, Clayton B, Bowton D, Chilton FH. Inhibition of leukotriene biosynthesis by a novel dietary fatty acid formulation in patients with atopic asthma: a randomized, placebo-controlled, parallel-group, prospective trial. *Clin Ther.* 2003 Mar;25(3):972-9; Surette ME, Stull D, Lindemann J. The impact of a medical food containing gammalinolenic and eicosapentaenoic acids on asthma management and the quality of life of adult asthma patients. *Curr Med Res Opin.* 2008 Feb;24(2):559-67; Lindemann J, David Pampe E, Peterkin JJ, Orozco-Cronin P, Belofsky G, Stull D. Clinical study of the effects on asthma-related QOL and

asthma management of a medical food in adult asthma patients. *Curr Med Res Opin*. 2009 Dec;25(12):2865-75.

52. Covar R, Gleason M, Macomber B, Stewart L, Szefler P, Engelhardt K, Murphy J, Liu A, Wood S, DeMichele S, Gelfand EW, Szefler SJ. Impact of a novel nutritional formula on asthma control and biomarkers of allergic airway inflammation in children. *Clinical & Experimental Allergy*, 40, 1163–1174.

53. Biltagi MA, Baset AA, Bassiouny M, Kasrawi MA, Attia M. Omega-3 fatty acids, vitamin C and Zn supplementation in asthmatic children: a randomized self-controlled study. *Acta Paediatr*. 2009 Apr;98(4):737-42.

54. Cui L, Morris A, Huang L, Beck JM, Twigg HL 3rd, von Mutius E, Ghedin E. The microbiome and the lung. *Ann Am Thorac Soc*. 2014 Aug;11Suppl 4:S227-32; van Woerden HC, Gregory C, Brown R, Marchesi JR, Hoogendoorn B, Matthews IP. Differences in fungi present in induced sputum samples from asthma patients and non-atopic controls: a community based case control study. *BMC Infect Dis*. 2013 Feb 5;13:69.

55. West CE. Gut microbiota and allergic disease: new findings. *Curr Opin Clin Nutr Metab Care*. 2014 May;17(3):261-6.

56. Fujimura KE, Demoor T, Rauch M, et al. House dust exposure mediates gut microbiome Lactobacillus enrichment and airway immune defense against allergens and virus infection. *Proc Natl Acad Sci U S A*. 2014;111:805–10.

57. Chen YS, Jan RL, Lin YL, Chen HH, Wang JY. Randomized placebo-controlled trial of lactobacillus on asthmatic children with allergic rhinitis. *Pediatr Pulmonol*. 2010 Nov;45(11):1111-20.

58. Miraglia Del Giudice M, Maiello N, Decimo F, Fusco N, D'Agostino B, Sullo N, Capasso M, Salpietro V, Gitto E, Ciprandi G, Marseglia GL, Perrone L. Airways allergic inflammation and L. reuterii treatment in asthmatic children. *J Biol Regul Homeost Agents*. 2012 Jan-Mar;26(1 Suppl):S35-40.

59. O'Driscoll BR, Powell G, Chew F, Niven RM, Miles JF, Vyas A, Denning DW. Comparison of skin prick tests with specific serum immunoglobulin E in the diagnosis of fungal sensitization in patients with severe asthma. *Clin Exp Allergy*. 2009 Nov;39(11):1677-83.

60. Kabe J. Late asthmatic reactions to inhalation of fractions from extracts of Candida albicans and Asperguillus fumigatus. *Allerg Immunol* (Leipz). 1974-1975;20-21(4):393-401; Tsukioka K. Studies on the mechanism developing bronchial asthma due to Candida albicans. 3. Relationship between types of response after inhalation challenge with Candida albicans and type I, type III allergy. *Arerugi*. 1985 May;34(5):289-96.

61. Dhamgaye S, Devaux F, Vandeputte P, Khandelwal NK, Sanglard D, Mukhopadhyay G, Prasad R. Molecular mechanisms of action of herbal antifungal alkaloid berberine, in Candida albicans. *PLoS One*. 2014 Aug 8;9(8):e104554; Iwazaki RS, Endo EH, Ueda-Nakamura T, Nakamura CV, Garcia LB, Filho BP. In vitro antifungal activity of the berberine and its synergism with fluconazole. *Antonie Van Leeuwenhoek*. 2010 Feb;97(2):201-5;

Li Z, Geng YN, Jiang JD, Kong WJ. Antioxidant and anti-inflammatory activities of berberine in the treatment of diabetes mellitus. *Evid Based Complement Alternat Med.* 2014;2014:289264; Yang N, Wang J, Liu C, Song Y, Zhang S, Zi J, Zhan J, Masilamani M, Cox A, Nowak-Wegrzyn A, Sampson H, Li XM. Berberine and limonin suppress IgE production by human B cells and peripheral blood mononuclear cells from food-allergic patients. *Ann Allergy Asthma Immunol.* 2014 Nov;113(5):556-564.

62. Largest grant ever awarded to UW School of Medicine and Public Health will continue inner-city asthma research. *University of Wisconsin–Madison News,* November 10, 2014. http://www.news.wisc.edu/23279.

Chapter 13

1. Kern DG, Frumkin H. Asthma in respiratory therapists. *Annals of Internal Medicine.* 1989; volume 110: pp 767-773. *Am J RespirCrit Care Med;* Christiani DC, Kern DG. Asthma risk and occupation as a respiratory therapist. *Am Rev Respir Dis.* 1993 Sep;148(3):671-4.

2. Delclos GL1, Gimeno D, Arif AA, Burau KD, Carson A, Lusk C, Stock T, Symanski E, Whitehead LW, Zock JP, Benavides FG, Antó JM. Occupational risk factors and asthma among health care professionals. *Am J Respir Crit Care Med.* 2007 Apr 1;175(7):667-75; Dimich-Ward H, Wymer ML, Chan-Yeung M. Respiratory health survey of respiratory therapists. *Chest.* 2004 Oct;126(4):1048-53.

3. Grammatopoulou EP, Skordilis EK, Georgoudis G, Haniotou A, Evangelodimou A, Fildissis G, Katsoulas T, Kalagiakos P. Hyperventilation in asthma: A validation study of the Nijmegen Questionnaire—NQ. *J Asthma.* 2014 Oct;51(8):839-46; Gotshall RW. Airway response during exercise and hyperpnoea in non-asthmatic and asthmatic individuals. *Sports Med.* 2006;36(6):513-27 ("...dynamic exercise has consistently demonstrated improved airway calibre in asthmatic individuals. . . . the exercise has typically been less than 15 minutes. Data from longer duration exercise [20-30 minutes] . . . suggest declining pulmonary function over time during exercise in asthmatic individuals after the initial bronchodilation"); Ritz T, Kullowatz A, Bobb C, Dahme B, Magnussen H, Kanniess F, Steptoe A. Psychological triggers and hyperventilation symptoms in asthma. *Ann Allergy Asthma Immunol.* 2008 May;100(5):426-32.

4. Prem V, Sahoo RC, Adhikari P. Comparison of the effects of Buteyko and pranayama breathing techniques on quality of life in patients with asthma—a randomized controlled trial. *Clin Rehabil.* 2013 Feb;27(2):133-41; Cowie RL, Conley DP, Underwood MF, Reader PG. A randomised controlled trial of the Buteyko technique as an adjunct to conventional management of asthma. *Respir Med.* 2008 May;102(5):726-32; McHugh P, Aitcheson F, Duncan B, Houghton F. Buteyko Breathing Technique for asthma: an effective intervention. N Z Med J. 2003 Dec 12;116(1187):U710; Cooper S, Oborne J, Newton S, Harrison V, Thompson Coon J, Lewis S, Tattersfield A. Effect of two breathing exercises (Buteyko and pranayama) in asthma: a randomised controlled trial. *Thorax.* 2003 Aug;58(8):674-9; Opat AJ, Cohen MM, Bailey

MJ, Abramson MJ. A clinical trial of the Buteyko Breathing Technique in asthma as taught by a video. *J Asthma*. 2000;37(7):557-64; Bowler SD, Green A, Mitchell CA. Buteyko breathing techniques in asthma: a blinded randomised controlled trial. *Med J Aust*. 1998 Dec 7-21;169(11-12):575-8.

5. Celik M, Tuncer A, Soyer OU, Saçkesen C, Tanju Besler H, Kalayci O. Oxidative stress in the airways of children with asthma and allergic rhinitis. *Pediatr Allergy Immunol*. 2012 Sep;23(6):556-61; Westerveld GJ, Dekker I, Voss HP, Bast A, Scheeren RA. Antioxidant levels in the nasal mucosa of patients with chronic sinusitis and healthy controls. *Arch Otolaryngol Head Neck Surg*. 1997 Feb;123(2):201-4; Kassim SK, Elbeigermy M, Nasr GF, Khalil R, Nassar M. The role of interleukin-12, and tissue antioxidants in chronic sinusitis. *Clin Biochem*. 2002 Jul;35(5):369-75.

6. Zavorsky GS, Kubow S, Grey V, Riverin V, Lands LC. An open-label dose-response study of lymphocyte glutathione levels in healthy men and women receiving pressurized whey protein isolate supplements. *Int J Food Sci Nutr*. 2007 Sep;58(6):429-36.

7. Baumann JM, Rundell KW, Evans TM, Levine AM. Effects of cysteine donor supplementation on exercise-induced bronchoconstriction. *Med Sci Sports Exerc*. 2005 Sep;37(9):1468-73.

8. Rushworth GF, Megson IL.Existing and potential therapeutic uses for N-acetylcysteine: the need for conversion to intracellular glutathione for antioxidant benefits. *Pharmacol Ther*. 2014 Feb;141(2):150-9.

9. Carlsten C, MacNutt MJ, Zhang Z, Sava F, Pui MM. Anti-oxidant N-acetylcysteine diminishes diesel exhaust-induced increased airway responsiveness in persons with airway hyper-reactivity. *Toxicol Sci*. 2014 Jun;139(2):479-87.

10. Yamamoto M1, Singh A, Sava F, Pui M, Tebbutt SJ, Carlsten C. MicroRNA expression in response to controlled exposure to diesel exhaust: attenuation by the antioxidant N-acetylcysteine in a randomized crossover study. *Environ Health Perspect*. 2013 Jun;121(6):670-5.

11. Dabirmoghaddam P, Amali A, Motiee Langroudi M, Samavati Fard MR, Hejazi M, Sharifian Razavi M. The effect of N-acetyl cysteine on laryngopharyngeal reflux. *Acta Med Iran*. 2013;51(11):757-64.

12. Martinez-Losa M, Cortijo J, Juan G, O'Connor JE, Sanz MJ, Santangelo F, Morcillo EJ. Inhibitory effects of N-acetylcysteine on the functional responses of human eosinophils in vitro. *Clin Exp Allergy*. 2007 May;37(5):714-22.

13. Sugiura H, Ichikawa T, Liu X, Kobayashi T, Wang XQ, Kawasaki S, Togo S, Kamio K, Mao L, Ann Y, Ichinose M, Rennard SI. N-acetyl-L-cysteine inhibits TGF-beta1-induced profibrotic responses in fibroblasts. *Pulm Pharmacol Ther*. 2009 Dec;22(6):487–91.

14. Kirkham P, Rahman I. Oxidative stress in asthma and COPD: Antioxidants as a therapeutic strategy. *Pharmacology & Therapeutics* 111 (2006):476–494.

15. Nuttall SL, Khan JN, Thorpe GH, Langford N, Kendall MJ. The impact of therapeutic doses of paracetamol on serum total antioxidant capacity. *J Biol Regul Homeost Agents*. 2012 Jan-Mar;26(1 Suppl):S35-40.

16. Muc M, Padez C, Pinto AM. Exposure to paracetamol and antibiotics in early life and elevated risk of asthma in childhood. *Adv Exp Med Biol*. 2013;788:393-400; Lee SH, Kang MJ, Yu HS, Hong K, Jung YH, Kim HY, Seo JH, Kwon JW, Kim BJ, Kim HJ, Kim YJ, Kim HS, Kim HB, Park KS, Lee SY, Hong SJ. Association between recent acetaminophen use and asthma: modification by polymorphism at TLR4. *J Korean Med Sci*. 2014 May;29(5):662-8; Henderson AJ, Shaheen SO. Acetaminophen and asthma. *Paediatr Respir Rev*. 2013 Mar;14(1):9-15.

17. Stone J, Hinks LJ, Beasley R. et al. Reduced selenium status of patients with asthma. *Clin Sci*. 1989;77495-500; Flatt A, Pearce N, Thomson CD, et al. Reduced selenium in asthmatic subjects in New Zealand. *Thorax*. 1990;4595-99; Misso NL, Powers KA, Gillon RL, et al. Reduced platelet glutathione peroxidase activity and serum selenium concentration in atopic asthmatic patients. *Clin Exp Allergy*. 1996;26838-847; Hu G, Cassano PA. Antioxidant nutrients and pulmonary function: the Third National Health and Nutrition Examination Survey (NHANES III). *Am J Epidemiol*. 2000;151975-981; Soutar A, Seaton A, Brown K. Bronchial reactivity and dietary antioxidants. *Thorax*. 1997;52166-170.

18. Voicekovska JG, Orlikov GA, Karpovlu G, Teibe U, Ivanov AD, Baidekalne I, Voicehovskis NV, Maulins E. External respiration function and quality of life in patients with bronchial asthma in correction of selenium deficiency. *Ter Arkh*. 2007;79(8):38-41; Gazdik F, Kadrabova J, Gazdikova K. Decreased consumption of corticosteroids after selenium supplementation in corticoid-dependent asthmatics. *Bratisl Lek Listy*. 2002;103(1):22-5; Jahnova E, Horvathova M, Gazdik F, Weissova S. Effects of selenium supplementation on expression of adhesion molecules in corticoid-dependent asthmatics. *Bratisl Lek Listy*. 2002;103(1):12-6.

19. Galland L 2010; Britton J, Pavord I, Richards K, Wisniewski A, Knox A, Lewis S, Tattersfield A, Weiss S. Dietary magnesium, lung function, wheezing, and airway hyperreactivity in a random adult population sample. *Lancet*. 1994 Aug 6;344(8919):357-62; Kurys E, Kurys P, Kuźniar A, Kieszko R. Analysis of antioxidant enzyme activity and magnesium level in chronic obstructive pulmonary disease (COPD). *Ann Univ Mariae Curie Sklodowska Med*. 2001;56:261-6.

20. Bede O, Nagy D, Surányi A, Horváth I, Szlávik M, Gyurkovits K. Effects of magnesium supplementation on the glutathione redox system in atopic asthmatic children. *Inflamm Res*. 2008 Jun;57(6):279-86; Bede O, Surányi A, Pintér K, Szlávik M, Gyurkovits K. Urinary magnesium excretion in asthmatic children receiving magnesium supplementation: a randomized, placebo-controlled, double-blind study. *Magnes Res*. 2003 Dec;16(4):262-70.

21. Gontijo-Amaral C, Ribeiro MA, Gontijo LS, Condino-Neto A, Ribeiro JD. Oral magnesium supplementation in asthmatic children: a double-blind randomized placebo-controlled trial. *Eur J Clin Nutr*. 2007 Jan;61(1):54-60.

22. Kazaks AG, Uriu-Adams JY, Albertson TE, Shenoy SF, Stern JS. Effect of oral magnesium supplementation on measures of airway resistance and subjective assessment of asthma control and quality of life in men and women with mild to moderate asthma: a randomized placebo controlled trial. *J Asthma*. 2010 Feb;47(1):83-92.

23. Bodenhamer J, Bergstrom R, Brown D, Gabow P, Marx JA, Lowenstein SR. Frequently nebulized beta-agonists for asthma: effects on serum electrolytes. *Ann Emerg Med*. 1992 Nov;21(11):1337-42.

24. Cates CJ, Wieland LS, Oleszczuk M, Kew KM. Safety of regular formoterol or salmeterol in adults with asthma: an overview of Cochrane reviews. *Cochrane Database Syst Rev*. 2014 Feb 6;2:CD010314; Rodrigo GJ, Moral VP, Marcos LG, Castro-Rodriguez JA. Safety of regular use of long-acting beta agonists as monotherapy or added to inhaled corticosteroids in asthma. A systematic review. *Pulm Pharmacol Ther*. 2009 Feb;22(1):9-19.

25. Anis AH, Lynd LD, Wang XH, King G, Spinelli JJ, Fitzgerald M, Bai T, Paré P. Double trouble: impact of inappropriate use of asthma medication on the use of health care resources. *CMAJ*. 2001 Mar 6;164(5):625-31.

26. Hernandez M, Zhou H, Zhou B, Robinette C, Crissman K, Hatch G, Alexis NE, Peden D. Combination treatment with high-dose vitamin C and alpha-tocopherol does not enhance respiratory-tract lining fluid vitamin C levels in asthmatics. *Inhal Toxicol*. 2009 Feb;21(3):173-81.

27. Zal F, Mostafavi-Pour Z, Amini F, Heidari A. Effect of vitamin E and C supplements on lipid peroxidation and GSH-dependent antioxidant enzyme status in the blood of women consuming oral contraceptives. *Contraception*. 2012 Jul;86(1):62-6; Smith AR, Visioli F, Hagen TM. Vitamin C matters: increased oxidative stress in cultured human aortic endothelial cells without supplemental ascorbic acid. *FASEB J*. 2002 Jul;16(9):1102-4.

28. Horska A, Mislanova C, Bonassi S, Ceppi M, Volkovova K, Dusinska M. Vitamin C levels in blood are influenced by polymorphisms in glutathione S-transferases. *Eur J Nutr*. 2011 Sep;50(6):437-46.

29. Karam RA, Pasha HF, El-Shal AS, Rahman HM, Gad DM. Impact of glutathione-S-transferase gene polymorphisms on enzyme activity, lung function and bronchial asthma susceptibility in Egyptian children. *Gene*. 2012 Apr 15;497(2):314-9; Lima CS, Néri IA, Lourenço GJ, Faria IC, Ribeiro JD, Bertuzzo CS. Glutathione S-transferase mu 1 (GSTM1) and theta 1 (GSTT1) genetic polymorphisms and atopic asthma in children from Southeastern Brazil. *Genet Mol Biol*. 2010 Jul;33(3):438-41; Wang IJ, Tsai CH, Chen CH, Tung KY, Lee YL. Glutathione S-transferase, incense burning and asthma in children. *Eur Respir J*. 2011 Jun;37(6):1371-7; Tamer L, Calikoğlu M, Ates NA, Yildirim H, Ercan B, Saritas E, Unlü A, Atik U. Glutathione-S-transferase gene polymorphisms (GSTT1, GSTM1, GSTP1) as increased risk factors for asthma. *Respirology*. 2004 Nov;9(4):493-8.

30. Moreno-Macías H, Dockery DW, Schwartz J, Gold DR, Laird NM, Sienra-Monge JJ, Del Río-Navarro BE, Ramírez-Aguilar M, Barraza-Villarreal A, Li H, London SJ, Romieu I. Ozone exposure, vitamin C intake, and genetic susceptibility of asthmatic children in Mexico City: a cohort study. *Respir Res*. 2013 Feb 4;14:14.

Chapter 14

1.   Millichap JG, Yee MM. The diet factor in pediatric and adolescent migraine. *Pediatr Neurol.* 2003 Jan;28(1):9-15.

2.   Salfield SA, Wardley BL, Houlsby WT, Turner SL, Spalton AP, Beckles-Wilson NR, Herber SM. Controlled study of exclusion of dietary vasoactive amines in migraine. *Arch Dis Child.* 1987 May;62(5):458-60; Galland L, McEwen LM. A role for food intolerance in childhood migraine. *World Pediatrics and Child Care.* 1996;6:2-8.

3.   Schürks M, Buring JE, Kurth T. Migraine features, associated symptoms and triggers: a principal component analysis in the Women's Health Study. *Cephalalgia.* 2011 May;31(7):861-9.

4.   Alpay K, Ertas M, Orhan EK, Ustay DK, Lieners C, Baykan B. Diet restriction in migraine, based on IgG against foods: a clinical double-blind, randomised, cross-over trial. *Cephalalgia.* 2010 Jul;30(7):829-37; Galland and McEwen 1996; Martelletti P, Sutherland J, Anastasi E, Di Mario U, Giacovazzo M. Evidence for an immune-mediated mechanism in food-induced migraine from a study on activated T-cells, IgG4 subclass, anti-IgG antibodies and circulating immune complexes. *Headache.* 1989 Nov;29(10):664-70; Martelletti P. T cells expressing IL-2 receptor in migraine. *Acta Neurol* (Napoli). 1991 Oct;13(5):448-56; Mansfield LE, Vaughan TR, Waller SF, Haverly RW, Ting S. Food allergy and adult migraine: double-blind and mediator confirmation of an allergic etiology. *Ann Allergy.* 1985 Aug;55(2):126-9; Monro J, Carini C, Brostoff J. Migraine is a food-allergic disease. *Lancet.* 1984 Sep 29;2(8405):719-21.

5.   Ozge A, Ozge C, Oztürk C, Kaleagasi H, Ozcan M, Yalçinkaya DE, Ozveren N, Yalçin F. The relationship between migraine and atopic disorders—the contribution of pulmonary function tests and immunological screening. *Cephalalgia.* 2006 Feb;26(2):172-9; Mortimer MJ, Kay J, Gawkrodger DJ, Jaron A, Barker DC. The prevalence of headache and migraine in atopic children: an epidemiological study in general practice. *Headache.* 1993 Sep;33(8):427-31.

6.   Galland and McEwen 1996; Theodoropoulos DS, Katzenberger DR, Jones WM, Morris DL, Her C, Cullen NA, Morrisa DL. Allergen-specific sublingual immunotherapy in the treatment of migraines: a prospective study. *Eur Rev Med Pharmacol Sci.* 2011 Oct;15(10):1117-21.

7.   Kox M, van Eijk LT, Zwaag J, van den Wildenberg J, Sweep FC, van der Hoeven JG, Pickkers P. Voluntary activation of the sympathetic nervous system and attenuation of the innate immune response in humans. *Proc Natl Acad Sci USA.* 2014 May 20;111(20):7379-84.

8.   van Hemert S, Breedveld AC, Rovers JM, Vermeiden JP, Witteman BJ, Smits MG, de Roos NM. Migraine associated with gastrointestinal disorders: review of the literature and clinical implications. *Front Neurol.* 2014 Nov 21;5:241.

9.   Egger J. Psychoneurological aspects of food allergy. *Europ J Clin Nutr.* 1991;45(suppl 1):35-45.

10. Stevens LJ, Kuczek T, Arnold LE. Solving the puzzle of attention deficit hyperactivity disorder. *Nutr Rev.* 2011 Jul;69(7):383-4; Stevens LJ, Burgess JR, Stochelski MA, Kuczek T. Amounts of artificial food colors in commonly consumed beverages and potential behavioral implications for consumption in children. *Clin Pediatr* (Phila). 2014 Feb;53(2):133-40; Stevens LJ, Kuczek T, Burgess JR, Hurt E, Arnold LE. Dietary sensitivities and ADHD symptoms: thirty-five years of research. *Clin Pediatr* (Phila). 2011 Apr;50(4):279-93; Stevens LJ, Kuczek T, Burgess JR, Stochelski MA, Arnold LE, Galland L. Mechanisms of behavioral, atopic, and other reactions to artificial food colors in children. *Nutr Rev.* 2013 May;71(5):268-81.

11. Ahrne S, Hagslatt ML. Effect of lactobacilli on paracellular permeability in the gut. *Nutrients.* 2011 Jan;3(1):104-17.

12. Montenegro L, Losurdo G, Licinio R, Zamparella M, Giorgio F, Ierardi E, Di Leo A, Principi M. Nonsteroidal anti-inflammatory drug induced damage on lower gastro-intestinal tract: is there an involvement of microbiota? *Curr Drug Saf.* 2014;9(3):196-204.

13. Dagci H, Ustun S, Taner MS, Ersoz G, Karacasu F, Budak S. Protozoon infections and intestinal permeability. *Acta Trop.* 2002 Jan;81(1):1-5; Maia-Brigagão C, Morgado-Díaz JA, De Souza W. Giardia disrupts the arrangement of tight, adherens and desmosomal junction proteins of intestinal cells. *Parasitol Int.* 2012 Jun;61(2):280-7; Lejeune M, Moreau F, Chadee K. Prostaglandin E2 produced by Entamoeba histolytica signals via EP4 receptor and alters claudin-4 to increase ion permeability of tight junctions. *Am J Pathol.* 2011 Aug;179(2):807-18; Frank CF, Hostetter MK. Cleavage of E-cadherin: a mechanism for disruption of the intestinal epithelial barrier by Candida albicans. *Transl Res.* 2007 Apr;149(4):211-22.

14. Neves AL, Coelho J, Couto L, Leite-Moreira A, Roncon-Albuquerque R Jr. Metabolicendotoxemia: a molecular link between obesity and cardiovascular risk. *J Mol Endocrinol.* 2013 Sep 11;51(2):R51-64.

15. Bode C, Bode JC. Effect of alcohol consumption on the gut. *Best Pract Res Clin Gastroenterol.* 2003 Aug;17(4):575-92.

16. Leclercq S, Cani PD, Neyrinck AM, Stärkel P, Jamar F, Mikolajczak M, Delzenne NM, de Timary P. Role of intestinal permeability and inflammation in the biological and behavioral control of alcohol-dependent subjects. *Brain Behav Immun.* 2012 Aug;26(6):911-8; Leclercq S, Matamoros S, Cani PD, et al. Intestinal permeability, gut-bacterial dysbiosis, and behavioral markers of alcohol-dependence severity. *Proc Natl Acad Sci USA.* 2014;pii:201415174.

17. Francavilla R, Miniello V, Magistà AM, De Canio A, Bucci N, Gagliardi F, Lionetti E, Castellaneta S, Polimeno L, Peccarisi L, Indrio F, Cavallo L. A randomized controlled trial of Lactobacillus GG in children with functional abdominal pain. *Pediatrics.* 2010 Dec;126(6):e1445-52.

18. Majamaa H, Isolauri E. Probiotics: a novel approach in the management of food allergy. *J Allergy Clin Immunol.* 1997 Feb;99(2):179-85.

19. Rosenfeldt V, Benfeldt E, Valerius NH, Paerregaard A, Michaelsen KF. Effect of probiotics on gastrointestinal symptoms and small intestinal permeability in children with atopic dermatitis. *J Pediatr.* 2004 Nov;145(5):612-6.

20. Ahrne S, Hagslatt ML. Effect of lactobacilli on paracellular permeability in the gut. *Nutrients.* 2011 Jan;3(1):104-17.

21. Bergmann KR, Liu SX, Tian R, Kushnir A, Turner JR, Li HL, Chou PM, Weber CR, De Plaen IG. Bifidobacteria stabilize claudins at tight junctions and prevent intestinal barrier dysfunction in mouse necrotizing enterocolitis. *Am J Pathol.* 2013 May;182(5):1595-606.

22. Konieczna P, Akdis CA, Quigley EM, Shanahan F, O'Mahony L. Portrait of an immunoregulatory Bifidobacterium. *Gut Microbes.* 2012;3:261–6; Konieczna P, Groeger D, Ziegler M, Frei R, Ferstl R, Shanahan F, et al. Bifidobacterium infantis 35624 administration induces Foxp3 T regulatory cells in human peripheral blood: potential role for myeloid and plasmacytoid dendritic cells. *Gut.* 2012;61:354–66.

23. Ghosh SS, Bie J, Wang J, Ghosh S. Oral supplementation with non-absorbable antibiotics or curcumin attenuates western diet-induced atherosclerosis and glucose intolerance in LDLR-/- mice—role of intestinal permeability and macrophage activation. *PLoS One.* 2014 Sep 24;9(9):e108577.

24. Sergent T, Piront N, Meurice J, Toussaint O, Schneider YJ. Anti-inflammatory effects of dietary phenolic compounds in an in vitro model of inflamed human intestinal epithelium. *Chem Biol Interact.* 2010 Dec 5;188(3):659-67.

25. Yanaka A, Sato J, Ohmori S. Sulforaphane protects small intestinal mucosa from aspirin/NSAID-induced injury by enhancing host defense systems against oxidative stress and by inhibiting mucosal invasion of anaerobic enterobacteria. *Curr Pharm Des.* 2013;19(1):157-62.

26. Assa A, Vong L, Pinnell LJ, Avitzur N, Johnson-Henry KC, Sherman PM. Vitamin D deficiency promotes epithelial barrier dysfunction and intestinal inflammation. *J Infect Dis.* 2014 Oct 15;210(8):1296-305.

27. Rorie A, Goldner WS, Lyden E, Poole JA. Beneficial role for supplemental vitamin D3 treatment in chronic urticaria: a randomized study. *Ann Allergy Asthma Immunol.* 2014 Apr;112(4):376-82.

28. Cayir A, Turan MI, Tan H. Effect of vitamin D therapy in addition to amitriptyline on migraine attacks in pediatric patients. *Braz J Med Biol Res.* 2014 Apr;47(4):349-54.

29. Castro M, King TS, Kunselman SJ, Cabana MD, Denlinger L, Holguin F, Kazani SD, Moore WC, Moy J, Sorkness CA, Avila P, Bacharier LB, Bleecker E, Boushey HA, Chmiel J, Fitzpatrick AM, Gentile D, Hundal M, Israel E, Kraft M, Krishnan JA, LaForce C, Lazarus SC, Lemanske R, Lugogo N, Martin RJ, Mauger DT, Naureckas E, Peters SP, Phipatanakul W, Que LG, Sheshadri A, Smith L, Solway J, Sullivan-Vedder L, Sumino K, Wechsler ME, Wenzel S, White SR, Sutherland ER. Effect of vitamin D3 on asthma treatment failures

in adults with symptomatic asthma and lower vitamin D levels: the VIDA randomized clinical trial. *JAMA*. 2014 May;311(20):2083-91.

30. Baris S, Kiykim A, Ozen A, Tulunay A, Karakoc-Aydiner E, Barlan IB. Vitamin D as an adjunct to subcutaneous allergen immunotherapy in asthmatic children sensitized to house dust mite. *Allergy*. 2014 Feb;69(2):246-53; Majak P, Jerzyńska J, Smejda K, Stelmach I, Timler D, Stelmach W. Correlation of vitamin D with Foxp3 induction and steroid-sparing effect of immunotherapy in asthmatic children. *Ann Allergy Asthma Immunol*. 2012 Nov;109(5):329-35.

31. Tran CD, Hawkes J, Graham RD, Kitchen JL, Symonds EL, Davidson GP, Butler RN. Zinc-fortified oral rehydration solution improved intestinal permeability and small intestinal mucosal recovery. *Clin Pediatr* (Phila). 2014 Dec 16; pii: 0009922814562665; Alam AN, Sarker SA, Wahed MA, Khatun M, Rahaman MM. Enteric protein loss and intestinal permeability changes in children during acute shigellosis and after recovery: effect of zinc supplementation. *Gut*. 1994 Dec;35(12):1707-11.

32. Mahmood A, FitzGerald AJ, Marchbank T, Ntatsaki E, Murray D, Ghosh S, Playford RJ. Zinc carnosine, a health food supplement that stabilises small bowel integrity and stimulates gut repair processes. *Gut*. 2007 Feb;56(2):168-75.

33. Ghaffari J, Khalilian A, Salehifar E, Khorasani E, Rezaii MS. Effect of zinc supplementation in children with asthma: a randomized, placebo-controlled trial in northern Islamic Republic of Iran. *East Mediterr Health J*. 2014 Jun 18;20(6):391-6.

34. Russo F, Linsalata M, Clemente C, Chiloiro M, Orlando A, Marconi E, Chimienti G, Riezzo G. Inulin-enriched pasta improves intestinal permeability and modifies the circulating levels of zonulin and glucagon-like peptide 2 in healthy young volunteers. *Nutr Res*. 2012 Dec;32(12):940-6.

35. González-Hernández LA, Jave-Suarez LF, Fafutis-Morris M, Montes-Salcedo KE, Valle-Gutierrez LG, Campos-Loza AE, Enciso-Gómez LF, Andrade-Villanueva JF. Synbiotic therapy decreases microbial translocation and inflammation and improves immunological status in HIV-infected patients: a double-blind randomized controlled pilot trial. *Nutr J*. 2012 Oct 29;11:90.

Be Part of the Solution

1. Mark Drajem, "Climate Catastrophe Predicted by US as Obama Urges UN action," *Bloomberg News*, June 22, 2015. http://www.bloomberg.com/politics/articles/2015-06-22/climate-catastrophe-predicted-by-u-s-as-obama-urges-un-action.

2. "White House, EPA say climate change a dire threat to economy, human health," *USA Today*, June 23, 2015. http://www.usatoday.com/story/news/nation/2015/06/23/white-house-epa-climate-change-threats/29165589/.

3.   "Fact Sheet: Obama Administration Announces Actions to
     Protect Communities from the Health Impacts of Climate
     Change at White House Summit," June 23, 2015. https://
     www.whitehouse.gov/the-press-office/2015/06/23/
     fact-sheet-obama-administration-announces-actions-protect-communities.

4.   Amanda Stone, "Your Health and Our Environment: How Can We Protect
     Both?" White House blog, June 18, 2015. https://www.whitehouse.gov/
     blog/2015/06/18/public-health-climate-summit.

5.   Environmental Protection Agency, "Climate Action Benefits: Air Quality."
     http://www2.epa.gov/cira/climate-action-benefits-air-quality.

6.   The Lancet Commissions, "Health and climate change: policy responses to
     protect public health." http://press.thelancet.com/Climate2Commission.pdf.

INDEX

ACKNOWLEDGMENTS

The doctors, nurses, and health care professionals who daily confront the challenges of the allergy epidemic deserve special recognition.

We acknowledge the achievements of researchers from around the world who work to expand our understanding of the critical role allergies play in our health, and for underscoring the science that shows how we are all inextricably linked to the environment.

Reid Tracy provided outstanding leadership and support. Louise Hay lighted the way and encouraged our message of healing. Patty Gift's vision and commitment brought *The Allergy Solution* to publication.

We are extremely grateful to our editor, Anne Barthel, whose extraordinary talents and dedication expertly guided us through every step of the journey of crafting this book. With insight and wisdom she shaped the structure, content, and language in a way that was truly remarkable.

Marlene Robinson brought her skill and enthusiasm to important aspects of the production and launch of this book. We appreciate the contribution of copy editor Elise Marton. Thanks to Christy Salinas for her creativity in leading the design of the book.

A big thank you to Tiffini Alberto, Jamie Antoniou, Jo Burgess, Evan Christopher, Jessica Crockett, Perry Crowe, Tony Ford, Richelle Fredson, Alexandra Gruebler, Diane Hill, Dani Johnson, Amy Kiberd, Rakesh Kumar, Chelsey Larson, Shay Lawry, Lindsay McGinty, Monica Meehan, George Papakyriacou, Michelle Pilley, Diane Ray, Kate Riley, Aurora Rosas, Heather Tate, Ruth Tewkesbury, Neill Thompson, Nick Welch, Kathryn Wells, and the entire team at Hay House.

We had the great pleasure of working with Niki Vettel on *The Allergy Solution* special for public television. She captured our message of healing and brought it to a broader audience. Bob Comiskey and Scot Broderick added their vision and experience to the production. The talented teams at Twin Cities Public Television and Georgia Public Broadcasting made filming our show there a wonderful experience. We thank the public television stations across the country that share *The Allergy Solution* special with their viewers.

We want to acknowledge the important contributions of Barbara and Randall Smith, Edward Kaufman, Damon Giglio, Bonnie and Gary Vogel, Beth Olmstead, Sandy and David Epstein, Deana Lenz and Joan Davidson, and all the supporters who have generously championed our educational mission through the Foundation for Integrated Medicine.

We would like to thank Anna Williams for her enthusiastic support of our work.

We appreciate the thoughtfulness of Paulette Cole in advancing our message.

Thanks to Imelda Goldberg, Theresita Ibaretta, Sandra Tejada, and Maria Fernandez.

Our dear friend Helen Burgess has always been there for us, in so many ways.

Jordan and Jessica Galland contributed their creativity and passion to this project. Jefferson Ray offered valuable insight.

In loving memory of Christopher—you are always with us.

Leo Galland and Jonathan Galland

I am delighted to highlight the special contribution of the award-winning journalist Ma Guihua, who has traveled the world to report with courage and passion about women's rights, education, the environment, and health. She brings her journalistic skills and talent for nature photography to our websites, Facebook, and Twitter. Her encouragement, belief, and optimistic spirit are a constant source of light and inspiration. With love and gratitude.

Jonathan Galland

ABOUT THE AUTHORS

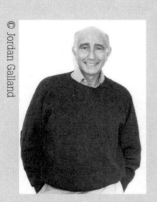

Dr Leo Galland, a board-certified internist, is recognized as the world leader in integrated medicine. Educated at Harvard University and the New York University School of Medicine, he won the Linus Pauling Award for his trailblazing vision that created a new way to practice medicine for thousands of doctors. Dr Galland has been featured in *The New York Times, The Wall Street Journal, Self* and *Men's Fitness* and has appeared on the *TODAY* show, *Good Morning America, The Dr. Oz Show,* and others. He is the author of *The Fat Resistance Diet, Power Healing* and *Superimmunity for Kids* and the director of the Foundation for Integrated Medicine.

www.drgalland.com

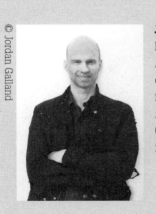

Jonathan Galland JD, a leader in integrated health education, writes for the *Huffington Post* and *MindBodyGreen*. Jonathan created over 100 recipes for *The Fat Resistance Diet,* featured in *Fitness* and *Woman's World,* on *The Dr. Oz Show* and in *The Washington Post.* He is CEO of pilladvised.com, which brings together integrated medicine and environmental health.

www.drgalland.com

Hay House Titles of Related Interest

YOU CAN HEAL YOUR LIFE, the movie, starring Louise Hay & Friends
(available as a 1-DVD programme and an expanded 2-DVD set)
Watch the trailer at: www.LouiseHayMovie.com

THE SHIFT, the movie,
starring Dr Wayne W. Dyer
(available as a 1-DVD programme and an expanded 2-DVD set)
Watch the trailer at: www.DyerMovie.com

~

*10 REASONS YOU FEEL OLD AND GET FAT . . . : And How YOU Can Stay
Young, Slim and Happy!,* by Dr Frank Lipman

*GODDESSES NEVER AGE: The Secret Prescription for Radiance, Vitality and
Well-Being,* by Dr Christiane Northrup

POWER UP YOUR BRAIN: The Neuroscience of Enlightenment,
by Dr David Perlmutter

All of the above are available at your local bookstore,
or may be ordered by contacting Hay House (see last page).

~

NOTES